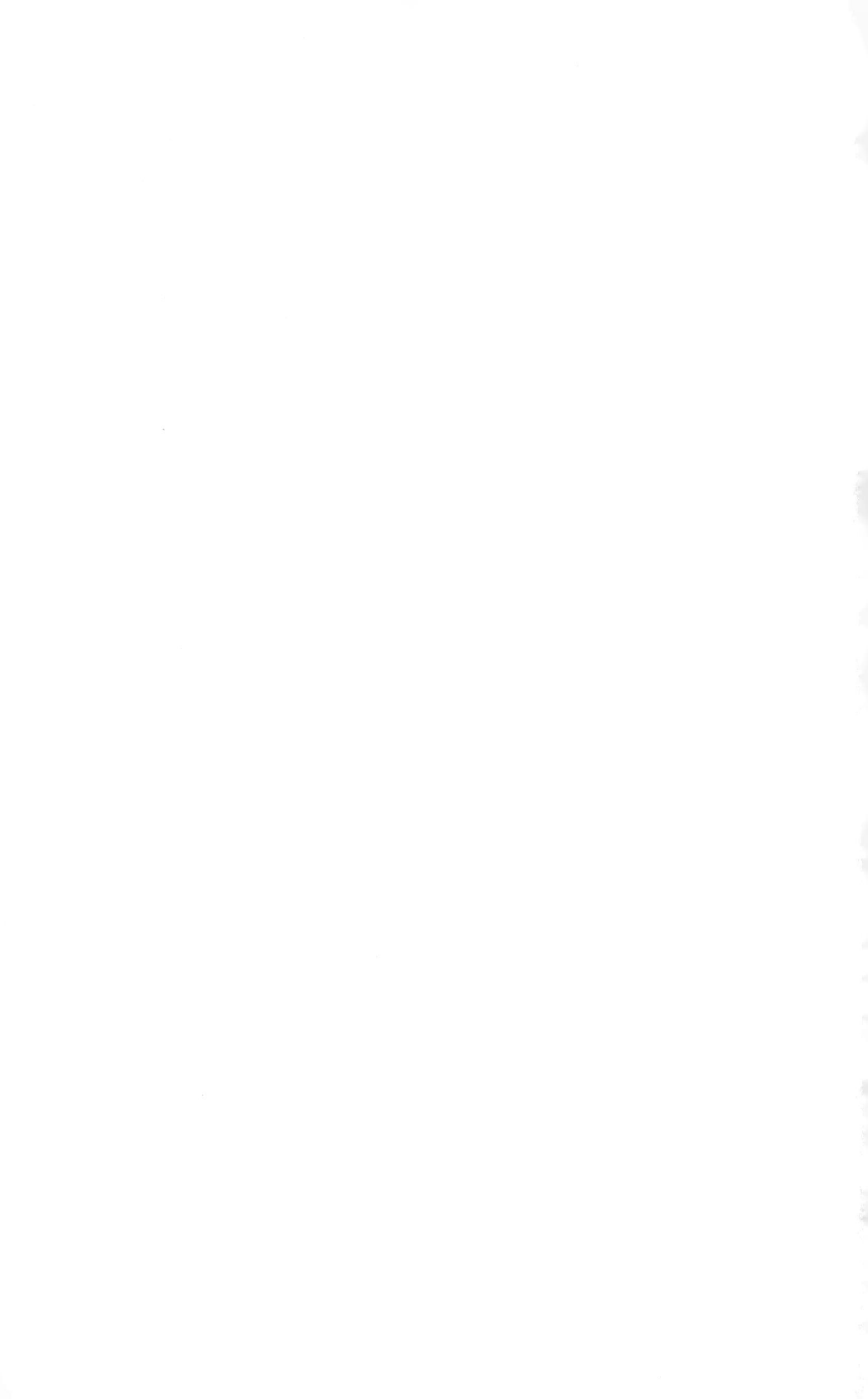

Care of People Living with HIV: Contemporary Issues

Editor

KARA S. MCGEE

NURSING CLINICS OF NORTH AMERICA

www.nursing.theclinics.com

Consulting Editor
BENJAMIN SMALLHEER

June 2024 • Volume 59 • Number 2

ELSEVIER

1600 John F. Kennedy Boulevard • Suite 1800 • Philadelphia, Pennsylvania, 19103-2899

http://www.theclinics.com

NURSING CLINICS OF NORTH AMERICA Volume 59, Number 2
June 2024 ISSN 0029-6465, ISBN-13: 978-0-443-13053-3

Editor: Kerry Holland
Developmental Editor: Malvika Shah

Nursing Clinics of North America (ISSN 0029-6465) is published quarterly by Elsevier Inc., 360 Park Avenue South, New York, NY 10010-1710. Months of issue are March, June, September, and December. Periodicals postage paid at New York, NY and additional mailing offices. Subscription price per year is, $168.00 (US individuals), $275.00 (international individuals), $231.00 (Canadian individuals), $100.00 (US and Canadian students), and $135.00 (international students). For institutional access pricing please contact Customer Service via the contact information below. To receive student/resident rate, orders must be accompanied by name of affiliated institution, date of term, and the signature of program/residency coordinator on institution letterhead. Orders will be billed at individual rate until proof of status is received. Foreign air speed delivery is included in all *Clinics* subscription prices. All prices are subject to change without notice. **POSTMASTER:** Send address changes to *Nursing Clinics*, Elsevier Health Sciences Division, Subscription Customer Service, 3251 Riverport Lane, Maryland Heights, MO 63043. **Customer Service: Telephone: 1-800-654-2452** (U.S. and Canada); **1-314-447-8871 (outside U.S. and Canada). Fax: 1-314-447-8029. E-mail: journalscustomerservice-usa@elsevier.com** (for print support) and **journalsonlinesupport-usa@elsevier.com** (for online support).

Nursing Clinics of North America is covered in *EMBASE/Excerpta Medica, MEDLINE/PubMed (Index Medicus), Social Sciences Citation Index, Current Contents, ASCA, Cumulative Index to Nursing, RNdex Top 100,* and Allied Health Literature and International Nursing Index (INI).

Contributors

CONSULTING EDITOR

BENJAMIN SMALLHEER PhD, RN, ACNP-BC, FNP-BC, CCRN, CNE, FAANP
Assistant Dean, Master of Science in Nursing Program, Associate Professor, Duke University School of Nursing, Durham, North Carolina

EDITOR

KARA S. MCGEE, DMS, MSPH, PA-C, AAHIVS
Associate Clinical Professor, Duke University School of Nursing, Duke University School of Medicine, Durham, North Carolina

AUTHORS

LISA L. ABUOGI, MD, MSc
Associate Professor, Department of Pediatrics, University of Colorado School of Medicine, Aurora, Colorado

DAVID AGOR, DNP, PMHNP-BC, HIVPCP
PhD Student, Department of Family and Community Health, University of Pennsylvania, School of Nursing, University of Pennsylvania Eidos Center, Philadelphia, Pennsylvania

EMILY A. BARR, PhD, RN, CPNP-PC, CNM, FAAN
Assistant Professor, University of Texas Health Science Center at Houston, Cizik School of Nursing, Houston, Texas

LACRECIA M. BELL, MSN, RN
Clinical Faculty, School of Nursing, Duke University School of Nursing, Durham, North Carolina

KRISTINE BUTLER, MSN, RN, FNP-BC
Instructor of Medicine, Division of General Cardiology, Oregon Health & Science University School of Medicine, Portland, Oregon

JARED CARTER-DAVIS, AGNP-C, MSN, AAHIVS
Principal Investigator, Medical Director, Ryan White Program Director, Division of Infectious Diseases, East Carolina University, ECU Adult Specialty Care, Greenville, North Carolina

JUSTIN COLE, MSN, APRN-CNP
Nurse Practitioner, Discreet NP, Norman, Oklahoma

AMY CULBERTSON, DNP, APRN, FNP-BC
Associate Professor, School of Nursing, Georgetown University, Washington, DC

KENNETH DAICI, BA
Research Assistant, Center for Sexual and Gender Minority Health Research, Columbia University School of Nursing, New York, NY

BRENICE DUROSEAU, MSN, FNP-C, RNC-OB, AAHIVS
PhD Candidate, Infectious Diseases Nurse Practitioner, Center for Infectious Disease and Nursing Innovation, Johns Hopkins School of Nursing, Baltimore, Maryland

DEVON FLYNN, PharmD, MPH, BCPS, AAHIVP
HIV Clinic Pharmacist, Oregon Health & Science University, Portland, Oregon

CHRISTOPHER B. FOX, MSN, RN, ANP-BC, AAHIVS
Assistant Professor of Medicine, Division of General Internal Medicine and Geriatrics, Oregon Health & Science University School of Medicine, Portland, Oregon

DOMINIQUE GUILLAUME, MSN, AGPCNP-BC, AAHIVE
PhD Candidate, Center for Infectious Disease and Nursing Innovation, Johns Hopkins School of Nursing, Global Women's Health Fellow, Johns Hopkins University, Baltimore, Maryland

SARAH E. JANEK, BSN, RN, ACRN
Clinical Instructor, School of Nursing, Duke University, Duke University School of Nursing, Durham, North Carolina

JENNA JANUSZKA, PharmD, BCPS, AAHIVP
Clinical Pharmacist, Department of Pharmacy, Duke University Hospital, Durham, North Carolina

BRANDON A. KNETTEL, PhD
Assistant Professor, Duke University School of Nursing, Duke Global Health Institute, Duke Global Mental Health Program, Duke University, Durham, North Carolina

ELIZABETH T. KNIPPLER, MPH
Program Coordinator, School of Nursing, Duke University, Duke University School of Nursing, Durham, North Carolina

ROBIN LENNON-DEARING, PhD, MSW, BSW
Professor, School of Social Work, University of Memphis, Memphis, Tennessee

ADAM LEONARD, MS, MPH, CPNP-PC, AAHIVS
PhD Student, Center for Infectious Disease and Nursing Innovation, Johns Hopkins School of Nursing, Baltimore, Maryland; Assistant Adjunct Professor, Community Health Systems, University of California, San Francisco School of Nursing, San Francisco, California

SERINA MADDEN, DNP, APRN-CNP, AAHIVM
Nurse Practitioner, Discreet NP, Norman, Oklahoma

KAREN McCREA, DNP, APRN, FNP-C
Assistant Professor, School of Nursing, Georgetown University, Washington, DC

STEVEN MEANLEY, MPH, PhD
Assistant Professor, University of Pennsylvania Eidos Center, University of Pennsylvania School of Nursing, Philadelphia, Pennsylvania

MARTA I. MULAWA, MHS, PhD
Assistant professor, School of Nursing, Duke University School of Nursing, Duke Global Health Institute, Duke University, Durham, North Carolina

ALI T. SASLAFSKY, BSN, RN, MSN, APRN, FNP-C
School of Nursing, Duke University, Duke University School of Nursing, Durham, North Carolina

ELLEN SEYMOUR, AGNP-C, MSN, MPH, AAHIVS, DNP Candidate
Infectious Disease Nurse Practitioner, Access Community Health Network, Chicago, Illinois

JENNY SHROBA, PharmD, BCIDP, AAHIVP
Clinical Pharmacist, Department of Pharmacy, Duke University Hospital, Durham, North Carolina

CHRISTIANA SMITH, MD, MSc
Associate Professor, Department of Pediatrics, University of Colorado School of Medicine, Aurora, Colorado

MELODY WILKINSON, DNP, APRN, FNP-C, FAANP
Associate Professor, School of Nursing, Georgetown University, Washington, DC

Contents

Integrase inhibitors and tenofovir alafenamide have become a mainstay in modern antiretroviral therapy; more recently, they have been implicated as causing increased weight gain beyond what may be expected with the "return to health" phenomenon. Some patients, namely those assigned female at birth, of the black race, or with lower baseline CD4 counts, may be more likely to experience weight gain. This review outlines existing evidence linking the agents to excessive weight as well as ongoing efforts to combat these effects.

Human immunodeficiency virus (HIV) criminalization is the prosecution of people with HIV using HIV-specific state statutes, sentence enhancements, and general criminal laws wherein otherwise legal conduct becomes criminalized based on a person's HIV diagnosis. HIV criminal laws perpetuate HIV stigma and discrimination, misrepresent how HIV is transmitted, and are a barrier to HIV prevention and care. Research has found that Black Americans are more likely to be arrested for and convicted of HIV-related offenses. The harm caused by HIV laws on already marginalized communities is long-lasting and severe.

People living with HIV (PLWH) have a risk of cardiovascular disease (CVD) that is 1.5 to 2 times higher than the general population owing to traditional risk factors, HIV-mediated factors like chronic inflammation and immune dysfunction, and exposure to antiretroviral therapy. Currently available CVD risk estimation calculators tend to underestimate risk in PLWH but can be useful when an individual's HIV history is considered. Improving modifiable risks is the primary intervention for reducing CVD risk in PLWH. Statin therapy is important for specific individuals, but attention should be given to drug interactions with antiretroviral agents used to treat HIV.

This scoping review identified contemporary stigma-reduction studies across US health-care settings. Despite the significance of this problem, only 3 intervention studies were identified in the past 5 years. These studies highlight the value of intervening during formative training experiences and the importance of including interprofessional health-care providers in interventions. The findings relate to the novel approaches (eg, virtual patient simulations) that are used in interventions. The importance of using a participatory approach to intervention design is noted. Critical gaps in human immunodeficiency virus (HIV) stigma measurement and the lack of interventions are identified, laying a foundation for future programs and research.

The transition of HIV into a chronic illness has brought to the forefront the pressing need to address the complex web of social determinants of HIV outcomes. A structured literature search and narrative review of studies describing intervention strategies for mental health among sexual/gender minority (SGM) older adults living with HIV (OALWH) published in the last decade identified 2 studies for inclusion. This narrative review identifies age-sensitive and culturally adapted therapies, mindfulness and meditation-based stress reduction, group therapy, digital mental health resources, and psilocybin-assisted group therapy as emerging intervention models tailored to meet the unique needs of SGM OALWH.

People living with human immunodeficiency virus (HIV) (PLWH) live near-normal life expectancies due to advances in antiretroviral therapy. PLWH are experiencing more non-HIV–related comorbidities and deaths. PLWH are diagnosed with cancer more often and experience worse cancer-related outcomes than the general population. Cancer prevention and screening in PLWH is essential and leads to earlier diagnosis and treatment which may result in improved health outcomes and increased long-term survival. Few cancer screening guidelines specific to PLWH exist. There are often discrepancies in general population cancer screening guidelines. Familiarity with the utilization of cancer screening guidelines in this population is imperative.

Human immunodeficiency virus (HIV) remains a significant public concern, with certain groups disproportionately impacted. Pre-exposure prophylaxis (PrEP) for HIV prevention was approved by the Food and Drug Administration in 2012. However, stark disparities persist in PrEP access and uptake, leaving those at highest risk of acquiring HIV without knowledge of, access to, and uptake of PrEP. Nurses play a key role in eliminating the causes of these disparities that occur at the individual, provider, and systemic level. It is imperative that we increase PrEP knowledge, access, and use, especially in groups most at risk for acquiring HIV.

NURSING CLINICS

SERIES OF RELATED INTEREST

Advances in Family Practice Nursing
www.advancesinfamilypracticenursing.com

THE CLINICS ARE AVAILABLE ONLINE!
Access your subscription at:
www.theclinics.com

Foreword

Navigating the Horizon of Progress in HIV/AIDS Care

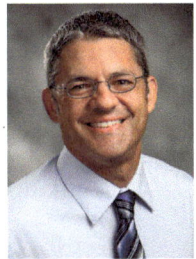

Benjamin Smallheer, PhD, RN, ACNP-BC, FNP-BC, CCRN, CNE, FAANP
Consulting Editor

Over the past few decades, the landscape of HIV/AIDS care has undergone a profound transformation, marked by persistent research, innovative therapies, and a deepened understanding of the virus and its impact on individuals and communities. Our commitment to advancing the battle against HIV/AIDS stands as a testament to human resilience, scientific ingenuity, and compassionate care.

As we embark on this exploration of advances in HIV/AIDS care, it is impossible to ignore the remarkable strides made in the field.

In retrospect, the initial decades of the HIV/AIDS epidemic were complicated by fear, stigma, and limited treatment options. However, the continued pursuit of knowledge has led to a paradigm shift in how we approach, manage, and ultimately combat HIV/AIDS. One of the most noteworthy advancements lies in antiretroviral therapy. The development and refinement of these medications have not only extended the lives of those living with HIV but also transformed the virus from a once-deadly diagnosis to a manageable chronic condition. The revolution of combination therapies can now suppress viral replication and boost immune function so that individuals diagnosed with HIV can lead fulfilling lives, with the virus controlled to undetectable levels, minimizing the risk of transmission to others.

Equally important is the evolving landscape of preventive strategies, such as preexposure prophylaxis and postexposure prophylaxis. These interventions have ushered in a new era of HIV prevention, offering more options to individuals at risk. This tireless work has played a pivotal role in dismantling the barriers of discrimination and health inequity. Disparities in health care access, persistent stigma, and the emergence of drug-resistant strains remind us that our journey is far from over.

This issue of *Nursing Clinics of North America* dives into the advances that have been made in HIV/AIDS care. We examine care of sexual and gender minorities, the

Nurs Clin N Am 59 (2024) xiii–xiv
https://doi.org/10.1016/j.cnur.2024.03.003
0029-6465/24/© 2024 Published by Elsevier Inc.

nursing.theclinics.com

transgender community, and adolescents and young adults living with HIV/AIDS. We also broach the topic of the criminalization of HIV in the United States.

As we delve into the pages ahead, let us celebrate the progress achieved, reflect on the lessons learned, and renew our commitment to ensure that every individual affected by HIV/AIDS receives the care, dignity, and hope they deserve.

Benjamin Smallheer, PhD, RN, ACNP-BC, FNP-BC, CCRN, CNE, FAANP
Duke University School of Nursing
307 Trent Drive
Box 3322, Office 3117
Durham, NC 27710, USA

E-mail address:
benjamin.smallheer@duke.edu

Preface

Care of People Living with HIV: Contemporary Issues

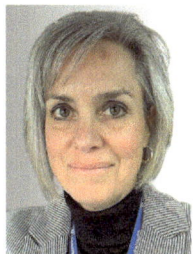

Kara S. McGee, DMS, MSPH, PA-C, AAHIVS
Editor

The landscape of HIV prevention and treatment has evolved significantly over the past few decades, and HIV is now a chronic, manageable illness. Medical advances in the treatment of HIV have translated to normal life expectancy for people living with HIV who are on effective treatment, and innovations in HIV prevention approaches means that we have the tools to significantly reduce the number of new HIV infections in the United States.

Despite significant scientific advancements in HIV treatment and prevention, HIV-related disparities persist in accessing care and achieving optimal health outcomes. The Southern United States faces a disproportionate burden of the HIV epidemic accounting for over 50% of new HIV cases annually. Black and Latinx communities continue to be disproportionately impacted by HIV. In 2019, Black people accounted for 42% and Latinx people accounted for 29% of the new HIV diagnoses in the United States.[1] These disparities arise from a complex interplay of factors, such as stigma and poverty, that are largely driven by structural racism perpetuating systemic inequities that impact access to HIV prevention and treatment services.[2] In addition, despite the biomedical advances in HIV treatment and prevention, HIV-related stigma continues to have significant impacts on the health and well-being of people with and at risk of HIV.

Nurses play an important role in assuring that people living with HIV receive appropriate treatment and health promotion and disease prevention services. In addition, it is critical that nurses and other healthcare professionals understand the unique needs of people living with HIV to ensure that they receive equitable and compassionate care in healthcare settings and in their communities.

This special issue provides an update on the epidemiology of HIV in the United States and contemporary care and treatment approaches for people living with and

Nurs Clin N Am 59 (2024) xv–xvi
https://doi.org/10.1016/j.cnur.2024.02.010
0029-6465/24/© 2024 Published by Elsevier Inc.

at risk of HIV. In addition, this issue includes discussion of the some of the unique issues faced by people living with HIV, including criminalization of HIV and experiences of stigma and discrimination in healthcare settings. All of the authors discuss the ongoing disparities and inequities faced by historically marginalized populations at risk for or living with HIV and offer suggestions for how health professionals can mitigate the impact of these inequalities.

DISCLOSURE

No commercial or financial conflicts of interest or funding sources.

Kara S. McGee, DMS, MSPH, PA-C, AAHIVS
Duke University School of Nursing
Duke University School of Medicine
307 Trent Drive
Box 3322
Durham, NC 27710, USA

E-mail address:
Kara.mcgee@duke.edu

REFERENCES

1. Centers for Disease Control and Prevention. Diagnoses of HIV infection in the United States and dependent areas, 2019. HIV Surveill Rep 2021;32.
2. Sullivan PS, Satcher Johnson A, Pembleton ES, et al. Epidemiology of HIV in the USA: epidemic burden, inequities, contexts, and responses. Lancet 2021; 397(10279):1095–106.

The Epidemiology of Human Immunodeficiency Virus
Reflections and Insights

Lacrecia M. Bell, MSN, RN

KEYWORDS

• HIV • PrEP • Vulnerable people • Health equity • Ending the HIV epidemic

KEY POINTS

- Individual factors cannot explain the ongoing human immunodeficiency virus (HIV)-related health disparities experienced by racial and ethnic minority groups in the United States
- Antiretroviral treatment adherence and viral suppression are key to increasing quality of life and decreasing transmission for those living with HIV.
- The development of innovative models of HIV care and prevention that improve outcomes and decrease disparities is the way forward to ending the HIV epidemic not just for some, but for all.

INTRODUCTION

The acquired immune deficiency syndrome (AIDS) was first discovered in the United States in June 1981.[1] Several previously healthy gay men living in California and New York were discovered to have *Pneumocystis carinii* and Kaposi's sarcoma, 2 rare opportunistic infections associated with compromised immunity. Following these reports, the Centers for Disease Control and Prevention (CDC) developed the task force on Kaposi's sarcoma and opportunistic infections. This new disease did not have a name and was only identified by the new occurrences of rare opportunistic infections. It was not until 1984 that the human immunodeficiency virus (HIV), the retrovirus responsible for AIDS, was named by Dr. Jay Levy, Dr. Robert Gallo, and Dr. Luc Montagnier.[2]

HIV is a retrovirus, affecting its human host by attacking the CD4, T helper white blood cells. It replicates, destroys the CD4 cells, and disables the body's infection-fighting capacity. HIV can be transmitted via blood, semen, breast milk, and vaginal and anal fluids that contain the virus. There is no cure for HIV. However, prevention, diagnosis, and treatment can make this a manageable chronic health condition.[3,4]

School of Nursing, Duke University School of Nursing, 307 Trent Drive, DUMC 3322, Durham, NC 27710, USA
E-mail address: lacrecia.m.bell@duke.edu

Nurs Clin N Am 59 (2024) 153–164
https://doi.org/10.1016/j.cnur.2024.01.011
nursing.theclinics.com

The World Health Organization 2025 target goals to address HIV include 95% of people living globally with HIV would know their status, 95% of people living globally with HIV would be on antiretroviral treatment (ART), and 90% of people on ART would be virally suppressed.[5–7] Globally, only 86% of people living with HIV (PLWH) are aware of their status, 89% of PLWH are receiving ART, and approximately 68% of people on ART are virally suppressed.[5–7] Countries that had seen a decline in new HIV diagnoses are currently seeing an increase with current rates of 1.5 million people acquiring HIV annually; 1 million greater than global targets.[5–7]

In 2021, it was estimated that over 1 million people were living with HIV in the United States.[8] Among them, 36,126 were new diagnoses (**Fig. 1**).[9] Although Black people represented only 12% of the U.S. population,[10] they comprised the largest percentage of new HIV diagnoses and HIV-related deaths in 2021.[11] With regard to new HIV diagnoses in 2021, 40% were among Black people, 29% among Hispanic people, and 25% among White people (**Fig. 2**).[12] In 2021, young people aged 13 to 34 years accounted for 58% of the new cases of HIV in the United States.[8] Black women are also greatly impacted by HIV as they account for the highest rates of new HIV diagnoses (54%) and HIV-related deaths (57%) among women.[13]

Individuals aged 55 years and older comprise 41% of PLWH in the United States.[8,11] Of those, Black people have the highest rates of new HIV diagnoses and death.[10,11] In 2021, more than 3900 adults aged 55 years and older were diagnosed with HIV, with the greatest number of new diagnoses in adults aged 55 to 59 years.[11,14] Among older adults who were newly diagnosed with HIV, 34% had a stage 3 HIV infection at the time of diagnosis.[11] Additionally, racial disparity persists among PLWH who are receiving ART treatment and have obtained viral suppression. Current data show that 62% of Black male individuals living with HIV were virally suppressed, the lowest percentage among Black, White, and Hispanic/Latino(e) persons.[13]

The incidence and impact of HIV is not only racial and ethnically disparate, but it also disproportionally impacts people living in the southern region of the United States. Despite only 38% of the U.S. population residing in the South, the 17 States that comprise the U.S. South have the highest rate of new and existing HIV

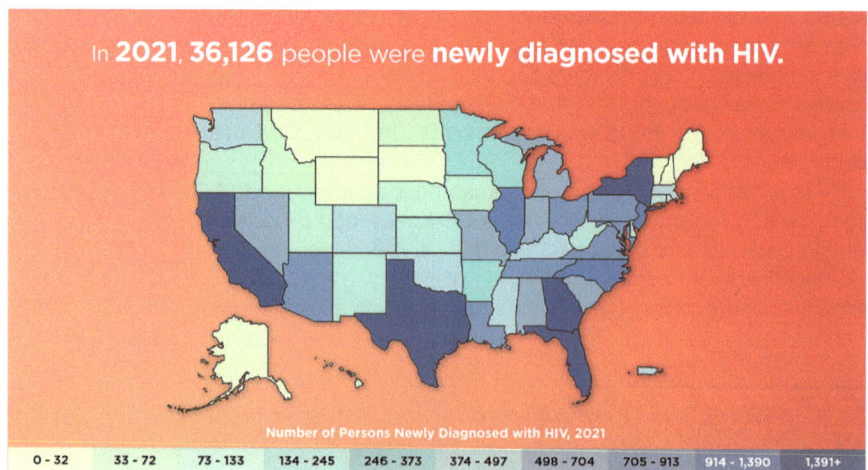

Fig. 1. Number of persons newly diagnosed with HIV, 2021. (Reprinted with permission from: AIDSVu, Center for Disease Control and Prevention.Emory University, Rollins School of Public Health.)

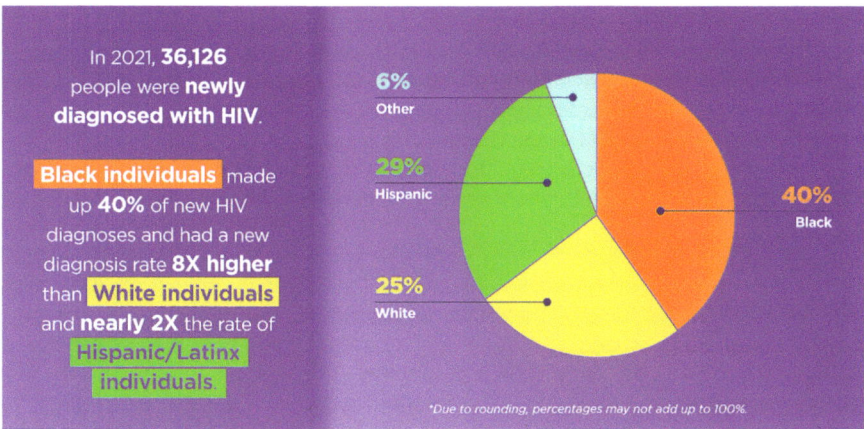

Fig. 2. Percentage of new HIV diagnoses by race/ethnicity, 2021. (Reprinted with Permission from: AIDSVu, Center for Disease Control and Prevention, Emory University, Rollins School of Public Health.)

diagnoses.[15] Furthermore, in 2021, Black and African Americans in the South accounted for approximately 48% of all persons newly diagnosed with HIV living in the South.[15,16]

Sexual and gender minority people are also disproportionately affected by HIV. It is estimated that there are 1.4 million transgender adults aged 18 years and older living in the United States.[17] Most recent estimates indicate that HIV prevalence is 14% among transgender women and 2% among transgender men.[17] More than 43% of transgender women living with HIV are Black and 26% are Hispanic/Latino(e).[11,13] Most transgender people diagnosed with HIV are Black, aged 25 to 35 years, and living in the South.[11,17]

Ending the Human Immunodeficiency Virus Epidemic

Several national initiatives have set goals to prioritize the prevention and treatment of HIV. The United States-based initiative, ending the HIV epidemic (EHE) was enacted in 2019 by then-U.S. President Donald Trump. The EHE goal was to end the HIV epidemic by 2030 with benchmarks of reducing new HIV infections by 75% in 5 years and by 90% in 10 years.[18] This initiative was designed to prioritize the testing, prevention, and treatment of people at risk of acquiring HIV, those living with HIV/AIDS, and those affected by HIV. The outlined strategy included early diagnosis, rapid and effective treatment with the goal of sustained viral suppression, evidence-based interventions to prevent new HIV transmission, and an expeditious response to actual and potential HIV clusters with prevention and treatment.[18,19]

The EHE goals are predicated on early diagnosis and rapid treatment. Yet, the lack of universal health care policies that include free universal HIV testing continues to be a barrier to early diagnosis and rapid treatment. The CDC recommends that all individuals aged 13 to 64 years have an HIV test as a part of routine health care.[19,20] However, many people living in the United States are uninsured or do not have a primary provider, making it difficult to obtain an HIV test.[19–21] These testing and treatment barriers are even more pronounced in rural areas where the ratio of primary care physicians per 100,000 residents is 38.9:100,000 in rural areas compared to 59.3 providers:100,000 residents in metropolitan areas.[22]

The Affordable Care Act

E HE and eradicating the disproportionate impact on Black and Brown people, necessitates Medicaid expansion in all 50 states. The Affordable Care Act (ACA) formally known as the Patient Protection and Affordable Care Act was signed into legislation in March 2010 by President Barack Obama. Also known as Obamacare, the ACA provided enhanced medical coverage to many Americans. The ACA was the most detailed health care reconstruction since Medicare and Medicaid were enacted in the 1960s.[23] Several of the benefits of the ACA include the protection of Americans from being denied or dropped from coverage because of pre-existing conditions like HIV, broader Medicaid eligibility, removal of lifetime financial cost caps on insurance benefits, lowered cost of prescription medications, the implementation of medical homes, and the expansion of community centers.[24] Many of the populations of PLWH and people at risk for HIV, including many gay, bisexual, and other men who have sex with men have been ineligible for Medicaid coverage making it challenging for them to access HIV prevention and treatment services.[25] Among the 40 states and the District of Columbia that have opted to expand Medicaid under the ACA, adults with income at or below 138% of the federal poverty level meet eligibility criteria. Currently, 10 states have not expanded Medicaid.[26]

The lack of Medicaid expansion disproportionately affects those who are lower income and people of color, as the rates of insurance coverage are often double the cost of insurance for people of color in states that have not expanded Medicaid.[27] On March 27, 2023, North Carolina became the 40th state to approve Medicaid expansion, providing health care to over 600,000 uninsured North Carolinians.[27] This provision raised the income cap on Medicaid eligibility and provide North Carolinians living with HIV and at risk of acquiring HIV access to comprehensive HIV prevention and HIV health care including prescription coverage, access to stable housing, and mental health services.[28,29] This legislation was implemented on December 1, 2023.[26]

RURALITY AND THE PREVENTION AND TREATMENT OF HUMAN IMMUNODEFICIENCY VIRUS

For PLWH in the South, there remains a dearth of education, psychological, and community support.[15] Disparities in HIV care access, treatment, and outcomes are even more pronounced in rural areas and in the South where 32% of PLWH have suboptimal access to HIV care providers, the highest percentage of any geographic region.[30] The journey toward EHE includes viral suppression for all PWLH. Compared to other regions of the United States, the South has the lowest rate of viral suppression (65%) among PLWH.[31]

Rural residence presents substantial risk of increased rates of mortality, and lower rates of HIV testing, diagnosis, and treatment.[32] There are significant socioeconomic and racial disparities between rural and urban communities. The largest gap between rural and nonrural wealth exists in the U.S. South. Current data demonstrate that Black rural residents have the poorest economic well-being when compared to native American, Hispanic, White, and Asian residents.[33] Comparing urban and rural dwellers living across the United States, rural dwellers living in the South have the highest overall mortality rates.[34]

Of the 17.9% of people living rurally, those living with HIV face numerous barriers to care.[35] There are few HIV care providers in rural areas to meet the needs of residents living with HIV. The Ryan White HIV/AIDS Program is the largest federal funder of HIV resources and provides care for over 500,000 clients, which is approximately 50% of PLWH in the United States. In 2020, 3.5% of the clients served by Ryan White programs resided in rural communities, and those clients received care from the 8.2% of Ryan White service providers practicing in rural areas.[35] Although the proposed fiscal year 2024 budget includes a 276 million dollar increase for HIV prevention, treatment, and care, this only represents a 3% in 2022 and 2023.[36,37] Many people who are affected by HIV are also affected by the structural inequities that make accessing health care, housing, food, and employment incredibly challenging.[34] Addressing HIV disparities and EHE requires a commitment from funding agencies and legislators to allocate much-needed funds to continue to address health disparities for people living with and affected by HIV.

The lack of investigations that include rurality leaves unanswered questions about how the challenges and barriers that rural residents face impact their experience of living with HIV. Many people living rurally chooses not to disclose their HIV status, live in secrecy, and fear the negative impact of stigma, all of which lead to isolation.[15] Even when people receive community support, many community workers are not trained to appropriately address the stigma associated with seeking HIV prevention and treatment.

The Role of Pre-exposure Prophylaxis in Ending the Human Immunodeficiency Virus Epidemic

In 2012, Truvada (emtricitabine coformulated with tenofovir disoproxil fumarate), an antiretroviral approved for HIV treatment in 2004, was approved by the U.S. Food and Drug Administration (FDA) as the first single tablet combination pre-exposure prophylaxis (PrEP) to prevent HIV.[38] When taken as prescribed, PrEP can reduce the risk of HIV from sex by 99% and the risk of HIV from injection drug use by greater than 70%.[32] The recent FDA approval of long-acting injectable PrEP, cabotegravir, has immense potential to be instrumental in changing the landscape of HIV prevention. Following 2 loading doses, cabotegravir, administered every 2 months as an intragluteal injection, reduces the pill burden that many recipients have, and decreases stigma associated with episodic or daily dosing of oral PrEP.[39]

We continue to make strides toward decreasing HIV in young male adults aged 13 to 24 years who identify as gay or bisexual. However, racial disparity persists even as HIV incidence declines. HIV incidence among White male adults has decreased by 45%, 36% among Hispanic/Latino male adults, and 27% among Black male adults.[40] The CDC estimates that 1.2 million people in the United States could benefit from PrEP but in 2021, only about 30% of people who could benefit were prescribed PrEP medication.[41] Although available as effective HIV prevention, there are many barriers and challenges that underscore the decreased rates of PrEP use. Although at disproportionate risk for HIV, Black sexual minority men living in the southern United States have low rates of PrEP usage. In 2022, only 13.6% of Black people who were eligible for PrEP were prescribed PrEP in comparison to 78% of White people.[42,43] The reasons for poor uptake are many and include distrust of the medical system, stigma, fear, and many other social determinants of health that, for African Americans, make engaging the health care system challenging.[44] Many PrEP eligible patients report barriers to receiving PrEP that include not knowing who to talk to about treatment, not understanding the benefits, and high cost.[45]

In 2019, the Biden administration launched the Ready, Set, PrEP campaign and provided free access to PrEP for those who receive Medicaid and are uninsured. This was beneficial for many, but there were large swaths of the population for which PrEP was unaffordable, leaving many with expensive medication and laboratory testing copays.[46] In 2021, people aged 13 to 24 years accounted for 19% of new HIV diagnoses.[47] These data highlight the imperative that young adults need access to PrEP education and prescriptions. Research studies identified that many primary care providers face barriers to prescribing PrEP to adolescents. If their colleagues were not prescribing PrEP, providers feared stigma related to prescribing PrEP.[45] Providers also reported challenges with liability laws, confidentiality, and insurance coverage as logistical hurdles that were often difficult to conquer. Most notably, in the South, where the number of PLWH is disproportionately high, sex education and/or sexually transmitted infection (STI)/HIV education in many K-12 school settings is not mandated.[48] In fact, several state laws penalize providers for providing sexual and reproductive health counseling and education.[45]

Transgender and gender-diverse persons are often overlooked and report not accessing PrEP because it can be difficult to see a provider that provides gender-affirming care. Misgendering or being asked irrelevant questions decreases health-seeking behavior and engagement with providers. Many gender diverse persons seeking PrEP report that providers are challenged with providing gender-affirming care as many providers have limited information about the interactions between hormone therapy and PrEP.[49]

AGING WITH HUMAN IMMUNODEFICIENCY VIRUS

Current CDC recommendations include HIV testing for adults aged 14 to 64 years.[18] Older adults living with HIV are often misdiagnosed or diagnosed late.[50,51] Late diagnosis is often related to apprehension of providers to initiate a conversation about sexual health and HIV risk. Many older adults remain sexually interested and active well into older adulthood.[52] When seeking health care, many report feeling comfortable discussing their sexual health, despite having to initiate these conversations with their health care providers (HCPs).[52]

Approximately 73% of older adults diagnosed with HIV are receiving HIV care.[53] Racial and socioeconomic disparity exists in older adults living with HIV as nearly half of all recipients of Ryan White Funding are over the age of 50 years, male, African American, and living at or below the federal poverty level.[54] Older adults living with HIV face unique challenges that include the risk of accelerated aging processes[55,56] and development of comorbid chronic health conditions.[15,57] The medical management of HIV and chronic illnesses like diabetes, dyslipidemia, and chronic kidney disease,[58,59] may precipitate polypharmacy[60] and contribute to pill burden.[58]

Policies and recommendations that advance the care of older adults living with HIV are needed. HCPs should receive ongoing training on how to screen older adults for HIV risk, initiate a sexual health history/screening,[52] and provide recommendations for HIV testing. Social isolation,[60] neurocognitive changes, depression, and stigma are significant factors that precipitate challenges with medication adherence and care engagement.

There is a great need for HCP education on the unique physiologic and psychosocial challenges that older adults living with HIV face. HCP training should be developed and executed with attention to cultural relevance and humility, especially when engaging minoritized communities[61] with diverse sexuality, gender identity, ethnicity, culture, race, language, and immigration status. It is time for the CDC recommendations to include HIV testing for all adults, regardless of age.

NOVEL APPROACHES TO PROVIDING CULTURALLY RELEVANT CARE

EHE begins and ends with reducing HIV-related disparities and health inequities. As we consider strategies to end the HIV epidemic, it is important to consider novel ways of providing HIV prevention, testing, and treatment. One strategy includes employing nurse-led models of care that allow and promote nurse practitioners to practice within the full extent of their training. Nurse-led models of care may provide telehealth, mobile care, or at-home laboratory testing. Nurses can coordinate mail-order prescriptions and other services that decrease patient challenges with transportation costs and logistics, scheduling nightmares that often accompany face-to-face office visits and the stigma that may be associated with taking PrEP. Keys to successful PrEP initiation, especially in Black, Southern, and rural communities where HIV treatment is the most disparate, include identification of eligibility, PrEP awareness, education, and same-day prescriptions.[62]

Telehealth can expand the reach of health professionals and give isolated rural communities greater access to health care.[63] Access to broadband services is a social determinant of health. Individuals living in rural communities who face stigma, discrimination, and transportation barriers[64] may be able to access health services in the privacy of their homes. This has significant implications for reducing disparities for people living in rural communities with chronic illnesses like HIV. However, many families living in rural communities do not have access to broadband Internet nor telehealth services.[64] Addressing upstream factors of infrastructure, allocation of funding, and community support must be addressed to implement widespread broadband access and improve health.

For many PLWH, access, treatment, and outcome inequities exist at the intersection of race, gender, and geography. Many Southern states where HIV incidence is increased are in the "Bible Belt." The "Bible Belt" is characterized by southeastern states where socially conservative and evangelical religious beliefs are predominant.[65] Over 60% of Black people who reside in the "Bible Belt" have a relationship with a historical Black church or Faith Based Organization (FBO).[66] Although Black organizations of faith have been facilitators of community engagement, they are underutilized in HIV education and prevention. Barriers for Black FBOs include stigma, homophobia, transphobia, and discomfort with discussing human sexuality. Strategies to increase HIV awareness include developing culturally relevant, engaging partnerships with FBOs to promote testing, and education in a way that aligns with the organization's values and beliefs and prioritizes a commitment to improve HIV outcomes for Black people living in the South.[66,67]

Historically Black colleges and universities (HBCUs) are pivotal to increasing the number of HIV resources available to Black youth living in the South, as more than 90% of all HBCUs are located in the South.[68] The Human Rights Campaign Foundation's PREP Ambassador Program is committed to reducing stigma and offering HIV education, testing, and resources for treatment.[69] Students attending HBCUs are trained as peer educators to provide peers with in-person and telehealth, culturally relevant HIV resources.[70] The inaugural cohort of peer educators began their work in 2022. In this setting, peer educators are often seen as a resource for sexually and gender-diverse students who report challenges obtaining culturally relevant resources.[71]

SUMMARY

Individual factors cannot explain the ongoing HIV-related health disparities experienced by racial and ethnic minority groups in the United States. There are systemic social and structural factors that contribute to the disparity in incidence and outcomes.[72] Unarguably, ART adherence and viral suppression are key to increasing quality of life and decreasing transmission for those living with HIV. Access to HIV prevention services is essential. However, as we advance in HIV treatment and prevention, we must continue to illuminate and address the social drivers that are inextricably linked to disparities in HIV outcomes, prevalence, incidence, and mortality.[73] The development of innovative models of HIV care and prevention that improve outcomes and decrease disparities is the way forward to EHE not just for some, but for all.

CLINICS CARE POINTS

- Ensure that every person aged 13 years and older knows their HIV status.
- Perform a sexual health history during annual well visits, and with increased frequency for those with increased HIV/STI risk.
- Increase awareness of PrEP by posting infographics in clinical offices and examination rooms.
- Take inventory of posted illustrations and infographics to ensure that they represent racial, ethnic, sexual, and gender diversity.
- Consider the myriad of challenges and barriers that PLWH may be facing. Avoid a paternalistic approach and lead with listening and resources.
- Advocate for nurse-led models of care that will reduce inequities in HIV treatment and prevention.

DISCLOSURE

The author has no conflict of interest to disclose.

REFERENCES

1. A timeline of HIV and AIDS. HIV.gov. Available at: https://www.hiv.gov/hiv-basics/overview/history/hiv-and-aids-timeline/#year-1981. [Accessed 12 August 2023].
2. Discovery of HIV. National Institutes of Health. Available at: https://history.nih.gov/display/history/Discovery+of+HIV. [Accessed 5 September 2023].
3. HIV and AIDS. Newsroom. 2023. World Health Organization. Available at: https://www.who.int/news-room/fact-sheets/detail/hiv-aids. [Accessed 12 August 2023].
4. Deeks SG, Lewin SR, Havlir DV. The end of AIDS: HIV infection as a chronic disease. Lancet 2013;382(9903):1525–33.
5. HIV and AIDS: Key Facts. 2023 World Health Organization. Available at: https://www.who.int/news-room/fact-sheets/detail/hivaids?gclid=EAlalQobChMIgKDD2_D4gAMVUjfUAR3uQwCTEAAYASAAEgJdI_D_BwE. [Accessed 25 August 2023].
6. UNAIDS. Global HIV & AIDS statistics — Fact sheet 2023. 2023. Available at: https://www.unaids.org/sites/default/files/media_asset/UNAIDS_FactSheet_en.pdf. [Accessed 28 September 2023].
7. Global Statistics. HIV.gov. Updated July 20, 2023. Available at: https://www.hiv.gov/hiv-basics/overview/data-and-trends/global-statistics/. [Accessed 15 October 2023].
8. U.S. Statistics. HIV.gov. Updated October 3, 2023. Available at: https://www.hiv.gov/hiv-basics/overview/data-and-trends/statistics/. [Accessed 15 October 2023].
9. AIDSVu, Center for Disease Control and Prevention. Map Displaying the Number of Persons Newly Diagnosed with HIV, 2021. Emory University, Rollins School of Public Health. Updated August 29, 2023. Available at: https://aidsvu.org/aidsvu-releases-2021-data-and-interactive-maps-visualizing-hiv-data-across-the-u-s/. [Accessed 21 November 2023].

10. 10. Black/African American Health. U.S. Department of Health and Human Services Office of Minority Health. Available at: https://minorityhealth.hhs.gov/blackafrican-american-health. [Accessed 30 October 2023].

11. Centers for Disease Control and Prevention, National Center for HIV, Viral Hepatitis, STD, and TB Prevention AtlasPlus. Chart displaying the number of HIV diagnoses and HIV related deaths among African Americans in 2021. Available at: https://www.cdc.gov/nchhstp/atlas/index.htm. [Accessed 1 November 2023].

12. AIDSVu, Center for Disease Control and Prevention. Chart displaying the Percentage of New HIV Diagnoses by Race/Ethnicity, 2021. Emory University, Rollins School of Public Health. Updated August 29, 2023. Available at: https://aidsvu.org/resources/deeper-look-hiv-in-black-communities/. [Accessed 21 November 2023].

13. AIDSVu, Center for Disease Control and Prevention. HIV in Black Communities. Emory University, Rollins School of Public Health. Updated August 29, 2023. Available at: https://aidsvu.org/resources/deeper-look-hiv-in-black-communities/. [Accessed 21 November 2023].

14. Budak J, Spach D. Core Concepts - HIV in Older Adults - Key Populations - National HIV Curriculum. National HIV Curriculum. August 8, 2023. Available at: https://www.hiv.uw.edu/go/key-populations/hiv-older-patients/core-concept/all. [Accessed 4 January 2024].

15. Sprague C, Brown SM, Simon S, et al. Towards ending the US HIV epidemic by 2030: Understanding social determinants of health and HIV in Mississippi. Global Publ Health 2020;5(1).

16. HIV in the United States by Region: HIV Diagnoses. 2022. Centers for Disease Control and Prevention. Available at: https://www.cdc.gov/hiv/statistics/overview/diagnoses.html. [Accessed 15 September 2023].

17. Rosen JG, Malik M, Cooney EE, et al. Antiretroviral Treatment Interruptions Among Black and Latina Transgender Women Living with HIV: Characterizing Co-occurring, Multilevel Factors Using the Gender Affirmation Framework. AIDS Behav 2019;23(9):2588–99.

18. National HIV/AIDS Strategy for the United States 2022-2025. The White House. Available at: https://files.hiv.gov/s3fs-public/NHAS-2022-2025.pdf. [Accessed 15 August 2023].

19. Ending the HIV Epidemic in the U.S. by 2030.Centers for Disease Control and Prevention. Updated June 9, 2023. Available at: https://www.cdc.gov/endhiv/index.html. [Accessed 21 August 2023].

20. HIV Testing. Centers for Disease Control and Prevention. Updated June 9, 2022. Available at: https://www.cdc.gov/hiv/testing/index.html. [Accessed 12 August 2023].

21. HIV Surveillance Report. 2022. Centers for Disease Control and Prevention. Available at: https://www.cdc.gov/hiv/pdf/library/reports/surveillance/cdc-hiv-surveillance-report-2020-updated-vol-33.pdf. [Accessed 8 September 2023].

22. About Rural Health Care. 2023. National Rural Health Care Association. National Rural Health Association. Available at: https://www.ruralhealth.us/about-nrha/about-rural-health-care. [Accessed 17 May 2023].

23. Obama B. United States Health Care Reform: Progress to Date and Next Steps. JAMA 2016;316(5):525–32.

24. Compilation of Patient Protection and Affordable Care Act. 2010. United States House of Representatives. Available at: http://housedocs.house.gov/energycommerce/ppacacon.pdf. [Accessed 25 April 2023].

25. HIV.gov. The Affordable Care Act and HIV/AIDS. Updated November 28, 2023. Available at: https://www.hiv.gov/federal-response/policies-issues/the-affordable-care-act-and-hiv-aids/. [Accessed 28 November 2023].

26. Status of state Medicaid expansion decisions: Interactive map. 2022. Kaiser Family Foundation; 2023. Available at: https://www.kff.org/medicaid/issue-brief/status-of-state-medicaid-expansion-decisions-interactive-map/. [Accessed 1 November 2023].

27. Artiga S, Hill L, Damico A. Health coverage by race and ethnicity, 2010-2021. Kaiser Family Foundation; 2022. Available at: https://www.kff.org/racial-equity-and-health-policy/issue-brief/health-coverage-by-race-and-ethnicity/. [Accessed 25 July 2023].

28. Francis A. AIDS United. March 28, 2023. North Carolina Medicaid expansion shows bipartisanship possible. Available at: https://aidsunited.org/north-carolina medicaid-expansion-shows-bipartisanship-possible/. [Accessed 3 May 2023].

29. Murphy T. HIV/AIDS providers are ecstatic about North Carolina finally expanding Medicaid. The Body. 2023. Available at: https://www.thebody.com/article/providers-ecstatic-north-carolina-expanding.medicaid. [Accessed 3 September 2023].

30. Masiano SP, Martin EG, Bono RS, et al. Suboptimal geographic accessibility to comprehensive HIV care in the US: regional and urban-rural differences. J Int AIDS Soc 2019;22(5):e25286.

31. Center for Disease Control and Prevention. Monitoring Selected National HIV Prevention and Care Objectives by Using HIV Surveillance Data—United States and 6 Dependent Areas. Supplemental Report 2021;28(4). Available at: https://www.cdc.gov/hiv/library/reports/hiv-surveillance/vol-28-no-4/index.html.

32. Schafer KR, Albrecht H, Dillingham R, et al. The Continuum of HIV Care in Rural Communities in the United States and Canada: What Is Known and Future Research Directions. J Acquir Immune Defic Syndr 2017;75(1):35–44.

33. O'Dell K. Economic Innovation Group. Redefining Rural: Towards a Better Understanding of Geography, Democracy and Economy in America's Rural Places. March 9, 2021. Available at: https://eig.org/redefining-rural-basics-and-well-being/. [Accessed 25 September 2023].

34. Miller AS, Krakower DS, Mayer KH. The Potential of Long-Acting, Injectable PrEP, and Impediments to its Uptake. J Urban Health 2023;100(1):212–4.

35. Health Resources and Services Administration. HRSA. Ryan white HIV/AIDS program. HIV care and treatment in rural communities. Available at: 2020 https://ryanwhite.hrsa.gov/sites/default/files/ryanwhite/resources/hiv-rural-communities-fact-sheet.pdf. [Accessed 27 June 2023].

36. HIV.gov. Funding for HIV Programs & Research in President Biden's FY24 Budget. March 23. 2023. Available at: https://www.hiv.gov/blog/funding-for-hiv-programs-research-in-president-biden-s-fy24-budget/. [Accessed 15 September 2023].

37. Ryan White HIV/AIDS Program Funding. Updated March 2023. Available at: https://ryanwhite.hrsa.gov/about/budget. [Accessed 19 June 2023].

38. Jones J, Zlotorzynska M, Villarino X, et al. Where is Rural? Examining the Effect of Rural Classification Method on Disparities in HIV and STI Testing Uptake Among Men Who Have Sex with Men in the United States. AIDS Behav 2022;26(9):2897–906.

39. U.S. Food & Drug Administration. FDA Approves First Injectable Treatment for HIV Pre- Exposure Prevention. Press Announcements. 2021. Available at: https://www.fda.gov/news-events/press-announcements/fda-approves-first-injectable-treatment-hiv-pre-exposure-prevention. [Accessed 25 September 2023].

40. Centers for Disease Control and Prevention. HIV and Gay and Bisexual Men. Available at: https://www.cdc.gov/hiv/group/gay-bisexual-men/index.html. [Accessed 15 October 2023].
41. Centers for Disease Control and Prevention. PrEP for HIV Prevention in the U.S. Updated September 29, 2023. Accessed December 1, 2023.
42. AIDSVu, Center for Disease Control and Prevention. National HIV/AIDS and Aging Awareness Day2023 Toolkit. 2023. Emory University, Rollins School of Public Health. Updated August 29, 2023. Available at: https://aidsvu.org/national-hiv-aids-and-aging-awareness-day-2023-toolkit/- aging citation goes somewhere. [Accessed 17 September 2023].
43. Centers for Disease Control and Prevention. HIV in the United States by Race and Ethnicity: PrEP Coverage. Available at: https://www.cdc.gov/hiv/group/racialethnic/other-races/prep-coverage.html. [Accessed 20 October 2023].
44. Brousseau NM, Driver R, Simon K, et al. PrEP-Related Interactive Toxicity Beliefs: Associations With Stigma, Substance Use, and PrEP Uptake. AIDS Educ Prev 2023;35(2):114–25.
45. Owens C, Gray SJ, Carter K, et al. Implementation Facilitators and Barriers for Primary Care Providers Prescribing Daily Oral PrEP to Adolescents in the United States. AIDS patient care and STDs 2023;37(8):379–93.
46. Kay ES, Pinto RM. Is Insurance a Barrier to HIV Preexposure Prophylaxis? Clarifying the Issue. American journal of public health 2020;110(1):61–4.
47. U.S. Food and Drug Administration. Truvada for PrEP Fact Sheet: Ensuring Safe and Proper Use. July, 2012. Available at: https://www.fda.gov/files/drugs/published/Truvada-for-PrEP-Fact-Sheet–Ensuring-Safe-and-Proper-Use.pdf. [Accessed 25 August 2023].
48. Sex Ed for Social Change. The SIECUS State Profiles. Available at: https://siecus.org/state-profiles/. [Accessed 12 October 2023].
49. Hanna-Walker V, Simon KA, Lawrence SE, et al. Black Sexual Minority Men's Stigma-Based Experiences Surrounding Pre-exposure Prophylaxis in the Southern United States. LGBT Health 2023;10(3):245–51.
50. Justice AC, Goetz MB, Stewart CN, et al. Delayed presentation of HIV among older individuals: a growing problem. Lancet HIV 2022;9(4):e269–80.
51. Yasin F, Rizk C, Taylor B, et al. Substantial gap in primary care: older adults with HIV presenting late to care. BMC Geriatr 2020;20(1):438.
52. Agochukwu-Mmonu N, Malani PN, Wittmann D, et al. Interest in Sex and Conversations About Sexual Health with Health Care Providers Among Older U.S. Adults. Clin Gerontol 2021;44(3):299–306.
53. AIDSVu, Center for Disease Control and Prevention. HIV Care Continuum Among people aged 55 and older. Emory University, Rollins School of Public Health. Updated August 29, 2023. Available at: https://aidsvu.org/resources/#/infographics?infographic_types=aging. [Accessed 21 November 2023].
54. HRSA. Ryan White HIV/AIDS Program. Older Adult Clients: HRSA's Ryan White HIV/AIDS Program, 2021. Population Fact Sheet | March 2023. Available at: https://ryanwhite.hrsa.gov/sites/default/files/ryanwhite/resources/population-factsheet-older-adults.pdf. [Accessed 2 January 2024].
55. Siddiqi KA, Ostermann J, Zhang J, et al. Ageing with HIV in the United States: Changing trends in inpatient hospital stays and comorbidities, 2003–2015. HIV Med 2023;24(1):93–103.
56. Martínez-Sanz J, Serrano-Villar S, Vivancos MJ, et al. HIV-associated comorbidities Study Group. Management of Comorbidities in Treated HIV Infection: A Long

Way to Go: HIV, comorbidities, and aging. Int J Antimicrob Agents 2022;59(1): 106493.

57. Petroll AE, Quinn KG, John SA, et al. Factors associated with lack of care engagement among older, rural-dwelling adults living with HIV in the United States. J Rural Health 2023;39(2):477–87.

58. Smith L, Letendre S, Erlandson KM, et al. Polypharmacy in older adults with HIV infection: Effects on the brain. J Am Geriatr Soc 2022;70(3):924–7.

59. Webel AR, Schexnayder J, Cioe PA, et al. A Review of Chronic Comorbidities in Adults Living With HIV: State of the Science. J Assoc Nurses AIDS Care 2021; 32(3):322–46.

60. Brennan-Ing M. Diversity, stigma, and social integration among older adults with HIV. Eur Geriatr Med 2019;10(2):239–46.

61. Harris LM, Crawford TN, Kerr JC, et al. African American Older Adults Living with HIV: Exploring Stress, Stigma, and Engagement in HIV Care. J Health Care Poor Underserved 2020;31(1):265–86. https://doi.org/10.1353/hpu.2020.0022.

62. Hollcroft MR, Gipson J, Barnes A, et al. PrEP Acceptance among Eligible Patients Attending the Largest PrEP Clinic in Jackson, Mississippi. J Int Assoc Provid AIDS Care 2023;22. 23259582231167959.

63. Vilme H, Duke NN, Muiruri C, et al. Using Telehealth to Disseminate Primary, Secondary, and Tertiary CVD Interventions to Rural Populations. Curr Hypertens Rep 2019;21(12):92.

64. Graves JM, Abshire DA, Amiri S, et al. Disparities in Technology and Broadband Internet Access Across Rurality: Implications for Health and Education. Fam Community Health 2021;44(4):257–65.

65. Abadi M, Gal S, Lee L. MAP: From the Bible Belt to the Rust Belt, the United States has 13 distinct 'belts'. Business Insider. Updated February 20, 23. Available at: https://www.businessinsider.com/regions-america-bible-belt-rust-belt-2018-4. [Accessed 5 January 2024].

66. Nunn A, Jeffries WL 4th, Foster P, et al. Reducing the African American HIV Disease Burden in the Deep South: Addressing the Role of Faith and Spirituality. AIDS Behav 2019;23(Suppl 3):319–30.

67. Bradley ELP, Sutton MY, Cooks E, et al. Developing FAITHH: Methods to Develop a Faith-Based HIV Stigma-Reduction Intervention in the Rural South. Health Promot Pract 2018;19(5):730–40.

68. HBCU List Map. HBCU First. Available at: https://hbcufirst.com/resources/hbcu-list-map. [Accessed 20 October 2023].

69. Keller J. Human Rights Campaign HBCU Program Announces New Cohort of PrEP Ambassadors. Human Rights Campaign. August 25, 2023. Available at: https://www.hrc.org/press-releases/human-rights-campaign-hbcu-program-announces-new-cohort-of-prep-ambassadors. [Accessed 20 October 2023].

70. Brewer R, Daunis C, Ebaady S, et al. Implementation of a Socio-structural Demonstration Project to Improve HIV Outcomes Among Young Black Men in the Deep South. J Racial Ethn Health Disparities 2019;6(4):775–89.

71. Spitalniak L. Stigma is still killing students': Inside a student-driven program to prevent HIV at HBCUs. Higher Ed Dive. May 2, 2023. Available at: https://www.highereddive.com/news/hrc-prep-education-ambassadors-hbcus/648546/. [Accessed 20 October 2023].

72. Carter JW Jr, Flores SA. Improving the HIV Prevention Landscape to Reduce Disparities for Black MSM in the South. AIDS Behav 2019;23(Suppl 3):331–9.

73. Kalichman SC. Ending HIV Hinges on Reducing Poverty. AIDS Behav 2023; 27(1):1–3.

The Impact of Human Immunodeficiency Virus on Women in the United States

Dominique Guillaume, MSN, AGPCNP-BC, AAHIVE

KEYWORDS

- HIV • HIV prevention • HIV treatment • Women • Women living with HIV
- Ending the HIV epidemic

KEY POINTS

- Women experience the highest burden of HIV globally. In the United States, women account for nearly a quarter of all new HIV infections with the southern United States comprising the majority of new infections.
- Clinicians in both HIV-based and non-HIV-based settings should be readily aware of the unique risk factors that propel HIV risk among women, along with the variables that contribute to suboptimal treatment outcomes for women on preexposure prophylaxis and antiretroviral therapy.
- In prioritizing well-being among women living with HIV and women at risk of HIV, clinicians must go beyond solely biomedical approaches and also address underlying financial and social forces that can adversely affect health outcomes.

INTRODUCTION

Women's HIV incidence rates currently surpass that of men worldwide.[1,2] Among the approximately 1.2 million people living with HIV in the United States, 23% are cisgender women, in which we define as those whose gender identity aligns with the sex they were assigned at birth (ie, being born with female sex organs and identifying as female).[3] In the United States, substantial improvements have been made in reducing HIV incidence rates among women, with HIV diagnoses decreasing among women by 6% from 2015 to 2019.[4] These successes are critical to acknowledge given the severe inequities women have faced throughout the HIV epidemic. Although current trends have been favorable, it will be imperative for HIV prevention and treatment efforts to be amplified in order to successfully meet the Center for Disease Control Ending the HIV Epidemic (EHE) targets, which involve reducing new HIV infections by 90% by 2030 through proper diagnoses, treatment, prevention, and response.[5]

Center for Infectious Disease and Nursing Innovation, Johns Hopkins School of Nursing, Johns Hopkins University, 525 North Wolfe Street, Baltimore, MD 21205, USA
E-mail address: dguilla2@jhu.edu

Nurs Clin N Am 59 (2024) 165–181
https://doi.org/10.1016/j.cnur.2024.01.003
0029-6465/24/© 2024 Elsevier Inc. All rights reserved.

Meeting these pillars will require examining and addressing the powerful social, economic, and structural forces that promote the demographic distribution of HIV among women in the United States.[6] In this article, we discuss recent trends in women's HIV incidence and prevalence rates, along with implications HIV has on health, social, and financial well-being for women living with HIV (WLWH) and for women at risk for HIV.

RECENT TRENDS IN WOMEN'S HUMAN IMMUNODEFICIENCY VIRUS INCIDENCE AND PREVALENCE

HIV is a disease that is entrenched in numerous inequities, with data indicating HIV incidence and prevalence being strongly linked to sociodemographic variables such as age, race, and poverty level. Throughout the HIV epidemic, it has been well documented that women have faced numerous barriers in accessing resources for HIV prevention and treatment. Barriers such as socioeconomic status, education, housing, stigma, gender inequality, poverty, and intimate partner violence (IPV) result in a constellation of vulnerabilities that can predispose women to HIV and can affect treatment outcomes for those already living with HIV.[7] These barriers negatively influence women's experience throughout the HIV care continuum (**Fig. 1**) and are critical to acknowledge when contextualizing the HIV disparities that women experience.

Human Immunodeficiency Virus Incidence and Prevalence

The most common routes of HIV transmission among women include heterosexual contact (85%) and injection drug use (16%).[8] However, variances exist in HIV transmission among different subgroups of women. For instance, Black women have the largest percentage of HIV infection attributable to heterosexual transmission (92%), whereas American Indian/Alaskan Native women (43%) and White women (45%) are more likely to acquire HIV through injection drug use.[8] These varied epidemiologic patterns are critical to acknowledge in addressing HIV risk and developing prevention measures among diverse communities.

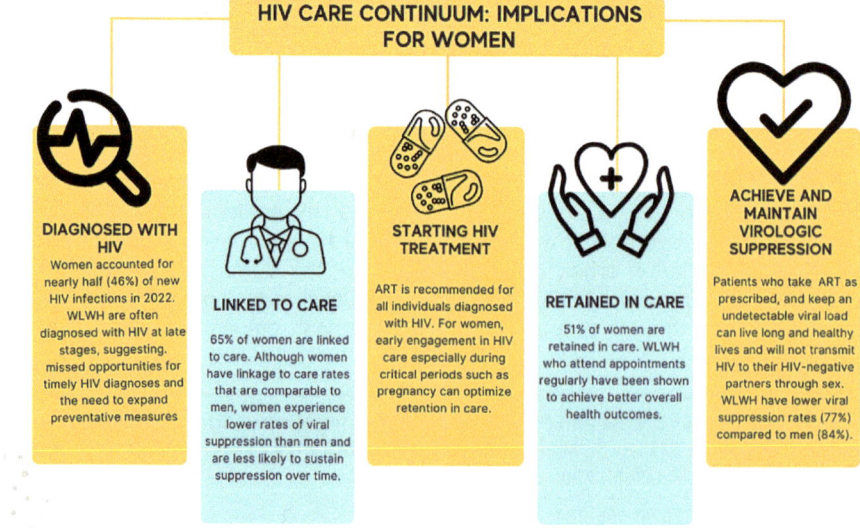

Fig. 1. HIV care continuum: implications for women.

In addition, HIV diagnoses are unevenly distributed among women, with certain subgroups of women experiencing higher burdens of HIV. In the United States, Black women have unequal HIV incidence and prevalence rates compared with women of other racial groups. Despite only comprising 13% of the female population, Black women account for 54% of new HIV diagnoses.[4] Studies have also indicated absolute and relative disparity values and trends in HIV diagnosis among immigrant women living in the United States. Although the relative disparity in HIV incidence rates has primarily declined for US born-Black women, it has increased for Caribbean, African, and all non-US-born Black women.[9] HIV-related disparities simultaneously exist for Hispanic women who are 4 times more likely to have HIV compared with their White counterparts.[4] Current data show that the likelihood of a woman being diagnosed with HIV in their lifetime is significantly higher for Black women (1 in 54) and Hispanic women (1 in 256) compared with that of White women (1 in 941).[4,10]

Regional differences exist in HIV incidence and prevalence rates among women across the United States. Among female adults and adolescents, the southern United States accounts for highest rates of new HIV infections compared with any other region of the United States, with Black women who live in the South having the highest rates of HIV.[8] In the Southern United States, White women are more likely to be diagnosed with HIV compared with any other region.[8] These regional nuances largely differ for Hispanic women in which the Northeastern United States accounts for the highest rates of new HIV infections among Hispanic women.[8] Accounting for these contexts are important for health-care providers to consider when addressing HIV risk, prevention, and treatment across the HIV care continuum for women.

DISCUSSION
Health Considerations

Health practitioners who provide care to WLWH and those at risk for HIV must be aware of the unique health challenges this population faces as a complex interplay of biological and psychosocial factors influence their health and well-being. In the following sections, we highlight key comorbidities that have received heightened attention for WLWH (**Table 1**). We also discuss preexposure prophylaxis (PrEP) considerations for women at risk for HIV.

Differences in Antiretroviral Therapy Adherence Among Women Living with Human Immunodeficiency Virus

Although women have linkage to care rates that are comparable to men, women experience lower rates of viral suppression than men and are less likely to sustain suppression over time.[11,12] For WLWH and who are on ART differences have been noted in the use of ART and treatment outcomes among racial groups. Correlates of virologic failure, which perpetuate HIV transmission, have been found to vary based on women's race, ethnicity, socioeconomic status, access to health insurance, drug use, and their mental health status. Black WLWH have been found to present with more advanced stages of HIV infection at the time of diagnosis, are slower in initiating ART, and experience higher rates of discontinuing ART with resulting virologic failure.[13,14] Income below the poverty line, depressive symptoms, and tobacco use have been found to have a stronger association with discontinuing ART among Black WLWH, compared with Hispanic and White WLWH.[15,16] Hispanic WLWH with a history of recent drug use are more likely to discontinue ART compared with Black and White WLWH.[15,16] In comparison to Black WLWH, Hispanic and White WLWH who have no health insurance are more likely to present with virologic failure.[15,16] Thus, for WLWH who are

Table 1
Clinical implications for health concerns pertaining to WLWH and women at risk for HIV

Health Concern	Key Highlights	Clinical Implications
Mental health	WLWH experience mental health disorders at higher rates than the general population Mental health disorders contribute to worsening medical appointment adherence and reduced adherence to antiretroviral therapy (ART) thus hastening the progression to AIDS In many settings, access to comprehensive mental health treatment that are tailored to the needs of WLWH are inadequate	Integrating psychosocial and cognitive-behavioral components (eg, behavioral therapy and motivational interviewing) within ART adherence and self-management interventions should be prioritized Clinicians must address WLWH's unique needs including decisions pertaining to HIV disclosure, stigma, coping, advocacy, and building strong support networks Selective serotonin reuptake inhibitors are often used for depression among WLWH and have a safe profile in pregnancy, breastfeeding, and in combination with ART[1]
Human papilloma virus (HPV)-associated cancers	The incidence of cervical cancer and anal cancer, have continued to increase among WLWH even in the presence of ART WLWH have worse outcomes for cervical neoplasia, with high rates of treatment failure and recurrence WLWH are more likely to have persistent HPV infections leading to anal high-grade squamous intraepithelial lesions (HSIL), which can ultimately progress to anal cancer	Clinicians must ensure eligible WLWH receive the Gardasil 9-valent HPV vaccine for primary prevention against high-risk oncogenic HPV strains that can cause cervical cancer and anal cancer, in addition to other HPV-associated cancers Clinicians should follow guidelines for cervical cancer screening. For WLWH ≤30 y, Pap tests should be conducted. WLWH ≥30 y can be screened with either pap tests only, or pap tests coupled with HPV cotesting. Screening should occur annually until 3 consecutive Pap tests are normal; afterward screening can be conducted once every 3 y[3]
		Clinicians must ensure WLWH receive primary prevention against high-risk oncogenic HPV strains that can cause anal cancer using the Gardasil 9-valent HPV vaccine National guidelines for anal cancer screening for WLWH do not exist. For clinicians who decide to screen WLWH, further evaluation of screen positives with high-resolution anoscopy to detect HSIL should be considered[4]

Obesity	Women have more pronounced weight gain than the general population with HIV Studies have implicated the role of specific ART drug-classes in contributing to weight gain	In selecting ART regimens, clinicians should consider their patient's baseline weight and underlying comorbidities that could worsen in the presence of weight gain Lifestyle interventions (eg, diet, physical activity, and behavioral skills) focused on weight loss should be promoted for WLWH
Cardiovascular disease	The relative risk of both myocardial infarction and stroke is significantly greater among WLWH compared with men living with HIV Sex-based differences in immune mechanisms can contribute to heightened cardiovascular disease risk among WLWH	Aggressive lipid management is essential for primary and secondary cardiovascular disease prevention Statins are commonly used for treating dyslipidemia. Pitavastatin has shown clinical efficacy in reducing cardiovascular disease risk for people living with HIV. Clinically relevant drug–drug interactions exist between statins and certain antiretroviral drugs; thus clinicians should refer to a drug interaction database before prescribing statins with ART Health practitioners must address behavioral risk factors (eg, tobacco use, alcohol consumption, obesity, and mental health) that can severely affect cardiovascular health outcomes, which are often underassessed among WLWH Clinicians can consider modifying ART (eg, certain protease inhibitors) to reduce elevated triglyceride and low-density-lipoprotein (LDL)-cholesterol levels
PrEP	Only 10% of women who could benefit from PrEP are prescribed PrEP Two forms of PrEP are approved for cisgender women: the daily oral pill Truvada and the long-acting injectable Apretude Women who agree to take PrEP and who are prescribed PrEP have a greater propensity in discontinuing the medication compared with men	Clinicians working in both HIV and non-HIV settings should promote awareness and education toward PrEP for all women Increasing PrEP use among women will require for women to perceive PrEP to be a beneficial medication. Clinicians should provide comprehensive PrEP information while addressing concerns related to stigma and negative societal perceptions pertaining to PrEP use For women who prefer to keep their PrEP use discrete, clinicians can discuss the possibility of using the long acting injectable Apretude compared with the daily oral pill

prescribed ART, health-care providers and supportive staff must comprehensively assess the unique factors that may influence their risk of ART discontinuation and provide appropriate counseling and linkage to resources (eg, social services, mental health services, and case management) to aid in promoting ART adherence.

Mental Health for Women Living with Human Immunodeficiency Virus

Individuals living with HIV experience mental health disorders at higher rates than the general population. Compared with men living with HIV, WLWH are more likely to have worse overall mental health outcomes with concurrent mental and physical comorbidities.[17,18] It has been proposed that this may be due to women being in vulnerable positions associated with HIV acquisition (eg, IPV and poverty), which can lead to harmful consequences for social, occupational, and familial functioning.[17] A new HIV diagnosis can also exacerbate preexisting mental illness and contribute to mental illness symptomatology due to the stigma and psychological distress associated with the disease itself.[17] The pregnancy and postpartum phase are also critical periods that can result in an increased risk of developing mental health disorders particularly depression and anxiety, which can be exacerbated by stressors regarding the disclosure of one's HIV status, concerns regarding the prevention of mother to fetal transmission, along with stigma related to carrying a pregnancy while living with HIV.[17]

Depression is the most commonly diagnosed mental health disorder among WLWH, with the prevalence of depression being 3 times higher than the general population.[18,19] Depression along with other psychiatric illnesses can significantly worsen existing disease states, thus contributing to poorer health outcomes for WLWH. Depression and trauma have been found to be closely linked, with studies delineating a strong association between a history of childhood trauma, IPV, and depression among WLWH.[17] Mental health disorders including depression have been found to contribute to worsening medical appointment adherence and a reduced adherence to ART with resulting lower CD4 cell counts and higher viral loads, thus hastening the progression to AIDS and an elevated risk of mortality.[17–19] Less than half of WLWH are adequately treated for depression, thus making depression along with other mental health conditions a top priority for this population.[11] In many settings, access to comprehensive mental health treatment that are tailored to the needs of WLWH are inadequate, and interventions targeting mental health for specific groups of WLWH are lacking. Thus, a dire need exists for more research and evidence-based public health and clinical interventions to fill the gaps in mental health services for WLWH.

Human Papilloma Virus-Associated Cancers

Infection with HPV is etiologically responsible for nearly all cervical cancers and a subset of cancers of the anus, oropharynx, penis, vagina, and vulva.[20] HPV is a small, non-enveloped, double-stranded DNA virus with more than 100 different genotypes. The most common high-risk genotypes are 16, 18, 31, 33, 35, 39, 45, 51, 52, 56, 58, 59, and 68.[21] WLWH, even when effectively treated with ART, are more likely to be infected with high-risk oncogenic HPV strains that can result in a more rapid progression to malignancy. The incidence of HPV-related diseases for WLWH, particularly cervical cancer and anal cancer, has continued to increase compared with the incidence of other HIV-associated comorbidities even in the presence of ART.[20,22]

WLWH are disproportionately affected by cervical cancer, with cervical cancer being the most commonly diagnosed HPV-related cancer among WLWH. Compared with the general population, WLWH have worse outcomes for cervical neoplasia, with high rates of treatment failure and recurrence particularly among those with low CD4 cell counts.[23,24] Primary prevention through the HPV vaccine and secondary prevention through cervical cancer screening are paramount in reducing cervical cancer burdens in this high-risk population. Currently, the World Health Organization recommends a 3-dose HPV vaccination schedule for those aged 15 years and older and for individuals who are immunocompromised including those living with HIV.[25] There is strong evidence supporting the efficacy of a single HPV vaccine dose, with data indicating that one dose confers adequate protection that is equivalent to a multiple dose vaccine schedule.[25,26] However, as of date, no clinical trials have explored the immunogenicity of a single-dose schedule for WLWH. Similarly to persons who are HIV negative, seropositivity levels and antibody titers among those living with HIV gradually decline over time; however, the significance of these lower antibody levels for individuals living with HIV remains unclear.[27] In addition to the HPV vaccine for primary prevention, cervical cancer screening should be offered for secondary prevention. For WLWH aged younger than 30 years, Papanicolaou (pap) tests with cytology is recommended. WLWH aged older than 30 years can screen with either the pap test only, or pap testing coupled with HPV cotesting.[28] Data strongly indicate that WLWH who receive regular cervical cancer screenings have lower incidence rates of invasive cervical cancer.[29]

Anal cancer is an HPV-associated malignancy that has become increasingly common among individuals living with HIV. Persistent HPV infection can lead to anal HSIL, which can ultimately progress to anal cancer.[30] In a large cohort study conducted in the United States, WLWH had an anal cancer rate of 30 out of 100,000 person-years, whereas there were no observed cases for women without HIV.[31] Even in patients with a CD4 cell count above 500 mL for 2 years or more, the risk of anal cancer is 20-fold.[32] The incidence of anal cancer among WLWH has increased 800% since the advent of ART; however, researches on anal cancer prevalence and screening have primarily focused with men living with HIV.[33] Early detection and treatment of precancerous lesions among WLWH is a research priority and unmet need. Although precancerous HSIL can be detected through high-resolution anoscopy and anal cytology, no national guidelines exist for screening individuals living with HIV.[33] Thus, primary prevention through HPV vaccination remains paramount in reducing the incidence of anal cancer among WLWH, in addition to other HPV-related cancers.

Obesity

The degree of weight gain experienced by WLWH is out of proportion with that of the current obesity epidemic in the United States.[34] Compared with men living with HIV, WLWH experience a significantly greater increase in body mass index (BMI) following ART initiation.[35] Furthermore, women, Black individuals, and those with lower weight and CD4 counts before starting ART have more pronounced weight gain than the general population with HIV.[36,37] Although weight gain among WLWH has been widely documented, the mechanisms of associated weight gain remain poorly understood. Systemic inflammation and immune activation contributing to disordered inflammatory regulation have been well described among persons living with HIV and is more robust in those with low CD4 cell counts and high viral loads.[35] Adipose tissue is increasingly recognized as a metabolically active tissue that participates in inflammatory and immunity processes. It has been found that adipocytes induce the secretion of inflammatory cytokines and interleukins associated with increased mortality in individuals living with HIV.[35] More specifically, adipocytes secrete the proinflammatory adipokine leptin, which is associated with an inflammatory state in the setting of obesity, and its synthesis happens to be significantly increased in the presence of female sex hormones.[35,37] Other markers of immune activation have been reported to be higher in WLWH compared with men, with certain markers of inflammation being associated with more significant gains in fat among WLWH after ART initiation.[35,38]

Recent studies evaluating weight gain among individuals living with HIV have placed a heightened focus on distinct classes of antiretroviral drugs, specifically integrase inhibitors (INSTI), that contribute to weight gain.[39] In a retrospective observational cohort study, ART regimens containing dolutegravir contributed to higher amounts of weight gain among individuals living with HIV compared with protease inhibitors (PIs) and nonnucleoside reverse transcriptase inhibitor-based regimens.[40] Another longitudinal study reported significantly greater increases in BMI and weight gain among individuals initiated on regimens with the INSTI bictegravir.[41] These incidences of weight gain associated with integrase inhibitor use have been demonstrated in both treatment-naive patients, along with patients in switch-trials. The mechanisms through which these ARTs result in weight gain remain unclear; however, the relationship between weight gain and adverse health outcomes such as cardiovascular disease and diabetes should be of great concern to health-care providers.

Cardiovascular Disease

Because people with HIV continue to live longer due to the advent of ART, there is an increased concern regarding their cardiovascular disease risk. Concerningly, the relative risk of both myocardial infarction and stroke is significantly greater among WLWH compared with men living with HIV.[42] Compared with men with HIV, the risk of myocardial infarction, stroke, and heart failure is 1.5 to 2-fold higher among women after adjusting for demographic factors, stroke risk factors (eg, obesity, tobacco use, and hypertension), and sex-specific risk factors (eg, menopause status).[6,43] Although the pathophysiological mechanisms have not been fully understood, it has been elucidated that this increased risk is due to chronic inflammation characterized by dysregulated immune activity even after treatment with ART.[43] As women have shown to mount greater immune responses than men, researchers have also noted sex-based differences in immune mechanisms that can contribute to heightened cardiovascular disease risk among WLWH.[42] Even in the presence of virological suppression, markers of inflammation (eg, tumor necrosis factor [TNF]-α1, TNF-α2, interleukin [IL]-6, IL-4, and c-reactive protein [CRP]) and monocyte activation have been found to be elevated among WLWH, thus increasing the risk of cardiovascular disease incidence and mortality.[43–45]

HIV infection affects lipid metabolism due to chronic inflammation and immune activation, resulting in dyslipidemia and an increased risk of cardiovascular disease. Although treatment with ART can result in some improvement in reducing low high-density lipoprotein cholesterol, it does not completely normalize the lipid profile. Furthermore, certain antiretroviral drug classes, particularly PIs, may exacerbate dyslipidemia and cardiovascular risk.[45,46] Aggressive lipid management among WLWH is essential for primary and secondary cardiovascular disease prevention and optimizing wellness across the life span.[47] The REPRIEVE trial, which is the first large-scale randomized clinical trial to test a daily dose of pitavastatin in reducing cardiovascular disease risk among individuals living with HIV, demonstrated efficacy of pitavastatin in reducing the risk of a major adverse cardiovascular event over a median follow-up of 5.1 years.[48] Although this trial underscores the importance of biomedical approaches in reducing cardiovascular disease risk, health practitioners must also address behavioral risk factors (eg, tobacco use, alcohol consumption, obesity, and mental health) that can severely affect cardiovascular health outcomes, which are often underassessed among WLWH.

Preexposure Prophylaxis for Human Immunodeficiency Virus Prevention

PrEP is an effective means of reducing the risk of HIV acquisition for individuals who are HIV negative. Currently, 2 forms of PrEP are approved for cis-gender women: (1) a daily oral pill coformulated with tenofovir disoproxil fumurate/emtricitabine (Truvada) and (2) a long-acting injectable consisting of cabotegravir (Apretude). All sexually active women should be informed about PrEP for HIV prevention.

Although the EHE plan aims to have at least 50% of PrEP eligible people to be prescribed PrEP by 2025, there have been entrenched geographic, gender, and racial disparities in PrEP uptake. Only 10% of women who could benefit from PrEP are prescribed PrEP, with the majority of female PrEP users being White women.[49] This is concerning because Black women account for 54% of new HIV diagnosis despite only comprising 13% of the female population and have a lower rate of PrEP uptake despite their disproportionate risk.[4]

Numerous factors that contribute to low PrEP uptake among women. A major contributing factor is low awareness and knowledge regarding PrEP among women. Among high-risk women, only 14.9% had adequate knowledge of PrEP.[49,50] Even among women who have high PrEP awareness, knowledge toward PrEP has been found to be generally low, with women believing misconceptions such as PrEP being solely for individuals in the lesbian, gay, bisexual, transgender, and queer (LGBTQ) community.[51] Concerningly, studies have demonstrated that even when women are adequately informed of PrEP, many are not willing to use the drug due to not perceiving themselves to be at risk of HIV along with the stigma associated with PrEP use.[51] Women who agree to take PrEP and who are prescribed PrEP have a greater propensity in discontinuing the medication compared with men.[52,53] In a study exploring PrEP adherence with Truvada among 7148 patients through a large pharmaceutical chain, women aged between 18 and 24 years had the lowest proportion of persistent PrEP use.[52] Low subjective risk perception toward HIV coupled with stigma have been associated with low levels of PrEP uptake among women. For women, PrEP use has been linked to a range of negative judgements and social concerns, particularly the fear that others will perceive PrEP as HIV treatment and perceive PrEP users as being sexually irresponsible.[54] The lower rates of adherence to the daily oral pill Truvada for PrEP among women may suggest the need for health-care providers to explore patient preferences toward the long-acting injectable cabotegravir. The HPTN 084 study demonstrated that cabotegravir was superior to daily tenofovir disoproxil fumurate/emtricitabine (TDF/FTC) among cisgender women, and among nearly 2500 women, 78% preferred the injectable to the daily oral pill as women voiced wanting a discrete PrEP option.[55]

Growing evidence has indicated that health-care providers may exhibit considerable bias in HIV testing and prescribing PrEP for women, especially Black women, thus further amplifying their risk of acquiring HIV.[51,56–59] A recent study of claims data exploring characteristics of new PrEP users reported noticeable differences in the age and gender of newly initiated PrEP users.[60] Adults who initiated PrEP were predominantly men (91.0%), whereas the majority of adolescents who initiated PrEP (69.7%) were women[60]; thus indicating a gap in ensuring adult women who are at risk for HIV are also targeted by health-care providers for PrEP. Primary care centers, gynecology offices, family planning clinics, and health departments are important entry points for reaching women and promoting HIV prevention services such as HIV testing and PrEP. Leveraging these settings to promote PrEP awareness and uptake for women will be key toward reaching EHE targets.

FINANCIAL IMPACT OF HUMAN IMMUNODEFICIENCY VIRUS AMONG WOMEN
Health-Care Associated Costs

Significant financial implications exist for WLWH and for women at risk for HIV. As previously described, those aging with HIV have a significantly higher risk of developing

·chronic comorbidities leading to poorer health outcomes. Consequentially, this often results in significant financial costs for women due to greater health-care needs and utilization costs. The costs of HIV and associated treatments, adverse events, and comorbidities are estimated to amount to up to US$1.7 million per patient.[60] A recent study of individuals living with HIV who were Medicaid-insured and aged younger than 65 years reported a disproportionate number of comorbidities and use of concomitant medications, which contributed to a significantly rate of health-care utilization expenses.[60] Similarly, a study conducted with adolescents and young adults living with HIV reported that increased age was associated with a higher number of emergency department visits and inpatient days, resulting in greater health expenditures.[61]

Employment

There is consistent evidence to support the direct relationship between employment and HIV outcomes across the HIV care continuum. WLWH who are employed are more likely to engage in medical care including HIV testing, timely linkage to care, retention in HIV care, and ART adherence.[62] However, the negative effects that HIV can cause on physical and mental functioning can render challenges with consistent employment, thus negatively influencing WLWH's socioeconomic status.[63,64] Furthermore, disease severity (ie, low CD4 cell counts and high levels of viremia) and HIV-related work discrimination can increase the risk for employment loss among WLWH.[62–64]

For women at high-risk for HIV, data from the Women's Interagency HIV Study (WIHS) have indicated that employment was negatively associated with health-care utilization particularly for women of low socioeconomic status.[65] It has been proposed that this may be due to lower income high-risk women lacking flexibility in their jobs to maintain health-care appointments. Given the importance of preventive care, this highlights the need for health-care providers to develop innovative ways to offer preventive services to high-risk populations.[65]

Poverty and Housing

Financial security and stable housing have been strongly tied with successful HIV-related health outcomes including engagement in HIV testing, PrEP utilization, linkage to HIV treatment, and viral suppression.[66,67] Unstable housing and unsafe neighborhoods embedded in violence, coupled with issues pertaining to substance abuse have been found to positively correlate with HIV risk behaviors among women.[7,68,69] Poverty and challenges related to housing can predispose WLWH and those at risk for HIV to engage in certain high-risk behaviors such as unprotected transactional sex and can also predispose women to unsafe environments that can potentiate the risk of IPV, which is strongly associated with HIV risk.[7,67,70] For WLWH who are pregnant, poverty and housing instability has also been associated with failure to achieve virologic suppression during the perinatal period.

Considered together, the existing evidence demonstrates a critical need for HIV services that are targeted for women to consider the underlying issues of medical care expenses, financial stability, employment, and housing.[67] Health-care providers treating WLWH and those at risk for HIV must consider the use of integrated services that address women's social and financial concerns, in addition to meeting their HIV and overall health needs. The high costs of health care that patients will incur must be considered when developing efforts for adherence to treatment. This warrants the need for health-care providers to be aware of underlying factors that may play into successful adherence to both PrEP and ART. Health-care providers should collaborate with supportive services to meet patients where they are and to explore available re-sources in which patients can be referred to.

SOCIAL IMPACT OF HUMAN IMMUNODEFICIENCY VIRUS AMONG WOMEN
Women's Intersecting Roles Affecting Human Immunodeficiency Virus Self-Management

Numerous vulnerabilities within women's social context affect HIV self-manage-ment.[71] The cumulation of demanding social roles, poverty, and inadequate access to health care along with pervasive structural factors such as racism, sexism, imbal-anced gender dynamics, and stigma can subsequently affect women's uptake of HIV prevention and treatment services.[71] Consistent findings suggest that the multiple roles women have within their households, may lead to women prioritizing the care of their families over their own needs. For instance, WLWH who have children and func-tion as primary caregivers are more likely to be less adherent to their ART regimens, thus posing a major challenge for day-to-day HIV care, which must be considered by health-care providers.[72] Although PrEP and ART adherence are critical in improving health outcomes along the HIV care continuum, it is imperative to go beyond solely biomedical interventions to enhance women's overall well-being.

Stigma and Social Support

It has been well described that the stigma and discrimination often associated with HIV remains a major obstacle in achieving and sustaining optimal health and quality of life outcomes.[73] HIV-related stigma can serve as a significant deterrent and can affect women's decisions to engage in HIV prevention and treatment services. For women without HIV who are PrEP eligible, PrEP stigma has been widely documented as a factor undermining PrEP interest, uptake, and adherence. The negative societal perceptions pertaining to PrEP, including the fear that others will perceive PrEP users as being HIV positive, both directly and indirectly reflects HIV stigma.[54,74] Among WLWH, it has been argued that internalized and societal stigma may have a greater impact on women compared with men living with HIV. The presence of stigma can adversely result in emotional distress, social avoidance, and low self-worth, which are key characteristics of depression, thus ultimately affecting HIV and overall health outcomes.[11]

The presence of social support has been associated with augmented medical care adherence and an improved quality of life among people with HIV. It is important to highlight that WLWH and those at risk for HIV may have preexisting low social capital, resulting in lower levels of social support and social integration.[71] An analysis of the WIHS cohort found an association between the presence of emotional support on health-care utilization and increased ART adherence for WLWH of lower socioeco-nomic status.[65] However, for many WLWH, the presence of social support may not al-ways lead to positive outcomes because women may be less interested in caring for themselves due to perceived stigma regarding their HIV status.[65] Several studies have reported that WLWH who decide to disclose their HIV status to family and friends tend to be viewed differently and do not always receive support.[71,74] In the presence of such dynamics, stigmatization and lack of support from families and friends can further impair WLWH's ability to manage their HIV, resulting in low psychological and physical well-being.

Intimate Partner Violence

IPV disproportionately affects WLWH, with 55% of WLWH reporting IPV victimiza-tion.[75] In many instances, the factors that place women at risk for contracting HIV are similar to the vulnerabilities that predispose them to IPV.[75] IPV functions as a significant barrier throughout the HIV prevention and care continuum and is associated with an increased risk of HIV along with contributing to poor HIV treatment outcomes.[76] Women at risk of HIV and those living with HIV who experience IPV often report limited autonomy in making key decisions regarding their sexual health, thus increasing their risk of both acquiring and transmitting HIV.[76] A recent scoping review examining interventions addressing the intersecting epidemics of both IPV and HIV, reported a dearth of interventions that adequately targeted both HIV acquisition and transmission along with IPV prevention.[76] Although the US Preventative Services Task Force recommends clinicians to screen patients for IPV and refer them to appropriate resources, data indicate that many clinicians do not actively screen patients for IPV.[77] Various IPV screening tools exist, and health-care providers should investigate screening tools to determine which is most appropriate for the patient.

Addressing social support services for WLWH and vulnerable women at risk for HIV is critical in optimizing their health outcomes.[65] Individual and group-based interventions that go beyond education and focus on developing coping skills, facilitating empowerment that humanizes women, and allows for women to provide their unique insight into their vulnerabilities with respect to factors such as HIV stigma, social support, and IPV is key in enhancing women's well-being and can improve HIV prevention and treatment across the HIV care continuum.

SUMMARY

Reducing the burden of HIV among women and successfully reaching EHE targets will require a culmination of efforts that go beyond biomedical approaches and adequately address structural and social determinants. Clinicians in both HIV and non-HIV-based settings should be readily aware of the unique risk factors that can propel HIV risk among women, along with the variables that can contribute to suboptimal treatment outcomes for women who are on PrEP and ART. As WLWH live longer due to biomedical advances, clinicians who are caring for WLWH should monitor for comorbidities that are associated with both HIV and aging. Financial factors related to poverty, health-care utilization costs, employment, and housing along with social considerations related to the presence or absence of social support, IPV, and HIV-related stigma can have a monumental influence on the overall health and well-being of WLWH and women at risk for HIV. Clinical interventions must account for these aforementioned factors, in order to promote women's engagement in HIV prevention and treatment services and subsequently reduce women's burden of HIV in the United States.

CLINICS CARE POINTS

- PrEP uptake among women is suboptimal. Clinicians working in both non-HIV and HIV clinical settings should be comfortable in discussing sexual and reproductive health with their patients, and raising women's awareness toward PrEP for HIV prevention.

- HIV results in an increased risk of developing comorbidities that are also often seen with aging. Due to sex-based differences in immune mechanisms, women living with HIV have a heightened predisposition to worsened cardiovascular health outcomes, which clinicians must account for.

- The HPV vaccine is critical for primary prevention of HPV-related cancers, including cervical cancer and anal cancer. WLWH should undergo routine cervical cancer screening.

Although no guidelines exist for anal cancer screening, clinicians should consider anal cancer screening and linkage to care for the treatment of HSIL lesions for WLWH.

- WLWH have a high burden of mental health disorders. Clinicians should routinely screen all WLWH for depression and other mental health conditions, and adequately treat women while also referring them to appropriate resources.

- Financial and social factors largely influence women's ART and PrEP adherence. Health-care providers must comprehensively assess the unique factors that may influence women's risk of ART and PrEP discontinuation, and provide counseling and linkage to resources as necessary.

DISCLOSURE

The author has no conflicts of interest to disclose.

REFERENCES

1. Haley DF, Farel CE. Women, Epidemiology of HIV/AIDS. Encycl AIDS 2017;1–6.
2. Tian X, Chen J, Wang X, et al. Global, regional, and national HIV/AIDS disease burden levels and trends in 1990–2019: A systematic analysis for the global burden of disease 2019 study. Front Public Health 2023;11. https://doi.org/10.3389/FPUBH.2023.1068664/FULL.
3. Kaiser Family Foundation. Women and HIV in the United States | KFF. 2021. Available at: https://www.kff.org/hivaids/fact-sheet/women-and-hivaids-in-the-united-states/#footnote-452735-26. [Accessed 24 July 2022].
4. CDC. HIV and Women: HIV Diagnoses. 2022. https://www.cdc.gov/hiv/group/gender/women/diagnoses.html. [Accessed 12 September 2023].
5. Pillars CDC. | About EHE | Ending the HIV Epidemic in the U.S. Initiative | CDC. 2021. Available at: https://www.cdc.gov/endhiv/about-ehe/pillars.html. [Accessed 1 November 2023].
6. Adimora AA, Ramirez C, Poteat T, et al. HIV and women in the USA: what we know and where to go from here. Lancet 2021;397(10279):1107–15.
7. Frew PM, Parker K, Vo L, et al. Socioecological factors influencing women's HIV risk in the United States: Qualitative findings from the women's HIV SeroIncidence study (HPTN 064). BMC Publ Health 2016;16(1):1–18.
8. CDC. Diagnoses Of HIV infection in the United States and Dependent areas, 2018. 2020. Available at: https://www.cdc.gov/hiv/library/reports/hiv-surveillance/vol-31/content/women.html. [Accessed 19 September 2023].
9. Demeke HB, Johnson AS, Wu B, et al. Unequal Declines in Absolute and Relative Disparities in HIV Diagnoses Among Black Women, United States, 2008 to 2016. Am J Publ Health 2018;108(S4):S299–303.
10. Kaiser Family Foundation. Women and HIV in the United States | KFF. 2020. Available at: https://www.kff.org/hivaids/fact-sheet/women-and-hivaids-in-the-united-states/. [Accessed 12 September 2023].
11. Koenig LJ, O'Leary A. Improving health outcomes for women with HIV: The potential impact of addressing internalized stigma and depression. AIDS 2019;33(3):577–9.
12. Crepaz N, Tang T, Marks G, et al. Changes in viral suppression status among US HIV-infected patients receiving care. AIDS 2017;31(17):2421–5.
13. Lemly DC, Shepherd BE, Hulgan T, et al. Race and sex differences in antiretroviral therapy use and mortality among HIV-infected persons in care. J Infect Dis 2009;199(7):991–8.

14. Bhagwat P, Kapadia SN, Ribaudo HJ, et al. Racial Disparities in Virologic Failure and Tolerability During Firstline HIV Antiretroviral Therapy. Open Forum Infect Dis 2019;6(2).

15. McFall AM, Dowdy DW, Zelaya CE, et al. Understanding the disparity: Predictors of virologic failure in women using highly active antiretroviral therapy vary by race and/or ethnicity. J Acquir Immune Defic Syndr 2013;64(3):289–98.

16. Geter A, Sutton MY, Armon C, et al. Trends of racial and ethnic disparities in virologic suppression among women in the HIV Outpatient Study, USA, 2010-2015. PLoS One 2018;13(1):e0189973.

17. Waldron EM, Burnett-Zeigler I, Wee V, et al. Mental Health in Women Living With HIV: The Unique and UnmetNeeds. J Int Assoc Provid AIDS Care 2021;20. https://doi.org/10.1177/2325958220985665.

18. Rubin LH, Springer G, Martin EM, et al. Elevated depressive symptoms are a stronger predictor of executive dysfunction in HIV-infected women than men. J Acquir Immune Defic Syndr 2019;81(3):274.

19. Tran BX, Ho RCM, Ho CSH, et al. Depression among Patients with HIV/AIDS: Research Development and Effective Interventions (GAPRESEARCH). Int J Environ Res Publ Health 2019;16(10).

20. Lekoane KMB, Kuupiel D, Mashamba-Thompson TP, et al. The interplay of HIV and human papillomavirus-related cancers in sub-Saharan Africa: scoping review. Syst Rev 2020;9(1). https://doi.org/10.1186/S13643-020-01354-1.

21. Badial RM, DIas MC, Stuqui B, et al. Detection and genotyping of human papillomavirus (HPV) in HIV-infected women and its relationship with HPV/HIV co-infection. Med (United States) 2018;97(14).

22. Silverberg MJ, Chao C, Abrams DI. New insights into the role of HIV infection on cancer risk. Lancet Oncol 2009;10(12):1133–4.

23. Agarossi A, Delli Carpini G, Sopracordevole F, et al. High-risk HPV positivity is a long-term risk factor for recurrence after cervical excision procedure in women living with HIV. Int J Gynaecol Obstet 2021;155(3):442.

24. Liu G, Sharma M, Tan N, et al. HIV-positive women have higher risk of human papilloma virus infection, precancerous lesions, and cervical cancer. AIDS 2018;32(6):795–808.

25. WHO. One-dose Human Papillomavirus (HPV) vaccine offers solid protection against cervical cancer. 2022. Available at: https://www.who.int/news/item/11-04-2022-one-dose-human-papillomavirus-(hpv)-vaccine-offers-solid-protection-against-cervical-cancer. [Accessed 17 July 2022].

26. Whitworth HS, Gallagher KE, Howard N, et al. Efficacy and immunogenicity of a single dose of human papillomavirus vaccine compared to no vaccination or standard three and two-dose vaccination regimens: A systematic review of evidence from clinical trials. Vaccine 2020;38(6):1302–14.

27. Staadegaard L, Rönn MM, Soni N, et al. Immunogenicity, safety, and efficacy of the HPV vaccines among people living with HIV: A systematic review and meta-analysis. eClinicalMedicine 2022;52. https://doi.org/10.1016/j.eclinm.2022.101585.

28. gov HIV. Human Papillomavirus Disease | NIH. 2023. Available at: https://clinicalinfo.hiv.gov/en/guidelines/hiv-clinical-guidelines-adult-and-adolescent-opportunistic-infections/human-0. [Accessed 20 October 2023].

29. Castle PE, Einstein MH, Sahasrabuddhe VV. Cervical cancer prevention and control in women living with human immunodeficiency virus. Ca 2021;71(6):505.

30. Deshmukh AA, Cantor SB, Fenwick E, et al. Adjuvant HPV vaccination for anal cancer prevention in HIV-positive men who have sex with men: The time is now. Vaccine 2017;35(38):5102–9.

31. Silverberg MJ, Lau B, Justice AC, et al. Risk of anal cancer in HIV-infected and HIV-uninfected individuals in North America. Clin Infect Dis 2012;54(7):1026–34.
32. Piketty C, Selinger-Leneman H, Grabar S, et al. Marked increase in the incidence of invasive anal cancer among HIV-infected patients despite treatment with combination antiretroviral therapy. AIDS 2008;22(10):1203–11.
33. Higashi RT, Rodriguez SA, Betts AC, et al. Anal cancer screening among women with HIV: Provider experiences and system-level challenges. AIDS Care 2022; 34(2):220.
34. Chandiwana NC, Siedner MJ, Marconi VC, et al. Weight Gain After HIV Therapy Initiation: Pathophysiology and Implications. J Clin Endocrinol Metab 2023;32. https://doi.org/10.1210/CLINEM/DGAD411.
35. Bares SH, Smeaton LM, Xu A, et al. HIV-Infected Women Gain More Weight than HIV-Infected Men Following the Initiation of Antiretroviral Therapy. J Wom Health 2018;27(9):1162.
36. Bedimo R, Adams-Huet B, Taylor BS, et al. Integrase Inhibitor-Based HAART Is Associated with Greater BMI Gains in Blacks, Hispanics, and Women. Open Forum Infect Dis 2018;5(Suppl 1):S199, 538.
37. Koethe JR, Lagathu C, Lake JE, et al. HIV and antiretroviral therapy-related fat alterations. Nat Rev Dis Prim 2020;6(1):1–20.
38. Borges ÁH, O'Connor JL, Phillips AN, et al. Factors associated with D-dimer levels in HIV-infected individuals. PLoS One 2014;9(3).
39. Kumar S, Samaras K. The Impact of Weight Gain During HIV Treatment on Risk of Pre-diabetes, Diabetes Mellitus, Cardiovascular Disease, and Mortality. Front Endocrinol 2018;9:705.
40. Bourgi K, Rebeiro PF, Turner M, et al. Greater Weight Gain in Treatment-naive Persons Starting Dolutegravir-based Antiretroviral Therapy. Clin Infect Dis An Off Publ Infect Dis Soc Am 2020;70(7):1267.
41. Emond B, Rossi C, Côté-Sergent A, et al. Body mass index increase and weight gain among people living with HIV-1 initiated on single-tablet darunavir/cobicistat/emtricitabine/tenofovir alafenamide or bictegravir/emtricitabine/tenofovir alafenamide in the United States. Curr Med Res Opin 2022;38(2):287–98.
42. Klein SL, Flanagan KL. Sex differences in immune responses. Nat Rev Immunol 2016;16(10):626–38.
43. Kentoffio K, Temu TM, Shakil SS, et al. Cardiovascular Disease Risk in Women Living with HIV. Curr Opin HIV AIDS 2022;17(5):270.
44. Bahrami H, Budoff M, Haberlen SA, et al. Inflammatory Markers Associated With Subclinical Coronary Artery Disease: The Multicenter AIDS Cohort Study. J Am Hear Assoc Cardiovasc Cerebrovasc Dis 2016;5(6).
45. Titanji B, Gavegnano C, Hsue P, et al. Targeting Inflammation to Reduce Atherosclerotic Cardiovascular Risk in People With HIV Infection. J Am Heart Assoc 2020;9(3).
46. da Cunha J, Maselli LMF, Stern ACB, et al. Impact of antiretroviral therapy on lipid metabolism of human immunodeficiency virus-infected patients: Old and new drugs. World J Virol 2015;4(2):56.
47. Sarkar S, Brown TT. Lipid Disorders in People with HIV. *Endotext*. 2023. Available at: https://www.ncbi.nlm.nih.gov/books/NBK567198/. [Accessed 18 October 2023].
48. Grinspoon SK, Fitch KV, Zanni MV, et al. Pitavastatin to Prevent Cardiovascular Disease in HIV Infection. N Engl J Med 2023;389(8):687–99.
49. HIV CDC. Women: PrEP Coverage. 2021. Available at: https://www.cdc.gov/hiv/group/gender/women/prep-coverage.html. [Accessed 10 August 2021].

50. Ojikutu BO, Bogart LM, Higgins-Biddle M, et al. Facilitators and Barriers to Pre-Exposure Prophylaxis (PrEP) Use Among Black Individuals in the United States: Results from the National Survey on HIV in the Black Community (NSHBC). AIDS Behav 2018;22(11):3576–87.
51. Chandler R, Guillaume D, Wells J, et al. Let Me Prep You to PREP Me: Amplifying the Voices of Black Women and Their Providers to Consider PrEP as an HIV Prevention Option. Int J Environ Res Publ Health 2022;19(3):1414.
52. Coy KC, Hazen RJ, Kirkham HS, et al. Persistence on HIV preexposure prophylaxis medication over a 2-year period among a national sample of 7148 PrEP users, United States, 2015 to 2017. J Int AIDS Soc 2019;22(2):e25252.
53. Marcus JL, Hurley LB, Hare CB, et al. Preexposure Prophylaxis for HIV Prevention in a Large Integrated Health Care System: Adherence, Renal Safety, and Discontinuation. J Acquir Immune Defic Syndr 2016;73(5):540–6.
54. Calabrese SK. Understanding, Contextualizing, and Addressing PrEP Stigma to Enhance PrEP Implementation. Curr HIV AIDS Rep 2020;17(6):579–88.
55. Delany-Moretlwe S, Hughes JP, Bock P, et al. Cabotegravir for the prevention of HIV-1 in women: results from HPTN 084, a phase 3, randomised clinical trial. Lancet 2022;399(10337):1779–89.
56. Hull SJ, Tessema H, Thuku J, et al. Providers PrEP: Identifying Primary Health care Providers' Biases as Barriers to Provision of Equitable PrEP Services. J Acquir Immune Defic Syndr 2021;88(2):165–72.
57. Calabrese SK, Earnshaw VA, Underhill K, et al. The impact of patient race on clinical decisions related to prescribing HIV pre-exposure prophylaxis (PrEP): Assumptions about sexual risk compensation and implications for access. AIDS Behav 2014;18(2):226–40.
58. Bunting SR, Feinstein BA, Calabrese SK, et al. Assumptions about patients seeking PrEP: Exploring the effects of patient and sexual partner race and gender identity and the moderating role of implicit racism. In: Blumenthal J, editor. PLoS One 2022;17(7):e0270861.
59. Sales JM, Escoffery C, Hussen SA, et al. Pre-exposure Prophylaxis Implementation in Family Planning Services Across the Southern United States: Findings from a Survey Among Staff, Providers and Administrators Working in Title X-Funded Clinics. AIDS Behav 2021;25(6):1901–12.
60. Chen CY, Donga P, Campbell AK, et al. Economic Burden of HIV in a Commercially Insured Population in the United States. J Heal Econ outcomes Res 2023;10(1).
61. Neilan AM, Lu F, Gebo KA, et al. Higher acuity resource utilization with older age and poorer HIV control in adolescents and young adults in the HIV Research Network. J Acquir Immune Defic Syndr 2020;83(4):424.
62. Maulsby CH, Ratnayake A, Hesson D, et al. A Scoping Review of Employment and HIV. AIDS Behav 2020;24(10):2942.
63. Dray-Spira R, Gueguen A, Lert F, et al. Disease severity, self-reported experience of workplace discrimination and employment loss during the course of chronic HIV disease: differences according to gender and education. Occup Environ Med 2008;65(2):112.
64. American Psychological Association. HIV/AIDS and Socioeconomic Status. 2010. Available at: https://www.apa.org/pi/ses/resources/publications/hiv-aids. [Accessed 19 September 2023].
65. Chandran A, Benning L, Musci RJ, et al. The Longitudinal Association between Social Support on HIV Medication Adherence and Healthcare Utilization in the Women's Interagency HIV Study. AIDS Behav 2019;23(8):2014.

66. CDC. Issue Brief: The Role of Housing in Ending the HIV Epidemic | Policy and Law | HIV/AIDS | CDC. 2022. Available at: https://www.cdc.gov/hiv/policies/data/role-of-housing-in-ending-the-hiv-epidemic.html. [Accessed 27 September 2023].

67. Riley ED, Vittinghoff E, Koss CA, et al. Housing first: unsuppressed viral load among women living with HIV inSan Francisco. AIDS Behav 2019;23(9):2326.

68. Groves AK, Niccolai LM, Keene DE, et al. Housing Instability and HIV Risk: Expanding our Understanding of the Impact of Eviction and Other Landlord-Related Forced Moves. AIDS Behav 2021;25(6):1913.

69. Wainwright JJ, Beer L, Tie Y, et al. Socioeconomic, Behavioral, and Clinical Characteristics of Persons Living with HIV Who Experience Homelessness in the United States, 2015–2016. AIDS Behav 2020;24(6):1701–8.

70. Schwartz RM, Bruno DM, Augenbraun MA, et al. Perceived financial need and sexual risk behavior among urban, minority patients following sexually transmitted infection diagnosis. Sex Transm Dis 2011;38(3):230–4.

71. Webel AR, Cuca Y, Okonsky JG, et al. The Impact of Social Context on Self-Management in Women Living with HIV. Soc Sci Med 2013;87:147.

72. Merenstein D, Schneider MF, Cox C, et al. Association of child care burden and household composition with adherence to highly active antiretroviral therapy in the Women's Interagency HIV Study. AIDS Patient Care STDS 2009;23(4):289–96.

73. Andersson GZ, Reinius M, Eriksson LE, et al. Stigma Reduction Interventions in People Living with HIV to Improve Health-Related Quality of Life. lancet HIV 2020;7(2):e129.

74. Ho SS, Holloway A. The impact of HIV-related stigma on the lives of HIV-positive women: an integrated literature review. J Clin Nurs 2016;25(1–2):8–19.

75. Kaiser Family Foundation. HIV, Intimate Partner Violence (IPV), and Women: An Emerging Policy Landscape | KFF. 2019. https://www.kff.org/hivaids/issue-brief/hiv-intimate-partner-violence-ipv-and-women-an-emerging-policy-landscape/view/footnotes/#footnote-439078-14. [Accessed 31 October 2023].

76. Alexander KA, Mpundu G, Duroseau B, et al. Intervention Approaches to Address Intimate Partner Violence and HIV: a Scoping Review of Recent Research. Curr HIV AIDS Rep 2023;20(5):296–311.

77. Portnoy GA, Colon R, Gross GM, et al. Patient and provider barriers, facilitators, and implementation preferences of intimate partner violence perpetration screening. BMC Health Serv Res 2020;20(1):1–12.

Care of the Transgender Person Living with Human Immunodeficiency Virus

Serina Madden, DNP, APRN-CNP, AAHIVM[1], Justin Cole, MSN, APRN-CNP*

KEYWORDS

- HIV • Transgender • Care

KEY POINTS

- Transgender people at risk for and living with HIV face numerous barriers to receiving HIV prevention and treatment services.
- A potential higher rate of housing instability and poverty should be considered when attempting to meet the unique health care needs of this population.
- Assuring gender affirmation in health care settings, integrating HIV care with gender care, and using unique approaches likes peer navigation will help improve health outcomes for transgender people at risk for or living with HIV.
- Health care providers should continue to advocate for the necessity of gender-related health care and oppose laws that limit transgender people's access to the full range of health care services they need.

INTRODUCTION

HIV has been part of medicine in the western world for more than 40 years.[1] Many watched the discovery of the virus unfold in the 1980s when it was referred to as GRID, or Gay-Related Immune Deficiency. However, with time and research, the world soon renamed the virus, more appropriately, human immunodeficiency virus (HIV), and testing and treatment slowly became accessible to the general public. Over the decades, research has continued and science has developed antiretroviral therapy for treatment and prevention of HIV transmission; but, research in regard to the transgender community and other subpopulations is still limited and sparse.

According to the Centers for Disease Control and Prevention,[2] an estimated one million people identify as transgender in the United States, and transgender people make up 2% of new HIV infections in the United States yearly.[3] In addition, transgender women are 66 times more likely to contract HIV than transgender men.[4] These findings can be further complicated when considering racial and cultural factors.

Discreet NP, Norman, OK, USA
[1] Present address: 1215 Crossroads Boulevard, Suite 214, Norman, OK 73072.
* Corresponding author. 1215 Crossroads Boulevard, Suite 214, Norman, OK 73072.
E-mail address: Justin-cole@att.net

Nurs Clin N Am 59 (2024) 183–188
https://doi.org/10.1016/j.cnur.2024.01.012
0029-6465/24/© 2024 Elsevier Inc. All rights reserved.
nursing.theclinics.com

In this article, HIV care for transgender individuals is explored; in particular, the barriers to early diagnosis of HIV, access and engagement in care, and disease complications. The article also examines how Advanced Practice Nurse Practitioners and other health care providers are well-positioned to mitigate these obstacles to wellness.

In this article, the authors have utlized the HIV Care Continuum as a method to describe care of transgender people living with HIV. The HIV Care Continuum is tool that outlines steps from initial diagnosis, to linkage of medical care, to retention in medical care, and to the ultimate goal of viral suppression. The HIV Care Continuum[5] is a tool used to assess and outline the specific level of engagement in care and their associated outcomes. If used cohesively, the model will help ensure the linkage and engagement of care is well established.

HUMAN IMMUNODEFICIENCY VIRUS DIAGNOSIS

Recent estimates of HIV prevalence among transgender people are 16% to 14% among transgender women and 2% among transgender men.[6] Transgender people are disproportionately impacted by HIV. Although prevalence rates for US adults overall are less than 0.5%, rates for transgender people overall are 9.2%.[6]

Transgender persons often present for health care seeking only gender-affirming hormone therapy. This initial visit is the time for the provider to establish a safe environment that will provide the framework for developing a strong rapport. Each visit should be focused on providing a safe environment in which the person will begin to discuss sensitive topics, such as sexual health. The establishment of a safe environment is more than placing "transgender-focused" pictures on the wall in the examination room. Although this practice is recommended, the authors recommend starting with cultural humility from the provider and staff. The University of Oregon[7] defines "cultural humility as an ongoing process of self-exploration and self-critique with a willingness to learn from others by honoring their beliefs, customs, and values." Simply put, it means acknowledging differences and accepting the patient for who they are even when they may differ from you. This requires self-reflection. The provider must address any internal struggles and biases or misconceptions they may have about the community of patients they care for. Once cultural humility has been addressed, the provider should begin learning about the community. This includes the multiple facets of the community and the various definitions of gender and sexual identity that they will encounter.

Sexual identity means different things within the transgender community. This is important to understand as the provider begins to weave sexual health within the conversations after a relationship of trust has been established. Many transgender individuals will share intimate details, and this can help the provider educate, assess, and treat. Once this happens, the provider is primed to integrate a risk assessment and associated HIV testing in the plan of care as he or she addresses gender-affirming hormone care. This trust relationship is the foundation for all care. The diagnosis of HIV is life-altering, and if the topic of HIV is addressed without this foundation, the patient could immediately fall out of care once diagnosed. This is catastrophic for the patient and the community because viral suppression without regular health care touchpoints is not possible.

The University of California San Francisco[8] recommends incorporating the following ideas/practices into the office setting: cultural humility, addressing staff training, and understanding of terminology and gender identity data in medical records. In addition, unisex bathrooms are a way to establish a safe environment for both gender care and sexual health. It is common in practice to place transgender-friendly and sex-positive information in common areas, such as examination rooms. This practice of inclusion is important for connecting the patient with the clinic staff and provider so that testing, linkage of care, and prevention or treatment of HIV are seamless.

When these obstacles are addressed appropriately, it is perhaps the beginning of a journey to diagnosis and manage HIV for many transgender individuals. Because research is so sparse in the transgender community, it is important for providers to understand risks and potential ways to promote health. Being in touch with how to receive these individuals and deliver safe and effective care is a critical piece in the diagnosis and continuation of the HIV continuum.

LINKAGE AND RECEIPT OF CARE

The transgender community worldwide is subjected to violence, discrimination, and laws imposed by groups that place barriers to adequate health care. These obstacles marginalize transgender individuals and isolate them from health care. As a result, there can be a mistrust of health care providers owing to past experiences of discrimination and transphobia in health care settings. This ultimately impacts the linkage of care and delays diagnosis and treatment of those who need it. It can also impact the ability to stay in care for management of long-term health.[9]

Social stigmas and lack of adequate training about diverse patient populations within the health care community all provide barriers to linkage to care. Understanding some statistics about this group is important for health care providers to consider. The Center for Public Integrity published findings from a 2022 review, citing transgender individuals are at 50% higher rate of unemployment than others living in the LGBTQ+ community.[10] This same source explores that transgender individuals are twice as likely to experience poverty because of lower compensation and higher rates of unemployment.

When financial resources are limited, such as in poverty and unemployment, basic needs are challenged, and medical appointments and medications are viewed as less important. This perceived hierarchy of needs complicates care and often leaves the transgender person choosing to seek only hormone care. For many transgender people with HIV, gender-affirming therapy is more important than HIV treatment and care.[11]

The authors recommend starting with open-ended communication and connecting the patient with resources that will ensure that the cost of medical care is not a burden. In the authors' practice, they offer low-cost office visits or a flat-rate fee that includes laboratory tests as well as office visits. The authors also recommend establishing relationships with local organizations, such as Transpire, an Oklahoma-based organization that provides medical scholarships for transgender care. Once the diagnosis of HIV has been established, health care providers can connect the patient with local case managers who target HIV support, and will assist with linkage of care. Providers are able to weave transgender care and HIV care into one office visit; this allows the patient to get all their health care needs met in one setting. This approach of researching and understanding local resources and weaving transgender care with HIV care will help establish the linkage of care and meet the patient's goal of gender-affirming care while establishing a framework for retaining transgender individuals in health care.

RETENTION IN CARE

Because HIV management and support are lifelong, keeping someone engaged in their health journey is critical to promote viral suppression and assure good long-term health outcomes. Access to care that is discrimination free and in a safe space is critical for transgender people to feel valued, affirmed, and supported. However, in 2023, there were currently more than 100 different anti-trans bills to be considered across the United States.[12] With a recent 2022 court ruling allowing for insurances to choose if pre-exposure prophylaxis (or PrEP) and transgender care is covered by their insurance plans,[13] along with other legislation pending ,[14] it is within reason that a transgender person would feel discrimination and fear the cost of medical care. One in 3 transgender people already delay seeking health care because of discrimination and the costs of care.[15]

Although the future of the legal climate and payer source is unknown, the authors believe that focusing on strong relationships and providing access to mental health by providing access to resources within the community is imperative to retention in care. This can be established by a Peer-to-Peer navigation program. Having a Peer-to-Peer navigation program is a process in which a patient is linked to someone who can support wellness that looks like the patient and personally understands the struggles they face. This can help facilitate increased compliance in health goals[16] and retention in care.

HUMAN IMMUNODEFICIENCY VIRUS VIRAL SUPPRESSION

Keeping individuals engaged in their HIV care over a lifetime can be a challenge. Once someone's viral load is suppressed and wellness is achieved, continuing to meet quarterly or regularly is a reminder of a virus that some might not want to face. The social and medical complexity that transgender individuals experience during their lifetime can complicate care. In one survey of more than one hundred transgender people living with HIV, respondents' top health concern was receiving patient-centered health care without stigma; second, hormone therapy; and finally, mental health care.[17] Antiretroviral therapy was the fifth most important health priority. Developing a plan of care that addresses all the health concerns of transgender people in conjunction with HIV treatment can improve ongoing engagement and trust. This is true regarding all aspects of care. If the entire individual is treated with their priority of needs, health care workers in the United States can keep the patient in optimal health to quickly diagnose and treat HIV. Getting the patient engaged in their health care goals will only improve overall health care outcomes.

BRINGING IT ALL TOGETHER

Transgender people at risk for and living with HIV face numerous barriers to receiving HIV prevention and treatment services. Understanding that transgender individuals may have had prior negative experiences in health care settings owing to stigma is important when establishing a rapport with new patients. Considering a potentially higher rate of housing instability and poverty should be considered when attempting to meet the unique health care needs of this population. Assuring gender affirmation in health care settings, integrating HIV care with gender care, and using unique approaches like peer navigation will help improve health outcomes for transgender people at risk for or living with HIV.

In addition, Advanced Practice Nurse Practitioners and medical providers of various training backgrounds in Urgent Cares, Emergency Rooms, Family Practice offices, and Sexual Health Clinics must affirm their commitment to seeing patients of all cultures and gender diversity. Seeing the patient for who they are and meeting them with their desired health care goals is the beginning of forming a relationship that will contribute to transgender people trusting health care providers. Health care providers should continue to advocate for the necessity of gender-related health care and oppose laws that limit transgender people's access to the full range of health care services they need. HIV is best fought with all our resources, in the light of day, without judgment or fear. Only together can we properly diagnose and offer treatment for those most in need.

DISCLOSURE

The authors have no financial or commercial conflicts with content within document.

REFERENCES

1. Cisneros L. 40 Years of AIDS: A Timeline of the Epidemic | UC San Francisco. www.ucsf.edu. 2021. Available at: https://www.ucsf.edu/news/2021/06/420686/40-years-aids-timeline-epidemic. Accessed September 17, 2023.
2. CDC, Transgender people. Centers for disease control and prevention, Available at: https://www.cdc.gov/hiv/group/gender/transgender/index.html, 2019. Accessed September 19, 2023.
3. CDC, HIV and transgender people. Centers for disease control and prevention, Available at: http://www.cdc.gov/hiv/group/gender/transgender/index.html, 2023. Accessed September 20, 2023.
4. Trans women 66 times more likely to have HIV, with trans men nearly 7 times more likely, global analysis finds. aidsmap.com, Available at: https://www.aidsmap.com/news/mar-2022/trans-women-66-times-more-likely-have-hiv-trans-men-nearly-7-times-more-likely-global. Accessed October 15, 2023.
5. HIV Care Continuum. HIV.gov, Available at: https://www.hiv.gov/federal-response/policies-issues/hiv-aids-care-continuum/. Accessed October 18, 2023.
6. Becasen JS, Denard CL, Mullins MM, et al. Estimating the Prevalence of HIV and Sexual Behaviors Among the US Transgender Population: A Systematic Review and Meta-Analysis, 2006–2017. Am J Publ Health 2019;109(1):e1–8.
7. Foronda C, Baptiste DL, Reinholdt MM, et al. Cultural humility: A concept analysis. J Transcult Nurs 2016;27(3):210–7.
8. Creating a safe and welcoming clinic environment | Transgender Care. transcare.ucsf.edu, Available at: https://transcare.ucsf.edu/guidelines/clinic-environment. Accessed November 15, 2023.
9. Coleman E, Radix AE, Bouman WP, et al. Standards of care for the health of transgender and gender diverse people, version 8. International Journal of Transgender Health 2022;23(sup1):S1–259.
10. Jones J., Hunger, depression and unemployment: Trans adults are struggling. Center for Public Integrity, Available at: https://publicintegrity.org/inside-publici/newsletters/watchdog-newsletter/transgender-adults-struggling/, 2022. Accessed November 25, 2023.
11. Sevelius JM, Patouhas E, Keatley JG, et al. Barriers and facilitators to engagement and retention in care among transgender women living with human immunodeficiency virus. Ann Behav Med 2013;47(1):5–16.
12. Trans Legislation Tracker, Anti-trans bills: trans legislation tracker. translegislation.com, Available at: https://translegislation.com/, 2023. Accessed November 16, 2023.
13. A Texas judge rules coverage of anti-HIV medicine violates religious freedom. NPR.org, Available at: https://www.npr.org/2022/09/08/1121690478/a-texas-judge-rules-coverage-of-anti-hiv-medicine-violates-religious-freedom. Accessed November 20, 2023.

14. Zaliznyak M, Jung EE, Bresee C, et al. Which U.S. States' Medicaid programs provide coverage for gender-affirming hormone therapy and gender-affirming genital surgery for transgender patients?: a state-by-state review, and a study detailing the patient experience to confirm coverage of services. J Sex Med 2021. https://doi.org/10.1016/j.jsxm.2020.11.016.
15. James Sandy E., Herman Jody, Keisling Mara, et al., 2015 U.S. Transgender Survey (USTS). Inter-university Consortium for Political and Social Research [distributor], Available at: https://doi.org/10.3886/ICPSR37229.v1, 2019. Accessed November 19, 2023.
16. Dowshen N, Lee S, Franklin J, et al. Access to medical and mental health services across the hiv care continuum among young transgender women: a qualitative study. Transgend Health 2017;2(1):81–90.
17. Grant J.M., Mottet L.A., Tanis J., et al., National transgender discrimination survey report on health and healthcare- findings of a study by the national center for transgender equality and the national gay and lesbian task force, Available at: https://cancer-network.org/wp-content/uploads/2017/02/National_Transgender_Discrimination_Survey_Report_on_health_and_health_care.pdf, 2010. Accessed November 1, 2023.

Contemporary Treatment Approaches for Human Immunodeficiency Virus Infection
Association of Antiretrovirals with Weight Gain and Potential Solutions

Jenny Shroba, PharmD, BCIDP, AAHIVP*,
Jenna Januszka, PharmD, BCPS, AAHIVP

KEYWORDS

- Integrase inhibitors • Tenofovir alafenamide • Antiretrovirals • Weight gain

KEY POINTS

- Integrase inhibitors, most notably dolutegravir and bictegravir, and tenofovir alafenamide have been associated with increased weight gain when compared to other antiretrovirals (ARTs).
- Factors that may predispose patients to increased weight gain include being assigned female at birth, being black, and having lower baseline CD4 T-cell counts.
- Solutions to reverse ART-associated weight gain are currently being investigated, with several clinical trials ongoing.

INTRODUCTION

Persons living with human immunodeficiency virus (HIV) (PLWHs) are living longer with the advances of antiretroviral therapy (ART) transforming a universally fatal disease into a manageable chronic illness.[1] Though historic lipodystrophies and disturbances in fat distribution due to mitochondrial toxicities related to ART are not in the clinical forefront with the advent of integrase inhibitors (INSTIs) and thymidine analog–sparing regimens,[2–4] management of ART-associated weight gain remains a challenge.

Current practice guidelines describe gradual weight gain after the initiation of all ART regimens, specifically citing pronounced effects with dolutegravir (DTG), bictegravir (BIC) and tenofovir alafenamide (TAF).[5] Though many attribute weight gain after the initiation of ART as a "return to health" phenomenon, the significant weight gain

Department of Pharmacy, Duke University Hospital, 40 Duke Medicine Circle, Durham, NC 27710, USA
* Corresponding author.
E-mail address: jenny.shroba@duke.edu

Nurs Clin N Am 59 (2024) 189–200
https://doi.org/10.1016/j.cnur.2024.01.004
0029-6465/24/© 2024 Elsevier Inc. All rights reserved.

associated with INSTIs and TAF remains unclear.[6–11] With the increasing prevalence of overweight and obesity reported in PLWH potentiated by known structural and socioeconomic factors,[12–16] the consequential increased risk of cardiovascular and metabolic diseases associated with weight gain must be considered with ART selection.[5,17–20]

In this review, the authors seek to provide an overview of pertinent clinical trial and observational data regarding weight gain associated with INTSIs and TAF, with special focus on pharmacologic mitigation strategies for a PLWH with suspected ART-associated weight gain outside of traditional lifestyle and dietary interventions.

DISCUSSION
Clinical Trials

Integrase inhibitors

INSTIs are currently recommended as the anchor drug class for all first-line recommended ART regimens according to the Department of Health and Human Services guidelines for Antiretroviral Use in Adolescents and Adults with HIV[5] (**Table 1**). A meta-analysis of 8 studies ranked the INSTIs by probability of significant weight gain as follows: DTG (79.2%), BIC (77.9%), raltegravir (RAL) (33.2%), and elvitegravir (EVG) (9.7%).[21] Other analyses observed similar findings, stating that DTG and BIC have the greatest propensity for weight gain.[11,22]

In major clinical trials the effect of first-generation INSTIs, RAL and EVG, on body weight was not investigated; however, a substudy of AIDS Clinical Trials Group (ACTG) A5257 examined the effect of tenofovir disoproxil fumarate/emtricitabine (TDF/FTC) plus boosted-atazanavir (ATV/r), boosted-darunavir (DRV/r), or RAL on body composition of 328 treatment-naïve adults. At week 96 of follow-up, body

Table 1	
Recommended initial antiretroviral therapy regimens for most people with human immunodeficiency virus	
For people who do NOT have a history of long-acting cabotegravir use as human immunodeficiency virus pre-exposure prophylaxis, the following regimens are recommended:	
Generic name	*Brand name*
INSTI + 2 NRTIs:	
• Bictegravir-tenofovir alafenamide-emtricitabine	• Biktarvy™
• Dolutegravir-abacavir-lamivudine—only for individuals who are HLA-B*5701 negative and without chronic HBV coinfection	• Triumeq™
• Dolutegravir plus (tenofovir alafenamide or tenofovir DF) plus (emtricitabine or lamivudine)	• Tivicay™ plus Truvada™ or Descovy™
INSTI + 1 NRTI	
• Dolutegravir-lamivudine—except for individuals with HIV RNA>500,000 copies/mL, HBV coinfection, or in whom antiretroviral therapy is to be started before the results of HIV genotypic resistance testing for reverse transcriptase or HBV testing are available	• Dovato™

Abbreviations: HBV, hepatitis B virus; HIV, human immunodeficiency virus; INSTI, integrase strand transfer inhibitor; NRTI, nucleoside reverse transcriptase inhibitor; RNA, ribonucleic acid.

Panel on Antiretroviral Guidelines for Adults and Adolescents. Guidelines for the use of antiretroviral agents in adults and adolescents with HIV. Department of Health and Human Services. What to start: initial combination regimens for people with HIV. September 21, 2022.

mass index (BMI) increased significantly in each arm without significant differences between groups.[23] A retrospective analyses of the entire ACTG A5257 population (n = 1809) investigating severe increases in weight and BMI was presented at the Conference on Retroviruses and Opportunistic Infections (CROI) in 2017. In their adjusted analyses, RAL lead to more frequent severe weight gain, defined as an increase of $\geq$10%, compared to ATV/r and more severe change in BMI, defined as an increase by 1 or more categories, than DRV/r. Overall, changes in weight and BMI were more pronounced in patients with more severe disease at baseline, and predictors of weight/BMI gain were black race, higher baseline disease severity, and the use of RAL.[24]

Dolutegravir
DTG has been associated with the greatest amount of weight gain amongst INSTIs with several studies investigating this phenomenon. NAMSAL ANRS 12313 was an open-label, randomized, noninferiority trial in Cameroon comparing DTG to efavirenz (EFV) both in combination with TDF and lamivudine (3 TC) in 613 subjects.[25] In this study, DTG was found to be noninferior to EFV for virologic suppression at week 48. There was a significantly greater increase in body weight in subjects taking DTG (5.0 kg) compared to those on EFV (3.0 kg) (P < .001). Obesity was also more common in the DTG group than with EFV, occurring in 12.3% versus 5.4% of subjects in each group, respectively (P = .004). Similarly, the ADVANCE trial was a randomized, open-label study in South Africa that demonstrated the noninferiority of DTG and FTC with either TDF or TAF compared to EFV in combination with TDF/FTC.[26] A total of 1053 subjects were randomized to either the DTG/TDF, DTG/TAF, or EFV groups in a 1:1:1 ratio. Subjects had a mean age of 32 years and 59% were female. At week 48, the DTG/TAF group had experienced the most absolute weight gain (6 kg) and treatment-emergent obesity (14%). The DTG/TDF group also had higher weight gain and new onset obesity (6 kg and 7%) compared to the EFV group (1 kg and 6%). At week 96, treatment-emergent obesity was higher in women than men and was significantly higher in the DTG/TAF (28% female and 5% male) group compared to both DTG/TDF (18% female and 4% male) and EFV (12% female and 3% male) groups (P < .001).[27,28] Female subjects experienced much higher weight gain than males across all 3 groups through week 144 of the study (12.3 kg vs 7.2 kg). In this study, analysis of weight gain and emerging obesity was exploratory as opposed to being considered a true endpoint of the study, therefore necessitating further investigation of these results.

CHARACTERISE was a small, open-label, extension of the ADVANCE trial evaluating weight and other metabolic outcomes for at least 52 weeks of follow-up in patients taking DTG/3 TC/TDF.[29] A total of 70 patients originally randomized to DTG + FTC/TAF, 31 to EFV/FTC/TDF, and 71 to DTG + FTC/TDF were included. The majority had viral loads less than 50 copies/mL (98%), were black (100%), and were assigned female at birth (62%). For those switching from DTG + FTC/TAF to DTG/3 TC/TDF, a significant reduction of about 1.6 kg in weight (P = .125) and 0.57 kg/m^2 in BMI (P = .0106) was reported. Significant differences were not observed for either metric in males assigned at birth. Participants switched from EFV/FTC/TDF to DTG/3 TC/TDF experienced a median increase of 2.9 kg of body weight; this change was significant in males (P = .0464) in this study but not in females (P = .1127). A major limitation of the aforementioned trials is that they were all open-label by design which could have altered participants' perceptions of the study medication and its effect on their health; however, weight gain was also observed in later double-blinded studies comparing DTG to BIC.

Bictegravir and cabotegravir

Compared to the older INSTIs, there is a paucity of data from randomized, controlled trials for BIC and cabotegravir (CAB). In Gilead studies 1489 and 1490 comparing co-formulated BIC/FTC/TAF to co-formulated DTG/abacavir/3 TC and DTG plus FTC/TAF, respectively, found similar rates of weight gain amongst all study groups.[30] These results suggest BIC has the same propensity for weight gain as DTG, which is consistent with observations from meta-analyses and systematic reviews comparing weight-gain associated with each INSTI.[11,22]

Currently, the only randomized trials to investigate weight gain with CAB are HPTN 077 and SOLAR.[31,32] HPTN 077 was a phase 2a study that compared long-acting CAB to placebo providing the unique opportunity to study the difference in weight gain in patients on an INSTI alone compared to those not taking any ART.[31] A total of 146 subjects were randomized 3:1 to either CAB or placebo. The study population was, on average, 31.5 years of age; two-thirds were female, and 40% were black. The median baseline weight was 74.7 kg with a median BMI of 26.6. No significant differences in weight were seen, even in subgroups divided by race/ethnicity, sex at birth, or dose cohort. These findings suggest CAB is not associated with any increase in weight gain compared to the general population.

SOLAR is a randomized, phase 3b study that includes an investigation of weight gain and metabolic changes in patients on CAB presented at the CROI in 2023.[32] Patients randomized 2:1 were either switched to CAB plus rilpivirine long-acting injections every 2 months or to co-formulated BIC/FTC/TAF daily. Notably, about 59% of patients included in this study were overweight or obese at baseline which may have biased the results of this study; in previous literature, having a lower BMI at baseline was associated with increased weight gain.[24] Overall, changes in weight and BMI as well as the incidence of metabolic syndrome and insulin resistance were similar between both groups at months 6 and 12. The differences in findings between SOLAR and HPTN 077 regarding CAB's propensity to cause weight gain require further investigation.[31,32]

Tenofovir alafenamide

TAF is a component of many recommended first-line antiretroviral regimens and fixed-dose single-tablet regimen formulations. It has also been associated with weight gain compared to TDF, abacavir, and zidovudine.[11]

The DISCOVER trial compared TDF and TAF head-to-head in 5387 subjects for use as pre-exposure prophylaxis in which TAF was found to be noninferior to TDF for the prevention of HIV.[33] At baseline, about 50% of participants were overweight or obese, and the mean BMI of all subjects was 25.3 kg/m^3. Participants taking TAF experienced more weight gain when compared to those on TDF at week 96 (1.7 kg vs 0.5 kg, $P < .001$). The low weight gain seen with TDF in this trial mirrors the weight suppressive effects seen in previous PrEP trials; similarly, the weight gain in TAF is similar to the weight gain observed in the placebo groups of those trials.[34]

Observational Studies

INSTI-associated weight gain was not studied as extensively in clinical trials for the first-generation agents, RAL and EVG. However, large observational studies have been conducted describing weight gain associated with RAL, EVG, DTG, and less commonly BIC.

Data from the NA-ACCORD cohort for ART-naïve subjects initiating ART between January 1, 2007 and December 31 2016 were analyzed to assess the relationships between ART classes and weight gain in treatment-naïve subjects.[8] A total of 22,972 participants met inclusion criteria and were included in the analysis, of which 11,296 started a non-nucleoside reverse transcriptase inhibitor (NNRTI)–based regimen, 7038 started a protease inhibitor (PI)–based regimen, and 4638 started INSTI-based regimens, and most participants had TDF-based nucleoside reverse transcriptase inhibitor (NRTI) backbones. Subjects initiating either PIs or INSTIs had significantly more weight gain compared to those starting NNRTI-based regimens; however, there was not significant difference between PIs and INSTIs at both 2 (4.9 kg in both groups) and 5 years (5.5 vs 5.9 kg, respectively) after switch. At 2 years, subjects who started RAL and DTG gained significantly more weight than those starting EVG (5.8 kg, 7.2 kg, and 4.1 kg, respectively). Factors associated with an adjusted odds of a greater than 10% increase in weight included initiating an INSTI or PI-based regimen as well as a CD4 count less than 100 at baseline. Conclusions of this study were that INSTIs resulted in significantly more weight gain when compared to NNRTIs; however, given the overlap in confidence intervals for weight gain associated with PIs and INSTIs and the clear separation of NNRTIs and PIs, it would be more accurate to conclude from these findings that PIs and INSTIs are associated with increased weight gain.

The RESPOND cohort consortium is a multicohort collaboration including prospective data for over 29,000 PLWHs.[35] In an analysis that included 14,703 of these participants and defined weight gain as an increase of greater than 7% from their pre-ART BMI, lamivudine was used as a reference antiretroviral in this study as it has not been previously associated with weight gain. Overall, 7866 participants met the primary outcome on at least 1 occasion over a median of 18.4 months of follow-up. Patients starting RAL, DTG, and TAF were associated with a higher risk of weight gain with 16%, 13%, and 10% of subjects, respectively, within those groups experiencing weight gain within the first 3 months of therapy. After 3 months, subjects receiving RAL appeared to be more likely to experience more than a 7% increase in BMI at all time points as opposed to DTG and TAF that began to behave more similarly to those receiving 3 TC. An association with etravirine and increased weight gain was seen in this cohort; however, given the small sample size, this association should be interpreted with caution as this association has only been demonstrated in 1 other small cohort study in combination with RAL.[36] Limitations of this analysis include that it was strictly descriptive in nature and not adjusted for potential confounders. It was also conducted prior to the approval of co-formulated BIC/FTC/TAF, and therefore, the association between BIC and weight gain was not assessed. Moreover, it was unable to assess the trajectory of weight gain of these agents.

In a US-based cohort of 736 virologically suppressed subjects without INSTI experience, changes in BMI after switch were evaluated to assess differences in weight gain with regimens including INSTIs and/or TAF.[37] Subjects were followed on average for 7.23 years and no differences were seen in baseline demographics between patients on INSTI and non-INSTI-based regimens with the exception of age which was slightly higher in the INSTI-group (51.7 vs 50.0 years, $P = .02$). In subjects switched to INSTIs, a significantly more rapid weight gain was observed in the first 8 months post-switch compared to those on a non-INSTI-based regimen. Subjects switched to TAF also experienced more rapid weight gain that those switched to a non-TAF regimen over the same timeframe; however, this difference failed to reach significance. After the initial 8 months, weight difference in patients on INSTI-based regimens mirrored that of those on non-INSTI-based regimens; however, participants with a TAF-containing regimen continued to experience a slightly numerically greater rate of weight gain. Interpretation of these results is limited because details of the non-INSTI-based regimen anchor drug and non-TAF NRTI use are not provided. Therefore, the contribution of agents with weight-loss potential such as EFV and TDF cannot be evaluated.[38] Additionally, the study period for this analysis also almost entirely precluded the approval of BIC. Therefore, subjects switched to BIC-based regimens were underrepresented and made up only 3.4% of the INSTI group.

A larger analysis of 5479 virologically suppressed participants within the OPERA cohort who switched from TDF to TAF and maintained the anchor drug of their regimen showed a different pattern of weight gain associated with TAF.[39] An accelerated rate of weight gain was seen within the first 9 months of switch from TDF to TAF with an observed increase from 0.48 kg/year to 2.43 kg/year. Following the initial 9-month period, weight continued to increase but at a stable, slower rate of 0.24 kg/year. This suggests that the increase in weight gain is an independent effect of TAF, despite conflicting results from the DISCOVER trial.[33,39]

Finally, a retrospective cohort study of 1652 patients receiving TAF 10 mg, TAF 25 mg, or TDF was conducted to evaluate the effect of different TAF doses on weight gain.[40] At baseline, subjects were, on average, 49.7 years old and between 80 to 85 kg. When comparing TAF 10 mg to TAF 25 mg, the adjusted odds of "any" weight gain or BMI increase were significantly lower in the TAF group (adjusted odds ratio: 0.63, 0.43–0.93 and adjusted odds ratio: 0.66, 0.45–0.98, respectively). No significant differences were seen at any other time point throughout the study period. Confounders not identified in this study are that TAF 10 mg is used in combination with EVG, the INSTI associated with the least amount of weight gain, and DRV, a PI. TAF 25 mg was used in combination with BIC, which has been associated with similar amount of weight gain to DTG. Additionally, from a pharmacokinetic standpoint, the inhibition of P-gp transporters by cobicistat has been shown to increase TAF concentrations nearly 3-fold, and therefore TAF 10 mg co-administered with a booster would result in similar TAF-exposure to TAF 25 mg without a booster.[40–42] While it cannot be said definitively that TAF-associated weight gain is not dose-dependent, further investigation is warranted.

Possible Solutions

Integrase inhibitors or tenofovir alafenamide discontinuation

Data for the reversibility of INSTI-associated and TAF-associated weight gain are scarce and limited to case reports and preliminary data presented at international conferences.[43–45] One observational cohort study of 6245 virologically suppressed patients was presented at the CROI in 2023.[45] Investigators reported a total of 1440 participants gained at least 7% of their body weight within the first 24 months following a switch to TAF and/or an INSTI. In subjects who continued the TAF-based and/or INSTI-based regimen, weight gain appeared to stabilize after the initial gain of ≥7%. Only 69 participants subsequently discontinued TAF and/or the INSTI-based regimen. The only factor identified to be associated with weight loss following TAF and/or INSTI discontinuation was a baseline BMI of ≥30 kg/m². Within the first 12 months after discontinuation, average weight change was −1.30 kg, −2.55 kg, and − 1.69 kg, in patients stopping only TAF, only an INSTI, or both, respectively. These results should be interpreted with caution due to the small number of participants who discontinued TAF/INSTIs but may signal that weight gain due to these drugs is only partially reversible.

Doravirine

In clinical trials, doravirine (DOR), the newest NNRTI, was not associated with increased weight gain when compared to EFV and DRV/r. Several ongoing clinical trials are focusing on the switch to DOR as a solution to INSTI-associated weight gain.[46,47] DeLiTE is a phase 4 trial to investigate if INSTI-associated or TAF-associated weight gain can be reversed or at least slowed with a switch to co-formulated DOR/3 TC/TDF.[46] This regimen was chosen because it is a modern single-tablet regimen that does not contain TAF or an INSTI, is well-tolerated, and has limited drug-drug interactions. Similarly, The Do IT Study is an open-label, randomized trial in which patients are randomized to either continue their INSTI + FTC/TAF, switch to DOR and continue FTC/TAF, or switch to DOR and FTC/TDF.[47] This study aims to determine if obese PLWHs on an INSTI-containing regimen lose weight or at least reduce their rate of weight gain after switching to a DOR-containing regimen over a 48-week period. Participants cannot undergo any bariatric surgeries or plan to make significant lifestyle modifications that would affect weight.

AVERTAS-2 is an ongoing, randomized, open-label trial to determine if switching from DTG/TDF/3 TC to either DTG/3 TC or DOR/TDF/3 TC will affect weight changes with a primary outcome of a 2 kg difference in weight.[48] No exclusions with regard to other weight loss strategies exist; however, the outcome of interest in this study does not focus solely on weight gain unlike the previous trials. Lastly, DAWN is a phase 3, open-label study to compare the effects of DOR with or without TAF and BIC/FTC/TAF on weight changes in black or Hispanic females.[49] Again, the primary outcome is the change in BMI fat at week 48 from baseline without a specific emphasis on weight gain.

Glucagonlike peptide-1 receptor agonists

Glucagonlike peptide-1 receptor agonists (GLP-1RAs) stimulate insulin secretion, decrease insulin resistance, and slow gastrointestinal motility, each of which may target different proposed mechanisms for INSTI-associated weight gain, which are the alteration of glucose and lipid metabolism and the suppression of melanocortin which increases appetite.[50,51] Currently, data investigating a benefit of GLP-1RA for PLWH and ART-associated weight gain are limited to case reports and 1 small retrospective observational study.

Two case reports of PLWHs and comorbid type 2 diabetes mellitus have reported some weight loss as a result of GLP-1RA therapy.[52,53] The first was a 57 year old who had experienced a total 27 kg weight gain over 6 years for a total body weight of 116 kg.[52] Following the initiation of liraglutide, titrated to 1.8 mg/day, the patient experienced an initial 6 kg weight loss within the first 3 weeks. At month 4, body weight decreased to 102 kg, which increased to 108 kg at month 7. Although some weight gain was observed after several months of therapy, the patient did achieve a net weight loss of 8 kg during the reported follow-up period. The second patient was a 55-year-old who initiated dulaglutide for glucose management and cardiovascular benefit.[53] At initiation, the patient weighed 48.5 kg which decreased to 45.5 kg after 3 months of treatment, with a net weight loss of 3 kg. Of note, dulaglutide is not currently Food and Drug Administration–approved for the indication of weight loss, but weight loss has been observed in clinical trials.[54]

In addition to the earlier case reports, a small retrospective study was presented at IDWeek 2022 in Washington, DC.[55] A total of 35 PLWHs and type 2 diabetes mellitus patients on dulaglutide (37%), liraglutide (40%), and semaglutide (26%) were followed for an average of 20.6 months. They were, on average, 55.2 years of age with an average BMI of 35.7%, and 89% were on INSTI-based regimens. Two-thirds of the subjects experienced some weight loss with 31% losing at least 5% of their body weight. While this study shows promising results for the use of GLP-1RA on weight loss in PLWHs, including those on INSTI-based regimens, the use of GLP-1RA in the absence of type 2 diabetes is currently absent in the literature.

Currently, a phase 2, randomized, double-blinded, placebo-controlled trial is recruiting subjects to investigate if semaglutide once weekly via subcutaneous injection is efficacious in treating lipohypertrophy in PLWHs, without comorbid type 2 diabetes mellitus.[56]

SUMMARY

There is a growing body of evidence to support the association of INSTIs and TAF with weight gain. Second-generation INSTIs had a greater association with weight gain than their first-generation counterparts; however, BIC was underrepresented in the existing observational data and CAB was completely absent compared to the other INSTIs and TAF. Nonetheless, BIC was found to have a similar propensity to cause weight gain as DTG in a meta-analysis which is not surprising given their very similar chemical structures.[21]

Careful attention should be paid to the comparator groups when evaluating the total effect of these agents on weight. DTG was compared mostly to EFV and TAF to TDF, with both comparators being associated with weight-lowering effects. Additionally, in separate studies BIC was associated with similar rates of weight gain to DTG and CAB; however, in HPTN 077, no difference was found between those who received CAB and placebo.[30,31] Further real-world analyses comparing second-generation INSTIs to first-generation agents and antiretrovirals not associated with weight gain are necessary to truly investigate the second-generation agents' propensity for weight gain.

What these studies have found are patient-specific factors associated with a higher likelihood of weight gain, particularly patients of female sex and those concomitant INSTI and TAF administration. Additional risk factors for weight gain and increased BMI in most studies included black race and lower baseline CD4 counts. The increase in weight gain among those with low baseline CD4 counts is not surprising, as they have more advanced disease and are more likely to experience the return-to-health phenomenon.

The reversibility of ART-associated weight gain is not yet known, with potential solutions to combat this weight gain still under investigation. There is no one-size-fits-all approach and is more complicated than simply discontinuing the offending agent. Additional data surrounding these solutions are on the horizon.

CLINICS CARE POINTS

- Most first-line treatment options for HIV contain INSTIs and/or TAF.
- The possibility of weight gain associated with DTG, BIC, and TAF should be discussed with patients prior to initiation, particularly with those in groups more likely to experience weight gain, but it should not deter providers from utilizing them.
- Strategies to reverse weight gain associated with DTG, BIC, and TAF are still being evaluated.

DISCLOSURE

All authors: no reported conflicts of interest.

REFERENCES

1. Deeks SG, Lewin SR, Havlir DV. The end of AIDS: HIV infection as a chronic disease. Lancet 2013;382(9903):1525–33.
2. Knudsen AD, Krebs-Demmer L, Bjørge NID, et al. Pericardial adipose tissue volume is independently associated with human immunodeficiency virus status

and prior use of stavudine, didanosine, or indinavir. J Infect Dis 2020;222(1): 54–61.

3. Gelpi M, Afzal S, Fuchs A, et al. Prior exposure to thymidine analogs and didanosine is associated with long-lasting alterations in adipose tissue distribution and cardiovascular risk factors. AIDS 2019;33(4):675–83.

4. Mallon PW, Miller J, Cooper DA, et al. Prospective evaluation of the effects of antiretroviral therapy on body composition in HIV-1-infected men starting therapy. AIDS 2003;17(7):971–9.

5. Panel on antiretroviral guidelines for adults and adolescents. Guidelines for the use of antiretroviral agents in adults and adolescents with HIV. Department of Health and Human Services. Year. Available at: https://clinicalinfo.hiv.gov/en/guidelines/adult-and-adolescent-arv. Accessed September 04, 2023 Table 17h.

6. Spieler G, Westfall AO, Long DM, et al. Trends in diabetes incidence and associated risk factors among people with HIV in the current treatment era. AIDS 2022;36(13):1811–8.

7. Rebeiro PF, Jenkins CA, Bian A, et al. Risk of incident diabetes mellitus, weight gain, and their relationships with integrase inhibitor-based initial antiretroviral therapy among persons with human immunodeficiency virus in the United States and Canada. Clin Infect Dis 2021;73(7):e2234–42.

8. Bourgi K, Jenkins CA, Rebeiro PF, et al. Weight gain among treatment-naïve persons with HIV starting integrase inhibitors compared to non-nucleoside reverse transcriptase inhibitors or protease inhibitors in a large observational cohort in the United States and Canada. J Int AIDS Soc 2020;23(4):e25484.

9. Surial B, Mugglin C, Calmy A, et al. Weight and metabolic changes after switching from tenofovir disoproxil fumarate to tenofovir alafenamide in people living with HIV : a cohort study. Ann Intern Med 2021;174(6):758–67.

10. Milic J, Renzetti S, Ferrari D, et al. Relationship between weight gain and insulin resistance in people living with HIV switching to integrase strand transfer inhibitors-based regimens. AIDS 2022;36(12):1643–53.

11. Sax PE, Erlandson KM, Lake JE, et al. Weight gain following initiation of antiretroviral therapy: risk factors in randomized comparative clinical trials. Clin Infect Dis 2020;71(6):1379–89.

12. Adult Obesity Facts. Available at: https://www.cdc.gov/obesity/data/adult.html. [Accessed 4 September 2023].

13. Koethe JR, Jenkins CA, Lau B, et al. Rising obesity prevalence and weight gain among adults starting antiretroviral therapy in the united states and canada. AIDS Res Hum Retrovir 2016;32(1):50–8.

14. Bakal DR, Coelho LE, Luz PM, et al. Obesity following ART initiation is common and influenced by both traditional and HIV-/ART-specific risk factors. J Antimicrob Chemother 2018;73(8):2177–85.

15. Crum-Cianflone N, Tejidor R, Medina S, et al. Obesity among patients with HIV: the latest epidemic. AIDS Patient Care STDS 2008;22(12):925–30.

16. Tate T, Willig AL, Willig JH, et al. HIV infection and obesity: where did all the wasting go? Antivir Ther 2012;17(7):1281–9.

17. Willig AL, Overton ET. Metabolic consequences of HIV: pathogenic insights. Curr HIV AIDS Rep 2014;11(1):35–44.

18. Willig AL, Overton ET. Metabolic complications and glucose metabolism in HIV infection: a review of the evidence. Curr HIV AIDS Rep 2016;13(5):289–96.

19. Willig AL, Westfall AO, Overton ET, et al. Obesity is associated with race/sex disparities in diabetes and hypertension prevalence, but not cardiovascular disease, among HIV-infected adults. AIDS Res Hum Retrovir 2015;31(9):898–904.

20. Mirza FS, Luthra P, Chirch L. Endocrinological aspects of HIV infection. J Endocrinol Invest 2018;41(8):881–99.

21. Bai R, Lv S, Wu H, et al. Effects of different integrase strand transfer inhibitors on body weight in patients with HIV/AIDS: a network meta-analysis. BMC Infect Dis 2022;22(1):118.

22. Hester EK, Greenlee S, Durham SH. Weight changes with integrase strand transfer inhibitor therapy in the management of HIV infection: a systematic review [published online ahead of print, 2022 Feb 8]. Ann Pharmacother 2022. https://doi.org/10.1177/10600280211073321. 10600280211073321.

23. McComsey GA, Moser C, Currier J, et al. Body composition changes after initiation of raltegravir or protease inhibitors: ACTG A5260s [published correction appears in Clin Infect Dis. 2021 Jul 1;73(1):174]. Clin Infect Dis 2016;62(7):853–62.

24. Bhagwat P, McComsey GA, Brown TT, et al. Predictors of severe weight gain/body mass index gain following antiretroviral initiation. Seattle, WA: Paper presented at Conference on Retroviruses and Opportunistic Infections; 2017.

25. NAMSAL ANRS 12313 Study Group, Kouanfack C, Mpoudi-Etame M, et al. Dolutegravir-based or low-dose efavirenz-based regimen for the treatment of HIV-1. N Engl J Med 2019;381(9):816–26.

26. Menard A, Meddeb L, Tissot-Dupont H, et al. Dolutegravir and weight gain: an unexpected bothering side effect? AIDS 2017;31(10):1499–500.

27. Venter WDF, Moorhouse M, Sokhela S, et al. Dolutegravir plus two different prodrugs of tenofovir to treat HIV. N Engl J Med 2019;381(9):803–15.

28. Venter WDF, Moorhouse M, Sokhela C, et al. Phase III ADVANCE: 96-week primary efficacy analysis of DTG + FTC/(TAF or TDF) vs EFV/FTC/TDF in ART-naïve PWH in South Africa. Presented at AIDS;2020; Virtual.

29. Chen YW, Hardy H, Pericone CD, et al. Real-world assessment of weight change in people with hiv-1 after initiating integrase strand transfer inhibitors or protease inhibitors. J Health Econ Outcomes Res 2020;7(2):102–10.

30. Orkin C, DeJesus E, Sax PE, et al. Fixed-dose combination bictegravir, emtricitabine, and tenofovir alafenamide versus dolutegravir-containing regimens for initial treatment of HIV-1 infection: week 144 results from two randomized, double-blind, multicentre, phase 3, non-inferiority trials. Lancet HIV 2020;7(6):e389–400.

31. Landovitz RJ, Zangeneh SZ, Chau G, et al. Cabotegravir Is Not Associated With Weight Gain in Human Immunodeficiency Virus-uninfected Individuals in HPTN 077. Clin Infect Dis 2020;70(2):319–22.

32. Tan DHS, Antinori A, Eu B, et al. Weight and metabolic changes with cabotegravir and rilpivirine long-acting or bictegravir/emtricitabine/tenofovir alafenamide. Seattle, Washington: Paper presented at the Conference for Retroviruses and Opportunistic Infections; 2023.

33. Mayer KH, Molina JM, Thompson MA, et al. Emtricitabine and tenofovir alafenamide vs emtricitabine and tenofovir disoproxil fumarate for HIV pre-exposure prophylaxis (DISCOVER): primary results from a randomised, double-blind, multicentre, active-controlled, phase 3, non-inferiority trial. Lancet 2020;396(10246):239–54.

34. Grant RM, Lama JR, Anderson PL, et al. Preexposure chemoprophylaxis for HIV prevention in men who have sex with men. N Engl J Med 2010;363(27):2587–99.

35. Bansi-Matharu L, Phillips A, Oprea C, et al. Contemporary antiretrovirals and body-mass index: a prospective study of the RESPOND cohort consortium. Lancet HIV 2021;8(11):e711–22.

36. Assoumou L, Racine C, Fellahi S, et al. Fat gain differs by sex and hormonal status in persons living with suppressed HIV switched to raltegravir/etravirine. AIDS 2020;34(12):1859–62.

37. Palella FJ, Hou Q, Li J, et al. Weight gain and metabolic effects in persons with HIV who switch to ART regimens containing integrase inhibitors or tenofovir alafenamide. J Acquir Immune Defic Syndr 2023;92(1):67–75.

38. Erlandson KM, Carter CC, Melbourne K, et al. Weight change following antiretroviral therapy switch in people with viral suppression: pooled data from randomized clinical trials. Clin Infect Dis 2021;73(8):1440–51.

39. Mallon PW, Brunet L, Hsu RK, et al. Weight gain before and after switch from TDF to TAF in a U.S. cohort study. J Int AIDS Soc 2021;24(4):e25702.

40. Vemlidy (tenofovir alafenamide) [prescribing information]. Foster City, CA: Gilead Sciences, Inc.; 2020.

41. Descovy (emtricitabine, tenofovir alafenamide) [prescribing information]. Foster City, CA: Gilead Sciences, Inc.; 2019.

42. Symtuza (darunavir, cobicistat, emtricitabine, tenofovir alafenamide) [prescribing information]. Titusville NJ: Janssen Therapeutics; 2020.

43. Max B, DeMarais P. Elvitegravir/cobicistat/emtricitabine/tenofovir alafenamide discontinuation and return to normal weight. Int J STD AIDS 2021;32(1):92–5.

44. Saple D, Save S, Powar I. Reduction in the weight, gained due to dolutegravir, following switch to bictegravir. Indian J Sex Transm Dis 2022;43(1):27–9.

45. Verburgh ML, Wit FWNM, Boyd A, et al. Reversibility of TAF- and/or INSTI-associated weight gain. Seattle, Washington: Paper presented at the Conference on Retroviruses and Opportunistic Infections; 2023.

46. Wamsley S. Can INSTI-associated weight gain be halted or reversed with a switch to doravirine/lamivudine/tenofovir DF? (DeLiTE). clinicaltrials.gov identifier: NCT04665375. 2023. https://classic.clinicaltrials.gov/ct2/show/NCT04665375. [Accessed 14 November 2023].

47. Kudumu M. Doravirine for persons with excessive weight gain on integrase inhibitors and tenofovir alafenamide. clinicaltrials.gov identifier: NCT04636437. 2023. https://clinicaltrials.gov/study/NCT04636437. [Accessed 14 November 2023].

48. Benfield T. Changes in weight, body composition, and metabolic parameters after discontinuing dolutegravir or tenofovir disproxil (AVERTAS-2). ClinicalTrials.gov identifier: NCT04903847. 2021. https://clinicaltrials.gov/study/NCT04903847. [Accessed 14 November 2023].

49. Doravirine and Weight Gain in Antiretroviral Naïve (DAWN). ClinicalTrials.gov identifier: NCT05457530. 2023. https://clinicaltrials.gov/study/NCT05457530. [Accessed 14 November 2023].

50. Culha MG, Inkaya AC, Yildirim E, et al. Glucagon like peptide-1 receptor agonists may ameliorate the metabolic adverse effect associated with antiretroviral therapy. Med Hypotheses 2016;94:151–3.

51. Wood BR, Huhn GD. Excess weight gain with integrase inhibitors and tenofovir alafenamide: what is the mechanism and does it matter? Open Forum Infect Dis 2021;8(12):ofab542.

52. Diamant M, van Agtmael M. Liraglutide treatment in a patient with HIV and uncontrolled insulin-treated type 2 diabetes. Diabetes Care 2012;35(5):e34.

53. Dardano A, Aragona M, Daniele G, et al. Efficacy of Dulaglutide in a Patient With Type 2 Diabetes, High Cardiovascular Risk, and HIV: A Case Report. Front Endocrinol 2022;13:847778.

54. Trulicity (dulaglutide) [prescribing information]. Indianapolis (IN): Eli Lilly and Company; 2022.
55. Tauhid L, Fondong M, Lovett A, et al. 443. Do people living with HIV lose weight on GLP-1 agonist therapy? Open Forum Infect Dis 2022;9(Suppl 2). ofac492.518.
56. Effects of Semaglutide in HIV-Associated Lipohypertrophy. ClinicalTrials.gov identifier: NCT04019197. 2023. https://clinicaltrials.gov/study/NCT04019197. [Accessed 15 November 2023].

Criminalization of Human Immunodeficiency Virus in the United States

Robin Lennon-Dearing, PhD, MSW

KEYWORDS

- HIV criminalization • HIV stigma • Disparities • Black Americans • Black men
- Black women • Sex workers • Marginalized communities

KEY POINTS

- Human immunodeficiency virus (HIV) criminal laws present a very real racial and social justice issue.
- Disparities in HIV prevalence mean that HIV criminal laws disproportionately impact people of color and those with intersecting marginalized identities.
- Strong support for repeal of HIV criminalization laws has been expressed by numerous medical associations and governmental agencies for the good of all people with HIV and for the public's health.

INTRODUCTION

There are approximately 1.2 million people in the United States living with a diagnosis of human immunodeficiency virus (HIV), and in many states, there are laws and statutes that only apply to these individuals. These are laws that criminalize otherwise legal conduct due to a person's HIV status.[1] The purpose of this article is to describe the issue of HIV criminalization in the United States and how it affects people living with HIV, health-care providers, and the public.

In the early 1980s, when HIV first came to the public's attention, magazine headlines announced "AIDS: Fatal, Incurable, and Spreading" igniting fear and uncertainty across the United States.[2] AIDS was perceived as a gay disease and the term "gay plague" was commonly used.[3] Media played a significant role in perpetuating HIV stigma by portraying stereotyped depictions of the individuals and populations most affected by the acquired immunodeficiency syndrome (AIDS) epidemic.[4] However, when it became clear that women, children and heterosexual men were being diagnosed with the disease, people's fear turned to panic. Initially there was no treatment of HIV, before azidothymidine in 1987, and an AIDS diagnosis was considered a death sentence.[3]

School of Social Work, University of Memphis, Memphis, TN 38152, USA
E-mail address: rlnnndrn@memphis.edu

Nurs Clin N Am 59 (2024) 201–217
https://doi.org/10.1016/j.cnur.2024.01.001
0029-6465/24/© 2024 Elsevier Inc. All rights reserved.

nursing.theclinics.com

Although the Centers for Disease Control and Prevention (CDC) ruled out casual contact as a transmission route in 1983, this reassurance did not stop state lawmakers across the country from taking a punitive approach to keeping HIV out of their communities.[5] The first HIV exposure law was passed in 1987 in Louisiana. It imposed a sentence of up to 10 years in prison and a US$5000 fine on anyone who intentionally exposed a person to HIV without their knowing and lawful consent.[6]

In 1987, President Reagan formed the President's Commission on the HIV Epidemic as an advisory group that would recommend national strategies to address the AIDS pandemic. Remarkably, the Commission's report came out strongly against HIV stigma and discrimination of people living with HIV by calling for state and federal laws to provide uniform and strong legal antidiscrimination protection. However, the report also recommended that states hold people with HIV criminally liable for engaging in behaviors, which are likely to result in transmission of HIV. The use of criminal sanctions was to be "directed only towards behavior which is scientifically established as a mode of transmission and employed only when all other public health and civil actions fail to produce responsible behavior."[7(p139)] Anticipating possible obstacles, the Commission noted that criminalizing HIV transmission brings with it the danger of intrusive policing, "selective prosecution and misuse of the criminal law to harass unpopular groups."[7(p139)]

Congress passed the Ryan White Care Act[8] in 1990 to provide financial assistance to states for the delivery of essential services to people living with HIV. To receive assistance states had to certify that they had adequate laws in place to protect against intentional HIV transmission through donation of blood, semen or breast milk, sexual activity, or sharing hypodermic needles. The Act confirmed that a state's general criminal laws were sufficient if they could be used to apply to the conduct specified. This requirement was eliminated when the Ryan White Care Act was reauthorized in 2000.

The arrival of highly active antiretroviral therapy in 1996 transformed the treatment of HIV and led to such dramatic improvements in the health of patients with HIV that it was referred to as the "Lazarus effect."[9,10] Patients who had been on the verge of death made extraordinary recoveries and many returned to work. Treatment with new HIV drugs changed the outcome of an HIV diagnosis from certain death to living with a chronic treatable illness.[10] For people with HIV on long-term antiretroviral therapy, life expectancies are estimated to be close to those of the general population.[11] Because of the social history of HIV/AIDS and the lack of knowledge about the scientific advances in HIV care that have taken place since the epidemic began 40 years ago, society has not collectively embraced the new norm of HIV as treatable.

As new scientific evidence became available, medical experts issued statements that HIV criminal laws should be revised to ensure current scientific knowledge informs application of the law in cases related to HIV.[11,12] Disappointingly, many state legislatures have not revised their HIV laws despite these recommendations and calls to action from the scientific and medical communities.[13]

DISCUSSION
Human Immunodeficiency Virus Laws

HIV criminalization is the prosecution of people with HIV based on the person's HIV status. This is done with HIV-specific state statutes, sentence enhancements, and general criminal laws. HIV-specific laws are not uniform across the US Elected officials at the state level pass laws that establish what constitutes an HIV offense, which behaviors are prohibited and what the punishment will be for someone who is found guilty of those crimes.[14] These laws may be located in the state's criminal code or health code and carry felony or misdemeanor penalties. Several states have laws that fall into both the state's criminal code and its sexually transmitted disease (STD) or communicable disease law. STD laws apply to people living with HIV, even if HIV is not specifically identified, because HIV is a sexually transmitted infection.

One of the greatest concerns is that the intent to transmit HIV is not a required element of laws in many states. Most states' HIV-specific laws and sentence enhancements were created without a *mens rea* requirement, which distinguishes someone with the intent to harm another person from someone who did not mean to commit a crime.[15] HIV laws that require only general intent (ie, only that a person with HIV is aware of their HIV status) are particularly troubling from a health and equity perspective because they can be used to prosecute people with HIV regardless of whether the person intended to cause harm.[16] A document summarizing each state's HIV laws and their penalties has been created by The Center for HIV Law and Policy.[17] To find the HIV criminalization laws in your state access this link: https://www.hivlawandpolicy. org/rights-resources/find-laws-your-state.

State HIV statutes criminalize a spectrum of conduct and situations where a person living with HIV is required to disclose their status. A state's HIV law may make nondisclosure itself the activity that is being criminalized such that the failure to disclose one's status before engaging in certain conduct or failure to disclose to certain people (eg, sex partners and needle sharing partners) that will subject a person to prosecution. Alternately, a state's law may specifically reference some kind of exposure to HIV as criminal conduct for someone living with HIV unless the person has disclosed their HIV status. Exposure behaviors may be either narrowly defined in a state's statute or broadly inclusive of any HIV exposure. The typical exposure behaviors are (a) sexual activity; (b) exposure to bodily fluids; (c) needle sharing exposure; and (d) organ, tissue, blood, or semen donation.

Sexual activity exposure is described by several state statutes as sexual intercourse, intimate contact, and conduct that poses a substantial risk of transmitting HIV. Behavior such as sexual exposure to HIV is against the law in 19 states with a variety of caveats. Five of these states require actions with the intent to transmit (GA, IA, and MI) or intentional transmission (NV and WA) to face felony or misdemeanor charges. In 15 states sexual exposure to HIV is a felony (AR, FL, GA, ID, IN, IA, LA, MI, MS, ND, OH, OK, SC, SD, and TN). Four states have made this a misdemeanor (MD, NC, NV, and WA). For example, in South Carolina "it is unlawful for a person who knows that he is infected with HIV to: (1) knowingly engage in sexual intercourse, vaginal, anal, or oral, with another person without first informing that person of his HIV infection."[18]

Nonsexual exposure to bodily fluids (ie, spit, bite, and blood exposure) by a person with HIV is illegal in 12 states (AR, ID, IN, LA, MD, MS, NE, OH, OK, PA, SD, and UT). Bodily fluids may include all or some of the following: semen, blood, saliva, vaginal secretion, breast milk, urine, and feces. For example, Idaho criminalizes a person with HIV that exposes any person to bodily fluids (semen, blood, saliva, vaginal secretion, breast milk, and urine) "with the intent to infect."[19]

HIV statutes specifically people who inject drugs and others who share their needles and syringes. Needle sharing exposure to HIV is a felony in 6 states (ID, IN, ND, SC, SD, and TN) and a misdemeanor in North Carolina. For example, South Carolina criminalizes sharing a hypodermic needle or syringe with another person without disclosing their HIV status.[18] Additionally, 5 states have broadly written laws that could apply to any exposure including exposure by needle sharing (AR, IA, LA, MD, and MS). For example, in Maryland "an individual who has the human immunodeficiency virus may not knowingly transfer or attempt to transfer the human immunodeficiency virus to another individual."[20]

Donation of organs, tissue, blood, semen or bodily material from a person with HIV is illegal in some states. Notably, 10 states have laws that specifically criminalize blood donations by people living with HIV (FL, ID, IN, IA, MI, NC, OH, SC, SD, and TN).[21] Although prosecution is rare, there have been reported criminal cases of blood donation by people living with HIV in 3 states; Idaho, Indiana, and Missouri.[21] For example, it is a fourth-degree felony in Ohio for someone with HIV to "sell or donate his/her blood, plasma, or a product of his/her blood, if he or she knows or should know the blood, plasma, or product of his/her blood is being accepted for the purpose of transfusion to another individual."[22]

How have the state laws prohibiting donation of organs, blood, and semen affected the transplant community? People living with HIV in need of an organ transplant often have longer waitlists and lower access to receiving a transplant compared with people without HIV. To increase the number of possible organ donors the HIV Organ Policy Equity Act was passed in 2013, which allows HIV-to-HIV transplants under carefully designed clinical research protocols.[23] As of July 2021, 35 transplant centers in 21 states were operating with approval to perform HIV-to-HIV transplants, and there has been 300 kidney and 87 liver HIV-to-HIV transplants with 100% patient survival.[23]

The Health Resources Services Administration oversees the US Organ Donation and Transplantation program of human organs such as kidney, liver, heart, lung, or pancreas. The Food and Drug Administration is responsible for regulatory oversight of the US blood supply and human cells or tissues intended for human use. Examples of such tissues are bone, skin, corneas, heart valves, oocytes, and semen.[24] There are no known cases in which someone with HIV was prosecuted for donating organs for transplantation.[23] This may be because organ donation and transplantation services operate through health-care systems and have strict testing that follows all federal regulations.

There are a few states with HIV statutes that only apply in specific situations such as when a person with HIV is in custody. For example, in Utah, a person with HIV faces felony charges for assaulting a police or correctional officer with saliva or a substance that "carries an infectious agent."[25] Another example of a distinctive situation is in Arkansas where people living with HIV are required to disclose their HIV status to their physician or dentist before receiving medical or dental care.[26]

State prostitution laws, which are usually a misdemeanor, become felonies in 10 states when the accused person is living with HIV (FL, GA, KY, MO, OH, OK, PA, SC, TN, and UT). For example, in Tennessee, a person with HIV commits aggravated prostitution when engaging in sexual activity as a business.[27]

Sentence enhancement laws increase the sentence length when a person with HIV commits certain crimes, such as sexual offenses. These statutes are designed to result in harsher punishment for a criminal offense based on specific aggravating factors. HIV-specific sentence enhancements consider HIV exposure as an aggravating factor in 8 states (AK, CA, CO, IL, IN, TN, UT, and WI). For example, in Wisconsin a sentence enhancement law applies to a person with HIV who has been convicted of a serious sex offense in which "the victim of the serious sex crime was significantly exposed to HIV."[28]

HIV-specific statutes may provide for an affirmative defense that negates criminal liability of HIV exposure for individuals who disclose their status to partners. For example, in South Dakota it is an affirmative defense to HIV exposure if the person exposed to HIV "(1) was aware of the individual's HIV status, (2) knew that the sexual contact could result in HIV infection, and (3) consented to HIV exposure with knowledge of these risks."[29] Yet, facts such as having an undetectable viral load, use of risk reduction strategies such as condoms and/or that HIV is not transmitted are not typically affirmative defenses to a charge of HIV exposure in many states. Two states now identify an undetectable viral load as an affirmative defense: Kentucky and North Carolina.[30]

Ten states have general STD or communicable disease laws that do not identify HIV specifically but have criminal penalties for sexually transmitted infections. It is a misdemeanor in 6 states to knowingly expose another person to an STD (AL, AZ, NY, RI, VT, and WV). For example, in New York, "Any person who, knowing himself or herself to be infected with an infectious venereal disease, has sexual intercourse with another shall be guilty of a misdemeanor."[31] It is a felony in 4 states to willfully transmit a communicable disease (KS, MN, OR, and VI). For example, Kansas makes it a felony to expose another to a "life-threatening communicable disease."[32]

General Criminal Laws

States have used general felony laws to prosecute people living with HIV for attempted murder, aggravated assault, assault with a deadly weapon, and reckless endangerment for acts ranging from spitting on a police officer to having unprotected sex without prior disclosure.[1,33] A few recent examples of the use of non-HIV-specific laws to criminalize a person based on their HIV status originate in Hawaii, Texas, and Montana. A person in Hawaii was accused of spitting bloody mucus at a police officer and was charged with attempted murder.[34] A person in Texas was charged with harassment of a public servant for spitting on a police officer.[35] A person in Montana was charged with criminal endangerment for biting a hospital security guard.[36]

Enforcement of Human Immunodeficiency Virus Laws

Research on the enforcement of HIV criminalization examines how state HIV laws are implemented and enforced. Thousands of people have been prosecuted for HIV crimes. Most HIV laws do not require actual transmission of HIV, the intent to transmit, or even conduct that can transmit HIV. State-level studies on the enforcement of HIV laws have documented the demographic characteristics of people convicted of HIV crimes. When comparing demographics of people who have been convicted of an HIV crime with a state's population data, the disparities of HIV enforcement become clear.

Tennessee is an example of several trends observed in the data that Black Americans and women are disproportionately affected by HIV criminal laws. In 2022, 75% of people convicted of an HIV crime in Tennessee were Black Americans. Forty-six percent of statewide HIV convictions were women; 70% were Black women. A distinct pattern becomes apparent that people convicted of an HIV crime in Tennessee were Black and primarily Black women.[37] Unfortunately, data were unable to count the number of people who might identify as transgender. Research has found that the transgender community has been highly impacted by HIV laws in Tennessee.[38] Further indicators suggest that individuals convicted of an HIV crime in Tennessee may be suffering from unmet basic needs because 1 out of 5 people convicted were experiencing homelessness.[37]

In some states, HIV criminal arrests primarily originate from particular counties and law enforcement agencies. Differences in enforcement of HIV criminalization laws are found to be occurring based on geographic region in some states. For example, in Florida 53% of the state's HIV arrests occurred in 3 counties, Hillsborough, Duval, and Pinellas; yet, these counties account for only 16% of people with HIV throughout the state. In contrast, 7% of HIV-related arrests were in 2 counties, Miami-Dade and Broward, where 42% of people living with HIV reside.[39] In Nevada, 78% of all HIV-related arrests originated with the Las Vegas Metropolitan Police Department in Clark

County.[40] In Missouri, 61% of all HIV-related arrests came from St Louis City and St Louis counties.[41] In California, 57% of HIV-related arrests took place in Los Angeles County.[42] In Tennessee, 64% of people convicted for an HIV crime resided in Shelby County, which accounts for only 13% of the state's population and 37% of people living with HIV in the state.[37] Many state laws allow policing policies that permit a high degree of discretion, opening the possibility of discriminatory enforcement.[43]

Although people living with HIV were more likely to be arrested for an HIV-related crime in urban areas, that is not always the case. In Georgia, 36% of HIV-related arrests were in the metropolitan Atlanta area, and 64% were outside of urban counties. The counties with the highest arrest rates among people living with HIV were mostly rural counties clustered in the northern part of the state. This disparity may point to higher levels of HIV stigma in rural areas of Georgia.[44]

Patterns documenting the disproportionate impact HIV criminal laws are having among Black Americans have been found in many states (**Fig. 1**). For example, nearly 12% of Missouri residents are Black, 46% of Missourians living with HIV are Black, and 61% of people convicted of an HIV crime in Missouri were Black. More specifically, Black men are less than 6% of the state's population but account for 54.2% of those convicted of an HIV crime.[41]

Studies have found Black men overrepresented in enforcement of HIV criminal laws compared with their presence in the population of people with HIV. In Arkansas, Black men are 31% of people living with HIV and 44% of all HIV-related arrests.[45] In Virginia, Black men are 40% of people living with HIV and 59% of all HIV-related convictions.[46] In Ohio, Black men are 33% of people living with HIV and account for 62% of HIV-related arrests.[47] In Louisiana, Black men are 44% of people living with HIV and 91% of people arrested for an HIV crime.[48] When comparing the outcomes of HIV arrests for men in Georgia, Black men were nearly twice as likely to be convicted as White men (16% vs 9%, respectively).[44]

Women living with HIV are overrepresented in HIV criminal arrests and convictions. This is due to state laws that render sex work while living with HIV a felony. For

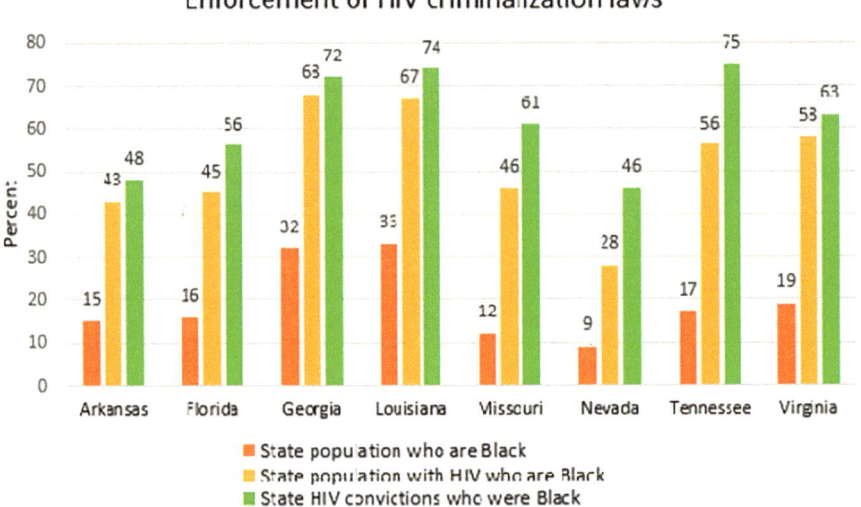

Fig. 1. Patterns documenting the disproportionate impact of HIV criminal laws among Black Americans. HIV Criminalization, UCLA School of law, The Williams Institute. Retrieved from: https://williamsinstitute.law.ucla.edu/issues/hiv-criminalization/.

example, in Kentucky, women were overrepresented in HIV-related arrests. Ninety-seven percent of arrests were crimes related to sex work and 59% of those arrested were White women despite only accounting for 8% of people living with HIV in Kentucky.[49]

In Florida, 56% of all HIV-related arrests were of women although only 27% of people living with HIV in Florida were women. Arrests were excessively high for White women, who accounted for 4% of people with HIV but 39% of all HIV-related arrests in Florida. Yet, when analyzing case outcomes Black women (60%) were the most likely to be convicted of an HIV-specific sex work offense.[39] In Georgia, White women accounted for only 3% of the population of people living with HIV but they were 11% of HIV-related arrests in the state. Whereas Black women accounted for 18% of people with HIV and 49% of Georgia's HIV-related arrests.[44]

In Shelby County Tennessee, the overwhelming majority of prostitution while living with HIV arrests (91%) were initiated by the Memphis Police Department's Organized Crime Unit during undercover sting operations on street-level sex workers. Seventy-five percent of those convicted for felony prostitution were Black women, 18% were Black men, and 7% were White women. Most of arrests (57%) occurred on Tuesdays and Wednesdays between 6 PM and midnight. In 95% of these arrests, the initial charge was for misdemeanor prostitution until the person's HIV status became known and then the charge became a felony. None of the 58 arrest reports alleged any actual sex acts. The arrests were mainly based on conversations between undercover officers and those they suspected of being sex workers and the proposed sex act in almost half of the arrests was for oral sex, which has no transmission risk.[37] It is important to note that criminal records do not separately identify gender identity and sex assigned at birth, so it is likely that most transgender people are miscoded as their sex assigned at birth rather than their current gender identity.

In California, Black women bear the heaviest burden of HIV criminalization.[50] Women account for less than 13% of people with HIV in California but between 2005 and 2013 made up 43% of people with an HIV-related charge. In terms of race/ethnicity Black women were 4% of people living with HIV, Hispanic women were also 4% of people with HIV and White women made up 3% of the population of people with HIV but 21%, 6%, and 15%, respectively of people in HIV arrests. By comparison, White men accounted for 16% of those who had an HIV arrest and make up 40% of the population of people with HIV in California. White men were significantly more likely to be released and not charged, compared with other groups. Ninety-five percent of HIV-related arrests in California were of sex workers living with HIV. Ninety-one percent of those convicted were sent to prison for an average of 2 years.[50]

Sentencing for an HIV conviction varies by state law. In Florida, the average sentence length for HIV convictions was 3.4 years.[39] In Georgia, the average sentence was 8.3 years.[44] HIV-related sentences in Virginia were an average of 2.1 years.[46] In Missouri, average sentences range from 2.9 to 10 years depending on the type of HIV crime.[41] In Tennessee, the average sentence for prostitution while living with HIV was 2.9 years and for criminal exposure to HIV was 3.7 years.[37] Louisiana had a median sentence of 4.3 years.[48] The combination of these 6 states together results in an average sentence length of 4.4 years for an HIV conviction.

State expenditures to enforce HIV criminal laws include surveillance, arrest, pretrial detention, prosecution, public defense, and incarceration.[43] The cost of incarceration varies by state based on the number of convictions and the length of prison sentences but conservative estimates have been published by the Williams Institute in state level HIV enforcement studies. Incarcerating people for HIV-related offenses has cost Virginia at least US$3.2 million, Tennessee US$3.8 million, Louisiana US$6.5 million, Georgia US$9.5 million, Missouri US$10.2 million, and Florida US$12 million.[37,39,41,44,46,48] These amounts do not include expenses related to policing, prosecuting, probation, or parole of people convicted for an HIV crime.

Changes in Human Immunodeficiency Virus Laws

Slowly, during the past 10 years, a few states have modernized or repealed their HIV criminalization laws. The scope of these reforms varies. Any changes made to laws go through the legislative body of each state. Outdated state HIV laws are not reviewed until a citizen, organization or advocacy group brings attention to the law and requests that they be updated. It has taken the partnership and advocacy work of state coalitions and national organizations working with state senators and representatives to bring about the recent changes in HIV statutes and to gain a modicum of progress toward accomplishing the goals set by the National HIV/AIDS Strategy for state HIV laws to be reformed or repealed.[51]

Two states have recently repealed all HIV criminal laws: they are New Jersey and Illinois.[30] Twelve states have made selected modifications to their HIV laws reflecting a better understanding of HIV science. Five states, California, Georgia, Kentucky, North Carolina, and Virginia, eliminated felony penalties for people with HIV who donate organs, skin, or other human tissue. Indiana now allows donation of blood, semen, or another body fluid for the purposes of research.[52] Three states, Nevada, California, and Colorado, removed felony status for sex work with HIV.[30]

Six states added a *mens rea* requirement for an HIV prosecution; 3 of these states also require HIV transmission for prosecution. Georgia, Iowa, and Michigan amended their statutes to require an intent to transmit HIV. Nevada, Virginia, and Washington require intent to transmit and HIV transmission.[30]

Regrettably, in the effort to modernize state laws and to remove the stigma of HIV from being singled out for criminalization, other diseases have been inadvertently criminalized. For example, in 2014, Iowa simultaneously repealed their HIV-specific criminalization law and adopted a new, more general contagious disease transmission law that criminalizes people with hepatitis, meningococcal disease, HIV, or tuberculosis.[53] Virginia amended its laws in 2021, and no longer has an HIV-specific criminal law but an STD law, infected sexual battery, that applies to all sexually transmitted infections. "A person with the intent to transmit a sexually transmitted infection and transmission of the infection to another person is guilty of a felony."[54]

Impact on Public Health

There are 3 ways HIV criminal laws negatively impact public health and are a barrier to HIV prevention and care: (1) perpetuating HIV stigma and discrimination, (2) misrepresenting how HIV is transmitted, and (3) diminishing people's willingness to get tested and if positive, to become linked to care.

The stigmatizing effect of HIV criminal laws cannot be over emphasized. Laws that single out HIV as a medical condition in which people living with HIV are potentially dangerous criminals negatively shape the public's opinion about people living with HIV. Laws that only apply to certain populations, for example, people living with HIV, send a clear message of disapproval to the public that people with HIV are unsafe and should be subject to different laws than the rest of the population.[55] Harmful and inaccurate beliefs about HIV are attributed to all people living with HIV.[56,57] Linking HIV with criminality makes living openly with HIV more difficult and increases the likelihood of secrecy and nondisclosure.[58] Research has found that people living with HIV fear being falsely accused of nondisclosure.[59] Criminalization may in fact discourage people from disclosing because they may not want to risk being placed in a position of vulnerability by a vindictive partner who knows their status.[60]

HIV criminal laws facilitate the spread of damaging stigma that may influence the mental health of persons living with HIV.[61] HIV laws erroneously label people with HIV as potential criminals and an HIV diagnosis as a death sentence. The detrimental impact of stigma and a discriminatory environment on the health and well-being of people living with HIV is exacerbated for people who may face intersecting forms of marginalization based on race, class, or gender. Disparaging attitudes and behaviors from friends, family, coworkers, and society about HIV can severely harm the mental and physical health, overall quality of life, economic stability, and access to care of those living with HIV.[62]

When health departments require newly diagnosed individuals to sign a form agreeing that they accept criminal liability for disclosing their status to all sexual and needle-sharing partners, it amplifies the negative stereotype that people with HIV have been marked and labeled as socially undesirable. This dehumanizing practice intensifies internalized stigma and creates barriers to engagement and linkage to care.[63]

Laws should protect people living with HIV against discrimination based on their HIV diagnosis. The federal Americans with Disabilities Act was created to provide legal protection against discrimination. HIV is a protected disability; however, HIV-specific criminal laws distinctly apply only to people with HIV, singling them out with different laws and policies and more severe punishment.[55] Laws targeting people living with HIV for different and harsher state statutes, solely due to HIV status, are not treating people equally and thus are discriminatory.[55]

The existence of and continued use of state HIV exposure laws perpetuate stereotypes and ignorance about people living with HIV and spread misinformation about how HIV is transmitted.[55] States are still criminalizing biting and spitting, despite scientific evidence that HIV cannot be transmitted through "saliva, tears, or sweat."[64] One study found that a majority of HIV exposure cases (73%) involved spitting, scratching, or blood spattering and occurred when individuals were resisting arrest and intoxicated, agitated, or otherwise impaired.[65] HIV laws are often enforced on individuals who are homeless or in prison during altercations with police officers.[66] Criminalizing conduct that poses no risk of transmission increases stigma and discrimination against all people living with HIV. It undermines scientific information about HIV prevention provided by public health agencies and promotes the myth that HIV is transmitted by casual contact.[67]

Laws criminalizing the donation of organs, blood, tissue, semen, or breast milk by people with HIV are misrepresenting the safety of these donation banks to the public because standard practices require that donations be screened and tested for HIV and other diseases before their use.[16] These criminal statutes may be unnecessarily limiting organs available to those who need transplants, people living with and without HIV.

HIV criminalization laws apply only when a person knows their HIV status thus individuals fearful of prosecution may refrain from HIV testing.[16] Laws that stigmatize or marginalize people with HIV undermine public health efforts to prevent the spread of HIV, making it less likely people will use services that support prevention, diagnosis, and treatment.[68] Research has found that people living in states with HIV criminal laws are less likely to get tested and know their HIV status when compared with states without HIV laws suggesting that such laws may be disincentivizing testing among those most at risk.[69]

Stigma is a well-documented barrier to health-seeking behavior, engagement in care, and adherence to treatment across a range of health conditions.[70] The fear of others learning their HIV status drives some people with HIV to self-isolate from friends, family, and community members to avoid being discriminated against or judged negatively if their status is revealed.[71] People may not want to attend care clinics or agencies that are associated with HIV because of the worry that people will see them at the location and deduce they are living with HIV.

People with HIV may experience anxiety in anticipation of stigmatizing responses from health-care providers, which may discourage them from seeking treatment or other support services, adversely affecting both their health and their quality of life.[58] They may limit the information they share with health-care providers fearing that they will report them for conduct that leads to an arrest.[56] People living with HIV were 6 times more likely to limit what they tell providers if they regarded them as caring more about enforcing HIV laws than about health.[72]

Impact on Marginalized Communities

The HIV prevalence rate for Black Americans is 7 times higher, and for Hispanic Americans, it is 3 times higher than for White Americans.[73] These disparities in HIV prevalence rates reflect other profound differences in people's experience based on the structural and social conditions in which people are born, grow, and live.[73] HIV criminalization exists in the context of many forms of structural inequalities that privilege some members of society at the expense of others.[55] Laws are a structural factor that influence, either positively or negatively, the health and well-being of citizens. When laws and policies are created to regulate and control members of specific groups structural inequality has been legally established.

The same communities most impacted by HIV are also disproportionately policed and incarcerated.[6] Black Americans are incarcerated in state prisons at 5 times the rate of White Americans and in jails an average of 4 times the rate of Whites.[74,75] Black Americans are disproportionally overrepresented across the criminal justice system in arrests, convictions, and harsher sentences than White Americans.[75] According to The Sentencing Project Black, women are almost twice as likely to be incarcerated as White women.[76]

The racial disparities that exist in the US criminal justice system hold true for HIV criminalization, which has been disproportionately applied to Black Americans. As described in a series of studies published by the Williams Institute, Black Americans are more likely to be arrested for and convicted of HIV-related offenses.[47] Disparities in HIV criminal enforcement multiply when considering the intersection of race, class, and gender.

Socioeconomic status is another source of inequality that makes a person with HIV vulnerable to criminalization. Research has found that people convicted of an HIV-related offense are more economically vulnerable when compared with others in the state. Up to 30% of HIV convictions in Tennessee were of persons that were homeless.[37,65] A lack of financial resources means that people who come into the criminal justice system because of an HIV-related charge are likely to be at a severe disadvantage. Access to justice is all too often contingent on being able to afford legal assistance.[77] Members of marginalized communities are most often reliant on the representation of a public defender. Without the financial ability to hire private counsel, unable to post bond, and unaware of the long-term consequences of a guilty plea, people who are impoverished are likely to plead guilty, even in cases where they do not believe themselves to be guilty. How often this situation happens is unknown but anecdotally it seems to be the norm.[38]

Over policing targets some of the poorest and most underserved communities, create opportunities for racial profiling and targeting specific communities, such as street-based sex workers and those experiencing poverty and homelessness, in enforcement of HIV laws. Sex workers are at heightened risk of HIV criminalization because of their stigmatized intersectional social identities, economic vulnerability, marginalization, societal disapproval, substance use disorders, and police profiling. The criminalization of sex work is much more likely to influence women, LGBTQ youth, transgender adults, and those who are homeless.[78] Transgender people of color in particular are more likely to report being involved in sex work as an economic necessity due to employment discrimination.[79] Most arrests for prostitution of people with HIV are a result of police stings making people engaged in street-based sex work easy targets. Police officers and prosecutors possess wide discretion to decide which laws to enforce and against whom.[57] HIV stigma is pervasive in all discretionary decisions in the criminal justice system.[57]

To understand the additional burden that HIV criminalization has on the lives of women, it is necessary to recognize women's unequal social and economic status in society.[6] In comparison to men, women (across racial groups) have lower earnings and higher poverty rates. A majority of women living with HIV in the United States are women of color and low-income women, and therefore also live with the compounding effects of sexism, racism, and limited financial resources in addition to HIV stigma.[80,81] Furthermore, being a Black transgender woman living with HIV, the added stigma of transphobia exponentially increases the levels of discrimination they face. Transgender people experience extreme and pervasive discrimination because of their gender identities, including physical violence, employment and housing discrimination, and harassment in school.

Women are less likely to be able to safely disclose their HIV status to sexual partners or negotiate condom use because of inequality in power relations, economic dependence, and risk of violence.[82] Women, particularly women of color and women of trans experience, may face violence if they disclose their HIV status. Disclosure creates power differentials in relationships wherein a person's HIV status can be used as a weapon by an abuser to threaten to falsely report nondisclosure, making it harder to leave violent, abusive, relationships.[6,81] In fact, strategic nondisclosure of HIV status by women has been identified as a source of empowerment giving women a sense of agency and power in their choices.[83]

Harms

Despite decades of HIV criminal laws, there is neither research evidence that supports it as a method to reduce the rate of HIV transmission nor any research demonstrating that it provides public health benefits. However, there is a body of research that describes and documents the harms caused by HIV laws.[38] Research into the firsthand perspective of individuals arrested for an HIV crime found that they experienced excessive and severe penalties causing them extreme harm and degradation that lasts a lifetime.[38]

Criminalizing individuals living with HIV who did not intend to transmit HIV nor transmitted it is particularly troubling because it results in a felony criminal record with numerous collateral consequences that are permanent. Even being arrested for an HIV crime, whether one is prosecuted, or the case is dismissed, exposes personal and private information about one's health diagnosis to the general public, which can be detrimental resulting in the loss of employment, housing, and straining relationships.[33,38] No other health condition requires the same invasion of privacy.[66]

Incarceration is a major life-altering event that creates obstacles to building a stable life in the community, gaining employment, and finding stable and safe housing after release. It also reduces lifetime earnings and negatively affects life outcomes among children of incarcerated parents.[75] On release, people may find themselves hampered by collateral consequences such as sex offender registration that dictates whether or where they will be able to find employment and housing, access public benefits, or reunite with their family. Five states require people convicted of an HIV crime to register as sex offenders (AR, LA, OH, SD, and TN). Sex offender status results in ongoing punishment and cruelty because it deprives a person living with HIV the ability to be self-supporting and independent. It comes with an onerous set of requirements that, if unheeded, can result in further prosecution and imprisonment.[55]

People who are prosecuted for HIV crimes are often experiencing numerous unmet needs such as for mental health care, substance use treatment, housing, and other basic needs. The criminal justice system does not provide people with HIV access to the services they need, instead criminalization results in further entrenching a person into poverty causing them more severe harm.[33,38] Without any change in circumstances or assistance the consequences of a felony criminal record may, for some, necessitate a return to sex work for economic reasons. These are incredibly high costs for anyone involved in the criminal legal system to pay.

SUMMARY

HIV laws have not kept pace with medical and scientific advancements regarding the transmission and treatment of HIV. As a result, they criminalize behaviors that pose little risk of transmission and punish people who cannot or do not infect others. Effective treatments for HIV mean that people with knowledge of their HIV status can receive medication that makes them unable to transmit the virus.[84] The reality is that for most people HIV is managed similar to other chronic health conditions.

Unfortunately, HIV criminal laws present a very real racial and social justice issue. Disparities in HIV prevalence mean that HIV criminal laws disproportionately influence people of color and those with intersecting marginalized identities. Research has found that the majority of people arrested under these laws are Black Americans, women, transgender and gender nonconforming people, the poor and homeless, and people experiencing substance use and mental health disorders. Arresting, prosecuting, and imprisoning individuals for HIV exposure crimes inflict further harm on already marginalized communities. Strong support for repeal of HIV criminalization laws has been expressed by numerous medical associations and governmental agencies for the good of all people with HIV and for the public's health.

CLINICS CARE POINTS

- Health-care providers need to know the HIV laws in the state in which they practice.
- Black Americans are more likely to be arrested for and convicted of HIV-related offenses.
- Disparities in HIV criminal enforcement multiply when considering the intersection of race, class, and gender.

REFERENCES

1. HIV Criminalization in the United States HIV Criminalization in the United States a Sourcebook on State and Federal HIV Criminal Law and Practice a Publication of the Center for HIV Law and Policy Third Edition. 2022. Available at: http://www.hivlawandpolicy.org/sourcebook. Accessed August 20, 2023.

2. Carlson P. AIDS: Fatal, incurable, and spreading. Published June 17, 1985. Available at: https://people.com/archive/aids-fatal-incurable-and-spreading-vol-23-no-24/. Accessed August 21, 2023.

3. Curran JW, Jaffe HW. AIDS: The early years and CDC's response. MMWR (Morb Mortal Wkly Rep) 2011;60(4):64–9.

4. Newell PW, Role of Media in Shaping Perceptions of HIV and Affecting Engagement in HIV Care. 2018. Master of Science Thesis, Trent University, Ontario, Canada.

5. Centers for Disease Control and Prevention. Current trends update: acquired immunodeficiency syndrome. MMWR (Morb Mortal Wkly Rep) 1983;32(35):465–7. Available at: https://www.cdc.gov/mmwr/preview/mmwrhtml/00000137.htm.

6. Brown R. When the body is a weapon: An intersectional feminist analysis of HIV criminalization in Louisiana. Berk J Gend Law Justice 2020;35(1):91–136.

7. Presidential Commission on the Human Immunodeficiency Virus. The Presidential Commission on the Human Immunodeficiency Virus Epidemic Report; 1988. Available at: https://files.eric.ed.gov/fulltext/ED299531.pdf. Accessed August 29, 2023.

8. Ryan White Comprehensive AIDS Resources Emergency (CARE) Act. 1990. Available at: https://ryanwhite.hrsa.gov/sites/default/files/ryanwhite/about-program/legislation-title-xxvi.pdf. Accessed June 4, 2023.

9. Fauci AS, Lane HC. Four Decades of HIV/AIDS — Much Accomplished, Much to Do. New England Journal of Medicine. 2020;383(1):1-4. Available at: https://doi.org/10.1056/nejmp1916753. Accessed September 14, 2023.

10. Scott S, Constantine LM. The Lazarus Syndrome: A Second Chance for Life with HIV Infection. J Am Pharmaceut Assoc 1999;39(4):462–6. https://doi.org/10.1016/s1086-5802(16)30464-8.

11. Barré-Sinoussi F, Abdool Karim SS, Albert J, et al. Expert consensus statement on the science of HIV in the context of criminal law. J Int AIDS Soc 2018;21(7). https://doi.org/10.1002/jia2.25161.

12. Harsono D, Galletly CL, O'Keefe E, et al. Criminalization of HIV Exposure: A Review of Empirical Studies in the United States. AIDS Behav 2016;21(1):27–50.

13. McArthur JB. As the tide turns: the changing HIV/AIDS epidemic and the criminalization of HIV exposure. PubMed 2009;94(3):707–42.

14. Montaldo C. The main classifications of criminal offenses. ThoughtCo; 2021. Available at: https://www.thoughtco.com/types-of-criminal-offenses-970835.

15. Intent. LII/Legal Information Institute. Available at: https://www.law.cornell.edu/wex/intent. Accessed July 28, 2023.

16. HIV Criminalization Legal and Policy Assessment Tool | Law | Policy and Law | HIV/AIDS | CDC. www.cdc.gov. Published January 6, 2023. Available at: https://www.cdc.gov/hiv/policies/law/hiv-criminalization-legal-and-policy-assessment-tool.html. Accessed September 29, 2023.

17. Find the Laws in Your State | The Center for HIV Law and Policy. Available at: www.hivlawandpolicy.org. Published August 24, 2022. Accessed October 1, 2023. https://www.hivlawandpolicy.org/rights-resources/find-laws-your-state.

18. S.C. CODE ANN. § 44-29-145.

19. ID Code Ann. § 39-608.

20. MD. CODE ANN., HEALTH-GEN. § 18-601.1.

21. Hatt E, Beaumont S, Bernard EJ. Bad Blood Criminalisation of Blood Donations by People Living with HIV.; 2022. Available at: https://www.hivjustice.net/wp-content/uploads/2022/09/Bad-Blood-September-2022.pdf. Accessed September 24, 2023.

22. OH Rev. Code § 2927.13.
23. Klitenic SB, Levan ML, Van Pilsum Rasmussen SE, et al. Science Over Stigma: Lessons and Future Direction of HIV-to-HIV Transplantation. Current Transplantation Reports 2021;8(4):314–23.
24. FDA. What does FDA regulate? U.S. Food and Drug Administration. Published 2019. Available at: https://www.fda.gov/about-fda/fda-basics/what-does-fda-regulate. Accessed July 6, 2023.
25. Utah Code Ann. § 76-5-102.6.
26. Ark. Code Ann. § 20-15-903.
27. Tenn. Code Ann. § 39-13-516.
28. Wis. Stat. § 973.017.
29. S.D. Codified Laws § 22-18-33.
30. Timeline of State Reforms and Repeals of HIV Criminal Laws, CHLP (updated 2022) | The Center for HIV Law and Policy. Available at: www.hivlawandpolicy. org. Published June 28, 2022. Accessed September 30, 2023. https://www. hivlawandpolicy.org/resources/timeline-state-reforms-and-repeals-hiv-criminal-laws-chlp-updated-2022.
31. NY PUB. HEALTH LAW § 2307.
32. KAN. STAT. ANN. § 21-5424.
33. Cross CK. Sex, Crime, and Serostatus. Washington and Lee Law Review 2021;78(1):71–153.
34. Police BJ. Attempted murder suspect with HIV spat on officer's face. Hawaii Tribune-Herald; 2022.
35. Man with AIDS sentenced to 12 years in prison after spitting in officer's face. kcentv.com. Published January 7, 2019. Available at: https://www.kcentv.com/article/news/local/man-with-aids-sentenced-to-12-years-after-spitting-in-officers-face/500-626803706. Accessed September 29, 2023.
36. Charges: Billings woman may have infected hospital employee with HIV through bite. KTVQ News, 2017. Available at: https://www.youtube.com/watch?v=Q_GjOXRxkPU.
37. Cisneros N, Sears B, Lennon-Dearing R. Enforcement of HIV criminalization in Tennessee. Los Angeles, CA: The Williams Institute; 2022. Available at: https://williamsinstitute.law.ucla.edu/publications/hiv-criminalization-tennessee.
38. Lennon-Dearing R, Hirschi M, Dill S, et al. "We all deserve justice": Perspectives on being arrested for aggravated prostitution. J HIV AIDS Soc Serv 2021;20(3):183–208.
39. Hasenbush A. HIV criminalization in Florida: penal implications for people living with HIV/AIDS. Los Angeles, CA: The Williams Institute; 2018. Available at: https://williamsinstitute.law.ucla.edu/publications/hiv-criminalization-fl/.
40. Cisneros N, Sears B. Enforcement of HIV criminalization in Nevada. Los Angeles, CA: The Williams Institute; 2021. Available at: https://williamsinstitute.law.ucla.edu/publications/hiv-criminalization-nevada.
41. Sears B, Goldberg SK, Mallory C. The criminalization of HIV and hepatitis B and c in Missouri. Los Angeles, CA: The Williams Institute; 2020. Available at: https://williamsinstitute.law.ucla.edu/publications/hiv-criminalization-mo.
42. Hasenbush A, Miyashita A, Wilson BD. HIV criminalization in California: penal implications for people living with HIV/AIDS. Los Angeles, CA: The Williams Institute; 2015. Available at: https://williamsinstitute.law.ucla.edu/wp-content/uploads/HIV-Criminalization-California-Updated-June-2016.pdf.

43. Lazzarini Z, Galletly CL, Mykhalovskiy E, et al. Criminalization of HIV Transmission and Exposure: Research and Policy Agenda. American Journal of Public Health 2013;103(8):1350–3.

44. Hasenbush A. HIV criminalization in Georgia: penal implications for people living with HIV/AIDS. Los Angeles, CA: The Williams Institute; 2018. Available at: https://williamsinstitute.law.ucla.edu/publications/hiv-criminalization-in-georgia/.

45. Cisneros N, Macklin ML, Tentindo W, et al. Enforcement of HIV criminalization in Arkansas. Los Angeles, CA: The Williams Institute; 2022. Available at: https://williamsinstitute.law.ucla.edu/publications/hiv-criminalization-ar.

46. Cisneros N, Sears B. Enforcement of HIV criminalization in Virginia. Los Angeles, CA: The Williams Institute; 2021. Available at: https://williamsinstitute.law.ucla.edu/publications/hiv-criminalization-va/.

47. HIV criminalization and race. The Williams Institute. Published December 2021. Available at: https://williamsinstitute.law.ucla.edu/wp-content/uploads/HIV-Crim-and-Race-Infographic.pdf. Accessed May 14, 2022.

48. Cisneros N, Sears B. Enforcement of HIV criminalization in Louisiana. Los Angeles, CA: The Williams Institute; 2022. Available at: https://williamsinstitute.law.ucla.edu/publications/hiv-criminalization-louisiana.

49. Cisneros N, Sears B. Enforcement of HIV criminalization in Kentucky. Los Angeles, CA: The Williams Institute; 2021. Available at: https://williamsinstitute.law.ucla.edu/publications/hiv-criminalization-ky.

50. Hasenbush A, Wilson BD, Miyashita A, et al. HIV criminalization and sex work in California. Los Angeles, CA: The Williams Institute; 2017. Available at: https://williamsinstitute.law.ucla.edu/wp-content/uploads/HIV-Criminalization-Sex-Work-CA-Oct-2017.pdf.

51. The White House. HIV/AIDS NATIONAL STRATEGY.; 2021. Available at: https://www.whitehouse.gov/wp-content/uploads/2021/11/National-HIV-AIDS-Strategy.pdf.

52. IND. CODE. §§ 35-45-21-1.

53. IOWA CODE § 709D.2.

54. VA. CODE ANN. § 18.2-67.4:1.

55. Blecher-Cohn J. Disability Law and HIV Criminalization. Yale Law J 2021;13(6): 1560–616.

56. Gagnon M. Toward a Critical Response to HIV Criminalization: Remarks on Advocacy and Social Justice. J Assoc Nurses AIDS Care 2012;23(1):11–5.

57. Novak A. Toward a Critical Criminology of HIV Criminalization. Crit Criminol 2021. https://doi.org/10.1007/s10612-021-09557-1.

58. Galletly CL, Pinkerton SD. Conflicting Messages: How Criminal HIV Disclosure Laws Undermine Public Health Efforts to Control the Spread of HIV. AIDS Behav 2006;10(5):451–61.

59. Mykhalovskiy E, Bernard E, Cameron S, et al. Using research in the fight against HIV criminalisation: a guide for activists. Amsterdam, The Netherlands: HIV Justice Network; 2019. Available at: https://www.hivjustice.net/publication/using-research-in-the-fight-against-hiv-criminalisation-a-guide-for-activists-hjn-2019/.

60. Adam BD, Elliott R, Corriveau P, et al. Impacts of Criminalization on the Everyday Lives of People Living with HIV in Canada. Sex Res Soc Pol 2013;11(1):39–49.

61. Siegler AJ, Komro KA, Wagenaar AC. Law Everywhere: A Causal Framework for Law and Infectious Disease. Publ Health Rep 2020;135(1_suppl):25S31S.

62. CDC. HIV-specific criminal laws. Centers for Disease Control and Prevention; 2023. Available at: https://www.cdc.gov/hiv/policies/law/states/exposure.html.

63. Ma A, Chambers BD, Jenkins Hall W, et al. Individual and structural factors influencing HIV care linkage and engagement: Perceived barriers and solutions

among HIV-positive persons. J HIV AIDS Soc Serv 2016;1–9. https://doi.org/10.1080/15381501.2015.1107799.

64. Centers for Disease Control and Prevention. Ways HIV is Not Transmitted | HIV Transmission | HIV Basics | HIV/AIDS | CDC. Available at: www.cdc.gov. Published April 21, 2021. https://www.cdc.gov/hiv/basics/hiv-transmission/not-transmitted.html.

65. Galletly CL, Lazzarini Z. Charges for Criminal Exposure to HIV and Aggravated Prostitution Filed in the Nashville, Tennessee Prosecutorial Region 2000–2010. AIDS Behav 2013;17(8):2624–36.

66. Perone A. From Punitive to Proactive: An Alternative Approach for Responding to HIV Criminalization that Departs from Penalizing Marginalized Communities. Hastings Wom Law J 2013;24(2):363.

67. Galletly CL, Pinkerton SD. Toward Rational Criminal HIV Exposure Laws. J Law Med Ethics 2004;32(2):327–37.

68. Sircar N. HIV Criminalization Laws and the Right to Health. Health and Human Rights Journal. Published August 18, 2017. Available at: https://www.hhrjournal.org/2017/08/hiv-criminalization-laws-and-the-right-to-health/. Accessed September 15, 2023.

69. Sah P, Fitzpatrick MC, Pandey A, et al. HIV criminalization exacerbates subpar diagnosis and treatment across the United States. AIDS 2017;31(17):2437–9.

70. Stangl AL, Earnshaw VA, Logie CH, et al. The Health Stigma and Discrimination Framework: a global, crosscutting framework to inform research, intervention development, and policy on health-related stigmas. BMC Med 2019;17(1). https://doi.org/10.1186/s12916-019-1271-3.

71. Audet CM, McGowan CC, Wallston KA, et al. Relationship between HIV Stigma and Self-Isolation among People Living with HIV in Tennessee. Kissinger P. PLoS One 2013;8(8):e69564.

72. The National HIV Criminalization Survey, 2021 Sero Project | 2. Available at: https://www.seroproject.com/wp-content/uploads/2023/03/Sero-Project-National-HIV-Criminalization-Survey-Report-2021.pdf. Accessed October 1, 2023.

73. Centers for Disease Control and Prevention. Estimated HIV incidence and prevalence in the United States, 2015–2019. HIV Surveillance Supplemental Report. 2021;26(1). Available at: http://www.cdc.gov/hiv/library/reports/hiv-surveillance.html.

74. Racial Disparities Persist in Many U.S. Jails. pew.org. Published May 16, 2023. Available at: https://www.pewtrusts.org/en/research-and-analysis/issue-briefs/2023/05/racial-disparities-persist-in-many-us-jails. Accessed September 20, 2023.

75. Nellis A. The Color of Justice: Racial and Ethnic Disparity in State Prisons. The Sentencing Project. Published October 13, 2021. Available at: https://www.sentencingproject.org/reports/the-color-of-justice-racial-and-ethnic-disparity-in-state-prisons-the-sentencing-project/. Accessed August 21, 2023.

76. The Sentencing Project. Incarcerated Women and Girls. The Sentencing Project. Published May 12, 2022. Available at: https://www.sentencingproject.org/fact-sheet/incarcerated-women-and-girls/. Accessed September 29, 2023.

77. Buckwalter3-Poza R. Center for American Progress. Published 2016. Available at: https://www.americanprogress.org/issues/criminal-justice/reports/2016/12/08/294479/making-justice-equal/. Accessed September 25, 2023.

78. Sears B, Goldberg S. HIV criminalization in Georgia: evaluation of transmission risk. Los Angeles, CA: The Williams Institute; 2020.

79. James SE, Brown C, Wilson I. 2015 U.S. transgender survey: report on the experiences of black respondents. Washington, DC and Dallas, TX: National Center for Transgender Equality, Black Trans Advocacy, & National Black Justice Coalition;

2017. https://www.transequality.org/sites/default/files/docs/usts/USTSBlackRespon dentsReport-Nov17.pdf.

80. Rice WS, Logie CH, Napoles TM, et al. Perceptions of intersectional stigma among diverse women living with HIV in the United States. Soc Sci Med 2018; 208:9–17.

81. Factsheet: Criminalization as Violence Against Women Living with HIV. Positive Women's Network - USA. Available at: https://www.pwn-usa.org/doa2016/ factsheet-doa2016/. Accessed September 30, 2023.

82. Bernard EJ, Symington A, Beaumont S. Punishing Vulnerability Through HIV Criminalization. American Journal of Public Health 2022;112(S4):S395–7.

83. Buseh AG, Stevens PE. Constrained But Not Determined by Stigma: Resistance by African American Women Living with HIV. Women Health 2007;44(3):1–18.

84. Evidence of HIV Treatment and Viral Suppression in Preventing the Sexual Trans- mission of HIV. CDC. Available at: www.cdc.gov. Published August 6, 2021. https://www.cdc.gov/hiv/risk/art/evidence-of-hiv-treatment.html. Accessed June 26, 2023.

Primary Prevention of Cardiovascular Disease for People Living with Human Immunodeficiency Virus

Christopher B. Fox, MSN, RN, ANP-BC, AAHIVS[a],*,
Kristine Butler, MSN, RN, FNP-BC[b],
Devon Flynn, PharmD, MPH, BCPS, AAHIVP[c]

KEYWORDS

- Human immunodeficiency virus • Primary prevention • Cardiovascular disease

KEY POINTS

- Cardiovascular disease (CVD) in people living with HIV is mediated by traditional risk factors, chronic inflammation, immune dysfunction, and exposure to antiretroviral therapy.
- CVD risk assessment calculators tend to underestimate risk in people living with HIV but are practical as long as HIV-specific risk factors are considered.
- Improving modifiable risks, particularly smoking cessation, is a key intervention for reducing CVD risk in people living with HIV.
- Statin therapy is the foundational pharmacologic intervention for CVD prevention for people living with HIV, but attention should be paid to drug-drug interactions with antiretrovirals.

INTRODUCTION

Since the advent of successful antiretroviral therapy (ART), HIV infection has become a chronic, manageable illness, leading to dramatically improved life expectancy, often allowing people living with HIV (PLWH) to live into old age. Most PLWH in the United States are now age 50 or older.[1] PLWH with sustained viral suppression on ART can now expect to live a near-normal lifespan, although they are likely to experience comorbidities like cardiovascular disease (CVD) at a younger age compared with

[a] Division of General Internal Medicine & Geriatrics, Oregon Health & Science University School of Medicine, 3270 Southwest Pavilion Loop, Mail Code: L-475, Portland, OR 97239, USA;
[b] Division of General Cardiology, Oregon Health & Science University School of Medicine, 3270 Southwest Pavilion Loop, Mail Code: L-475, Portland, OR 97239, USA; [c] Oregon Health & Science University, 3270 Southwest Pavilion Loop, PPV 350, Portland, OR 97239, USA
* Corresponding author.
E-mail address: christo@ohsu.edu

Nurs Clin N Am 59 (2024) 219–233
https://doi.org/10.1016/j.cnur.2023.12.001
0029-6465/24/© 2023 Elsevier Inc. All rights reserved.

people without HIV.[2] CVD has continued to be the leading cause of death in the US general population.[3] PLWH have a relative risk of myocardial infarction (MI) events that is estimated to be 1.5- to 2-fold higher than people without HIV,[4] as well as increased risk of ischemic stroke, heart failure (HF), pulmonary hypertension, and venous thrombosis.[5] The total cost of CVD to the US health care system in 2018 was $216 billion.[6] Although specific data on the annual cost of CVD in PLWH are not available, one can assume that the cost is substantial owing to the increased burden of CVD in the population of people with HIV. Given the impacts of CVD on PLWH, including longevity, quality of life, and cost to the health system, it is imperative for providers to prioritize prevention of CVD when caring for PLWH.

This article provides a review of primary prevention of CVD in PLWH. The authors discuss risk factors and HIV-specific mechanisms of CVD, review CVD risk assessment tools for PLWH, and identify both behavioral and pharmacologic strategies for reducing CVD in PLWH. Secondary CVD prevention is not the focus of this article, but many of the same principles apply, particularly regarding drug-drug interactions and selection of ART agents.

FACTORS ASSOCIATED WITH CARDIOVASCULAR DISEASE RISK IN PEOPLE LIVING WITH HUMAN IMMUNODEFICIENCY VIRUS

CVD risk in PLWH involves a combination of both traditional nonmodifiable and modifiable risk factors that are well-identified in the general population, as well as factors related to the HIV-disease process, exposure to antiretroviral medications, and common associated comorbidities.

Traditional nonmodifiable risk factors for CVD include age, gender, race, and family history of CVD. Modifiable factors include hypertension, hyperlipidemia, diabetes mellitus, and especially, tobacco use. Although tobacco use is on the decline in the United States, the prevalence of cigarette smoking in PLWH is more than 40%, and PLWH are twice as likely to smoke cigarettes compared with the general population.[7] In addition, they may smoke more cigarettes per day and be less successful at quitting.[7]

The role of the HIV-disease process in CVD risk is complex and not entirely understood. Uncontrolled HIV viremia, chronic immune activation and inflammation, and immune system dysfunction have all been implicated in the increased risk of CVD in PLWH. Although uncontrolled viremia is certainly a risk factor for MI and HF, chronic immune activation and inflammation persist even in the setting of viral suppression on ART.[8] Thus, successful ART does not negate CVD risk in PLWH. Many studies have shown that lower CD4 counts are associated with an increased risk of MI, suggesting that current and past cellular immunity may be an important marker of CVD risk.[5]

In the pre-ART era, AIDS-associated cardiomyopathy was common and continues to be in individuals without viral suppression. In the setting of persistent viral suppression, HF risk is likely related to atherosclerotic disease, increased myocardial fibrosis and steatosis, chronic inflammation and immune activation, and possibly substance use (alcohol, cocaine, and methamphetamine).[5,9]

Common comorbidities associated with HIV infection are known to increase CVD risk in PLWH. The metabolic complications of HIV disease and ART include insulin resistance, dyslipidemia, and lipodystrophy (including accumulation of visceral adipose tissue), all of which are associated with increased CVD risk.[5] The compounded inflammation of coinfections may also play a role in increased CVD risk. For example, PLWH who have chronic hepatitis C infection (HCV) have an increased risk of ischemic stroke compared with those without HCV.[10]

Fortunately, the primary first-line ART regimens available today are less associated with CVD risk enhancement compared with those used in the past. The mitochondrial toxicity caused by legacy nucleoside/nucleotide reverse transcriptase inhibitors (NRTIs)—zalcitabine, didanosine, stavudine, and zidovudine—has been connected to cardiomyopathy,[11] but these drugs are rarely used in practice today and should not be a part of a current ART regimen without an extremely compelling reason. Despite their absence from currently acceptable ART regimens, the lasting effects of legacy NRTI use should be considered in PLWH with past exposure. Another NRTI, abacavir, is still commonly used today, and there is inconsistent evidence that it increases MI risk, but not risk of HF.[12,13] The protease inhibitor (PI) class and efavirenz, a nonnucleoside reverse transcriptase inhibitor (NNRTI), have been associated with increased dyslipidemia including elevated triglycerides.[5] A landmark study also identified that each year of cumulative exposure to a PI (except atazanavir) is associated with a 10% increased risk of MI.[5,14]

ASSESSMENT OF CARDIOVASCULAR DISEASE RISK IN PEOPLE LIVING WITH HUMAN IMMUNODEFICIENCY VIRUS

Multiple factors need to be considered when choosing a method for assessing CVD risk in PLWH. To be useful, a CVD risk assessment tool must accurately predict observed risk over a period of time; accurately identify individuals at high, intermediate, and low risk; and have validity in the real world. Moreover, a risk estimation tool must be simple to use, easy for both patients and providers to understand, and use clinical data that are commonly measured as part of routine patient care.[15]

Many CVD risk estimators have been developed for use in clinical practice. All risk calculators identify low-density lipoprotein cholesterol (LDL-C) as a basic starting point for CVD risk assessment, and appropriate assessment of LDL-C is crucial for determining CVD risk in PLWH. Current ART management guidelines recommend obtaining a lipid profile at baseline, 1 to 3 months after initiation or changing ART, annually when CVD risk is increased, and at least every 5 years if there is no increased CVD risk.[16,17]

Although CVD risk calculators used in the general population tend to inadequately estimate the degree of risk in PLWH, for practical reasons, they are commonly used in clinical practice for the population of people with HIV. The 3 major risk calculators used in the general population are the Framingham Heart Study risk prediction model,[18] American Heart Association/American College of Cardiology (AHA/ACC) Pooled Cohort Equations (PCE) risk calculator,[19] and the Systematic Coronary Risk Evaluation[15] model, which is primarily used in the European Union. The PCE risk calculator is predominant in the United States (available online as the ASCVD Risk Estimator Plus, https://tools.acc.org/ascvd-risk-estimator-plus/#!/calculate/estimate/). Although the PCE calculator does not address HIV-specific risk factors, AHA/ACC do identify HIV infection as a potential "risk enhancer" when risk stratifying an individual person.[19]

The Data-Collection on Adverse Effects of Anti-HIV Drugs (D:A:D) study CVD risk equation was developed in 2010 and updated in 2016 to provide 5-year and 10-year CVD risk estimations for PLWH.[20] The equation is based on a large, primarily European and North American cohort of approximately 32,000 PLWH, most of whom were early middle age and white race. The equation variables include traditional CVD risk factors as well as HIV-specific datapoints: current treatment with abacavir, years of exposure to PIs and NRTIs, and CD4 cell count. **Table 1** contains a comparison between the PCE and the D:A:D risk estimation tools. Even by including HIV-specific risk factors, the D:A:D equation underestimated CVD risk in a Dutch cohort

Table 1
Comparison of cardiovascular disease risk calculators, American Heart Association/American College of Cardiology versus data-collection on adverse effects of anti-HIV drugs

Risk Calculator	Cohort Studied	CVD Risk Estimation	CVD Endpoints	CVD Risk Variables	Comments
AHA/ACC Pooled Cohort Equations Risk Calculator[a]	General population, ages 20–79	Lifetime risk (ages 20–59) and 10-y risk (ages 40–79)	Coronary death, nonfatal MI, fatal or nonfatal stroke	Age; sex; race; blood pressure; cholesterol (total, HDL-C, LDL-C); history of diabetes; history of smoking; current use of antihypertensives	HIV infection identified as a "risk enhancer"
D:A:D CVD Risk Equation[b]	People living with HIV, mostly early middle age (median age 39), mostly North Americans and Europeans of white race	5-y and 10-y risk	MI; invasive coronary artery procedure (including coronary artery bypass or angioplasty), stroke, carotid artery endarterectomy, or death from coronary heart disease	Age, gender, family history of CVD, systolic blood pressure, smoking status, cholesterol (total and HLD-C), diabetes, CD4 lymphocyte count, cumulative PI and NRTI exposure, current use of abacavir	Identification of cumulative PI and NRTI exposure may be challenging in routine clinical care

Abbreviation: HDL-C; high-density lipoprotein cholesterol.
[a] Adapted from the American Heart Association/American College of Cardiology Pooled Cohort Equations risk calculator.[19] Available at: https://tools.acc.org/ascvd-risk-estimator-plus/#!/calculate/estimate/.
[b] Adapted from the D:A:D CVD Risk Equation.[20] Available at: https://chip.dk/Resources/Clinical-risk-scores.

that had well-treated HIV.[15] Thus, without accounting for the chronic inflammation inherent in HIV, no risk equation is going to identify individuals who are at low risk by equation but still have a significant need for intensive primary prevention interventions. Identification of specific inflammatory markers for increased CVD risk that can be easily used in clinical practice is an area for research investigation.

Feinstein and colleagues[5] have proposed an algorithmic model for CVD risk estimation in PLWH who are on ART that uses the ACC/AHA risk calculator (or one of the alternative calculators) as well as accounting for specific HIV risk enhancement factors (history of delayed ART initiation or prolonged viremia, current or nadir CD4 cell count less than 350 cells/mm^3, history of ART failure or poor adherence) and the presence of certain comorbidities that are associated with increased CVD risk in PLWH (metabolic syndrome, fatty liver disease, lipodystrophy, and HCV virus coinfection). Furthermore, Feinstein and colleagues' approach accounts for initiation of ART early in HIV infection, which may be protective.[5] The algorithm accounts for the complexity of assessing risk in PLWH, while still offering a risk-assessment model that could potentially be used in clinical practice. The model also provides more nuance than the ACC/AHA's simple designation of HIV as an atherosclerotic cardiovascular disease (ASCVD) risk enhancer.[19]

The authors recommend an approach to CVD risk assessment similar to Feinstein and colleagues.[5] They use the ACC/AHA risk calculator to estimate the 10-year ASCVD risk based on risk factors shared by the general population. Then, the authors adjust the risk based on the patient's individual HIV history and comorbidities. In conversations with patients, providers must discuss the patient's 10-year estimated ASCVD risk but also educate patients on how their HIV history increases risk. The authors also agree with Feinstein and colleagues[5] that successful treatment of HIV precedes any risk assessment, because untreated HIV is well-known to potentiate very high-risk cardiovascular events like MI.

When CVD risk remains unclear—or in situations when a provider or patient may want more specific CVD risk data before choosing a primary prevention risk reduction strategy—the authors recommend ordering a computed tomography scan to calculate a coronary calcium score. They do not routinely order other blood markers, such as high-sensitivity C-reactive protein, lipoprotein (a), or apolipoprotein b.

The authors also recommend the use of an evidence-based decision aid when counseling patients on CVD risk and potential interventions, such as the Mayo Clinic's free online Statin Choice Decision Aid (https://statindecisionaid.mayoclinic.org/statin/index).

INTERVENTIONS TO REDUCE CARDIOVASCULAR DISEASE RISK IN PEOPLE LIVING WITH HUMAN IMMUNODEFICIENCY VIRUS
Lifestyle Management

Healthy lifestyle behaviors are the foundation of primary prevention of CVD in PLWH regardless of risk severity, just as in the general population. Lifestyle changes that reduce CVD risk include regular aerobic exercise and avoidance of a sedentary lifestyle, a healthy diet, maintaining a healthy weight, smoking cessation, and management of comorbidities like diabetes, hypertension, and alcohol and substance use disorders.[19]

Exercise and diet can positively alter the lipid profile and the cardiovascular system in general. The AHA/ACC recommends 150 minutes per week of moderate-intensity exercise or 75 minutes per week of vigorous exercise.[19] There are multiple diet plans with strong evidence for positively impacting cardiovascular health such as the DASH (Dietary Approaches to Stop Hypertension)[21] and Mediterranean diets.[22] However, the components and implementation of specific diet plans can be confusing for both patients and providers. Therefore, the AHA/ACC recommends counseling patients to eat a diet rich in fruits, vegetables, nuts, whole grains, legumes, and fish, while reducing or stopping sweetened beverages, avoiding highly processed foods, and reducing saturated fat (particularly in red meat and tropical oils) and eliminating trans fats.[19] Clinicians should ask patients about adherence to high animal protein popular diets like ketogenic ("keto"), paleolithic ("paleo"), or Atkins, which can increase LDL-C. Sweetened beverages should also be avoided. Consuming 1 to 2 daily sweetened beverages increases the risk of diabetes mellitus type 2 by 26%.[23]

The authors recognize that HIV affects many communities, and economic disparities are inherent in the United States. Counseling messages like "take a brisk walk in your neighborhood 3 to 4 times a week" may not recognize the lack of outdoor safety in some locations, and using the term "Mediterranean diet" may not resonate with the food traditions of diverse cultural backgrounds. Thus, the authors recommend that providers tailor their AHA/ACC–supported counseling regarding exercise and diet to fit an individual's life circumstances. Providers should also offer referrals to food banks or other nutrition assistance services to PLWH who would benefit.

Smoking Cessation

Given the high rates of cigarette smoking in PLWH,[7] attention to smoking cessation is key for reducing CVD risk and potentially the most important modifiable risk factor. There are many interventions to assist individuals in smoking cessation, including medication support (nicotine replacement products, varenicline, and bupropion) and various types of individual and group counseling.

Although only a handful of smoking cessation intervention strategies have been studied in PWLH, interventions that combine counseling and motivational interviewing with pharmacotherapy are most successful.[24] PLWH comprise a heterogenous group, and smoking cessation interventions that are tailored to the needs of individuals—such as women, people with mental illness, or other substance use—may be more successful than cookie-cutter approaches.[24]

Management of Comorbidities

Management of comorbidities is an essential component of reducing CVD risk in PLWH. Providers should follow evidence-based guidelines for management of hypertension[25] and diabetes.[26] For type 2 diabetes mellitus management specifically, the authors encourage the consideration of blood glucose-lowering agents that have a cardioprotective benefit like glucagon-like peptide 1 receptor agonists (GLP-1 RAs) and sodium-glucose transport protein 2 inhibitors. GLP-1 RAs have the added benefit of weight loss for individuals struggling with obesity.

Recognizing the often-suboptimal treatment of comorbidities like hypertension and dyslipidemia in PLWH, the authors recommend nurse-led interventions, such as the (A Nurse-Led Intervention to Extend the HIV Treatment Cascade for Cardiovascular Disease Prevention) EXTRA-CVD protocol, to support medication adherence and monitoring using telehealth and electronic health record tools.[27,28]

Heavy alcohol use and stimulant use, particularly methamphetamine, are known to increase CVD risk.[29,30] Although alcohol use disorder has many behavioral and pharmacologic treatment options,[29] treatment of methamphetamine use is primarily behavioral at this time.[31]

Statin Therapy

Hydroxymethylglutaryl-CoA reductase inhibitors, or statins, reduce LDL-C, total cholesterol, and triglycerides, while increasing high-density lipoprotein cholesterol. Statins are the pharmacologic foundation for reducing CVD morbidity and mortality in the general population and are recommended by the US Preventative Services Task Force[32] and the AHA/ACC.[19] Researchers have suggested that, in addition to lowering LDL-C, statins may also modulate the inflammatory and immunologic factors that increase CVD in PLWH.[33]

Although statin medications are a mainstay of LDL-C–lowering therapy, for many years there were no good trials to assess the impact of statin therapy on CVD risk in PLWH. The first of its kind, the Randomized Trial to Prevent Vascular Events in HIV (REPRIEVE) is a landmark phase 3 randomized trial to evaluate the impact of statins on CVD in PLWH who are low to moderate risk according to the AHA/ACC PCE risk estimator.[34] The investigators conducted the trial knowing that statins decreased LDL-C but also may have an impact on chronic inflammation and immune pathways. The trial used pitavastatin because it has fewer drug interactions with antiretrovirals,[34] and there is evidence from another trial that pitavastatin is superior to pravastatin at lowering LDL-C.[35] However, it should be acknowledged that pitavastatin is expensive, so it is rarely used in clinical practice. The investigators enrolled 7769 PLWH participants ages 40 to 75 years on ART. The participants were matched 1:1 to receive pitavastatin 4 mg daily or placebo and observed for more than 5 years. The primary endpoint was a composite cardiovascular event (cardiovascular death; MI; hospitalization for unstable angina; coronary, carotid, or peripheral artery revascularization; or death from undetermined cause). The trial was stopped early owing to efficacy, and statin therapy was shown to significantly decrease CVD risk, even in people who were low to moderate risk. The pitavastatin arm had 4.81 cardiovascular events per 1000 person-years versus 7.32 in the placebo arm, with a hazard ratio of 0.65 (95% confidence interval 0.48–0.90; $P = .002$).[34] The compelling results of the REPRIEVE trial have bolstered the argument for offering statin therapy to PLWH, even those at low or moderate CVD risk, and health care providers should counsel patients about this new evidence.

When prescribing statins to PLWH, clinicians should note that significant drug-drug interactions exist with some antiretroviral agents. Approximately 72% of statin adverse effects are muscular in nature, including risk of rhabdomyolysis.[36] Careful attention to these drug-drug interactions reduces the risk of a severe adverse event and helps patients with tolerance of more mild side effects. **Table 2** provides a comprehensive breakdown of statin dosing considerations when choosing a statin therapy in the setting of ART. The University of Liverpool HIV Drug Interaction Checker (available at https://www.hiv-druginteractions.org/) is also a helpful clinical resource.

Special attention should be given to drug-drug interactions when statins are prescribed with the pharmacokinetic enhancers, or "boosters," ritonavir and cobicistat. Simvastatin and lovastatin are contraindicated with boosters, and there are maximum dose limitations for atorvastatin and rosuvastatin when used with boosters. When used with darunavir 300 mg and ritonavir 100 mg twice daily, atorvastatin 10 mg daily achieves a similar area under the curve (a measure of total medication exposure throughout the dosing interval) as atorvastatin 40 mg alone.[37] Therefore, it is recommended to start atorvastatin at the lowest dose and titrate, as needed, up to a maximum dose of atorvastatin 20 mg when taken with darunavir/ritonavir or other boosted ART.[17]

Red yeast rice is an over-the-counter supplement that contains monacolin K (otherwise known as lovastatin) and is purported to have cholesterol-lowering effects.[38] Anecdotally, the authors have witnessed cases of patients who have experienced myalgia and elevated creatinine kinase (CK) when taking red yeast rice with pharmacokinetic enhancers, which highlights the need for clinicians to ask patients about the use of over-the-counter, herbal, or supplemental products when taking medical histories.

Table 2
Statin dosing and expected intensity of therapy when used with antiretroviral agents[a]

Antiretroviral agents	Low-Intensity Statin Therapy Daily dose lowers LDL-C on average <30%	Moderate-Intensity Statin Therapy Daily dose lower LDL-C on average 30%–49%	High-Intensity Statin Therapy Daily dose lowers LDL-C on average ≥50%
All NRTIs All NNRTIs INSTIs (except elvitegravir/cobicistat) Ibalizumab Maraviroc	Fluvastatin 20–40 mg Lovastatin 20 mg Pitavastatin 1 mg Pravastatin 10–20 mg Simvastatin 10 mg	Atorvastatin 10–20 mg Fluvastatin 40 mg BID Fluvastatin XL 80 mg Lovastatin 40 mg Pitavastatin 2–4 mg Pravastatin 40–80 mg Rosuvastatin 5–10 mg Simvastatin 20–40 mg	Atorvastatin 40–80 mg Rosuvastatin 20–40 mg
Cobicistat-boosted agents *Do not use lovastatin or simvastatin* *Use lowest effective dose of chosen statin* Atazanavir/cobicistat	 Pitavastatin 1 mg Pravastatin 10–20 mg	 Pitavastatin 2–4 mg Pravastatin 40–80 mg Rosuvastatin 5–10 mg *Do not use atorvastatin*	 Rosuvastatin up to 10 mg *Do not use atorvastatin*
Darunavir/cobicistat	Pitavastatin 1 mg Pravastatin 10–20 mg	Atorvastatin up to 10 mg Rosuvastatin 5–10 mg	Atorvastatin up to 20 mg Rosuvastatin up to 20 mg
Elvitegravir/cobicistat	Pitavastatin 1 mg (drug levels may be increased or decreased) Pravastatin 10–20 mg	Atorvastatin up to 10 mg Rosuvastatin 5–10 mg	Atorvastatin up to 20 mg Rosuvastatin 20–40 mg
Ritonavir-boosted agents *Do not use lovastatin or simvastatin* *Use lowest effective dose of chosen statin* Atazanavir with or without ritonavir	 Pravastatin 10–20 mg	 Atorvastatin 10–20 mg Pravastatin 40–80 mg Rosuvastatin 5–10 mg	 Atorvastatin 40–80 mg Rosuvastatin up to 10 mg
Darunavir/ritonavir	Pitavastatin 1 mg (drug levels may be reduced) Pravastatin 10–20 mg	Atorvastatin up to 10 mg Pitavastatin 2–4 mg (drug levels may be reduced) Pravastatin 40–80 mg (drug levels may be increased) Rosuvastatin 5–10 mg	Atorvastatin up to 20 mg Rosuvastatin 20–40 mg
Lopinavir/ritonavir	Pitavastatin 1 mg Pravastatin 10–20 mg	Atorvastatin up to 10 mg Pitavastatin 2–4 mg Pravastatin 40–80 mg Rosuvastatin 5–10 mg	Atorvastatin up to 20 mg Rosuvastatin up to 10 mg

Fostemsavir *Drug levels of statin may be increased* *Use lowest effective dose of chosen statin*	Fluvastatin 20–40 mg Lovastatin 20 mg Pitavastatin 1 mg Pravastatin 10–20 mg Simvastatin 10 mg	Atorvastatin 10–20 mg Fluvastatin 40 mg BID Fluvastatin XL 80 mg Lovastatin 40 mg Pitavastatin 2–4 mg Pravastatin 40–80 mg Rosuvastatin 5–10 mg[b] Simvastatin 20–40 mg	Atorvastatin 40–80 mg Rosuvastatin 20–40 mg[b]
Lenacapvir *Avoid lovastatin and simvastatin*	Fluvastatin 20–40 mg Pitavastatin 1 mg Pravastatin 10–20 mg	Atorvastatin 10–20 mg Fluvastatin 40 mg BID Fluvastatin XL 80 mg Pitavastatin 2–4 mg Pravastatin 40–80 mg Rosuvastatin 5–10 mg	Atorvastatin 40–80 mg Rosuvastatin 20–40 mg

Abbreviation: BID, twice daily.

[a] Derived from Table 3 in the American College of Cardiology/American Heart Association cholesterol management guidelines[19] and Tables 24a–24 g in the Department of Health and Human Services antiretroviral management guidelines.[17]

[b] Area under the curve increased 69% with rosuvastatin but may not be clinically relevant.

In addition, CK elevations can be seen with the integrase strand transfer inhibitor (INSTI) antiretroviral class.[39–43] Interestingly, the authors have seen a small number of patients develop muscle-related symptoms and elevated CK while taking a statin and INSTI. In these cases, the authors have chosen to stop the statin until CK normalizes and then restart statin therapy with the same agent or a more potent statin at the lowest dose. There have been no recurrences of muscle-related symptoms or CK elevation in these cases, even when the statin dose was increased slowly.

Other Lipid-Lowering Agents

Other LDL-C–lowering agents include ezetimibe, bile acid sequestrants, fibrates, niacin, proprotein convertase subtilisin/kexin type 9 (PCSK9) inhibitors, and dietary supplements. Ezetimibe, and less frequently bile acid sequestrants, can be used to augment statin therapy when LDL-C is resistant.[19] Fibrates and niacin, which are primarily used for treatment of hypertriglyceridemia, also lower LDL-C somewhat but are not recommended for augmenting statin therapy by the AHA/ACC.[19] PCSK9 inhibitors are primarily used for secondary CVD prevention, and in the authors' experience, are not covered by insurance payers without a cardiologist's prescription. The evidence to support dietary supplements like coenzyme Q10, red yeast rice, fish oil, multivitamins, and vitamin D is lacking.[19,44]

Antiplatelet Therapy

Historically, aspirin has been used for the primary prevention of CVD, but aspirin is no longer recommended by the USPFTF and AHA/ACC because of concerns that the cardiovascular benefit of preventing atherothrombosis is outweighed by increased bleeding risk.[19,45] Researchers have not yet determined if there is a subset of individuals who would benefit from antiplatelet therapy for primary prevention. A shared decision-making conversation about aspirin therapy is indicated for individuals who have high CVD risk, such as a coronary artery calcium score $\geq$ 100, including PLWH.[45,46]

Selection of Antiretroviral Agents

The primary goal when selecting an ART regimen is to achieve and maintain viral suppression, ideally with minimal impact on an individual's daily life. However, when multiple ART options are available, clinicians can consider the potential impact of specific agents on cardiovascular risk, both directly and indirectly by influencing factors associated with CVD risk.

As mentioned previously, the legacy NRTIs have been associated with direct effects on the myocardium owing to mitochondrial toxicity,[11] but this is less concerning with currently used NRTIs, with the possible exception of abacavir. In 2008, the D:A:D observational study identified an increased risk of MI, cardiovascular death, and invasive cardiovascular procedure with recent exposure to abacavir that was independent of metabolic risk factors.[47] Tenofovir disoproxil fumarate (TDF), another commonly used NRTI agent, was not included in the initial analysis. A follow-up publication with additional years of data in 2010 found no increased risk of MI associated with TDF but continued to find associations with abacavir.[48]

Several meta-analysis and retrospective observational studies have been conducted since the initial D:A:D Study results were published.[48,49] Findings have been conflicting regarding whether there is increased risk of cardiovascular events with abacavir, as well as whether the increased risk is limited to recent or cumulative exposure to the agent,[48] and the specific mechanism of increased risk of MI has not been definitively identified.[50] Therefore, in practice, the authors avoid using abacavir in PLWH who also have significant CVD risk whenever possible.

The PI antiretroviral class has been implicated in increased cardiovascular risk both directly and indirectly by increasing LDL-C and triglycerides. Compared with legacy PIs, atazanavir and darunavir are both considered to have less impact on lipids, but darunavir was shown to have an increased risk of cardiovascular events.[51] When reasonable alternatives exist, the authors avoid using PIs in PLWH who have increased risk of CVD.

There is emerging evidence from multiple trials that INSTIs and tenofovir alafenamide, possibly through associated weight gain, may increase risk of hypertension.[52,53] The clinical practice implications of this evidence are not yet clear, although these data highlight the need to monitor blood pressure and treat hypertension in PLWH.

Referral to Specialty Care

Generally, primary CVD risk in PLWH can be managed in primary care by a general practitioner or HIV specialist. A referral to a preventative or general cardiologist can be considered when there is a concern for familial hyperlipidemia, a strong history of premature CVD or cardiac death in a first-degree relative, or a need for assistance with lifestyle or pharmacologic interventions. A referral to cardiology is also indicated for severe statin intolerance when a PCSK9 inhibitor should be considered.

SUMMARY

In the era of highly successful ART, primary prevention of CVD is an essential component of health care for PLWH, just as it is in the general population. Clinicians should recognize the unique increase in CVD risk in PLWH and use evidence-based interventions to reduce risk. Improving modifiable risks is key, particularly smoking cessation. As the REPRIEVE trial results illustrate, statin therapy has an important role as well,[32] although attention should be paid to drug-drug interactions to prevent side effects and adverse events.

CLINICS CARE POINTS

- People living with HIV have a risk of cardiovascular events that is 1.5 to 2 times higher than people without HIV.

- Use an evidence-based cardiovascular disease risk calculator (such as the Pooled Cohort Equations) to assess risk in people with HIV, but adjust risk based on HIV-specific risk factors: delayed antiretroviral therapy initiation or prolonged viremia, current or nadir CD4 cell count less than 350 cells/mm^3, history of HIV treatment failure or poor adherence, and HIV-associated comorbidities.

- Smoking cessation is a key lifestyle intervention to reduce cardiovascular disease risk in people living with HIV, who have high rates of cigarette smoking.

- The landmark REPRIEVE trial has demonstrated that statin therapy significantly reduces incidence of cardiovascular death and myocardial infarction in people with HIV who are low to moderate risk for cardiovascular disease.

- When prescribing statin therapy, pay special attention to possible drug-drug interactions with antiretroviral agents.

- When possible, construct antiretroviral therapy regimens that avoid agents linked to increased cardiovascular risk, such as protease inhibitors, when individuals have heightened risk.

DISCLOSURE

C.B. Fox and D. Flynn have received research support to their institution from ViiV Healthcare, United Kingdom. K. Butler has no disclosures to report.

REFERENCES

1. Centers for Disease Control and Prevention. HIV Surveillance Report, 2021. Available at: http://www.cdc.gov/hiv/library/reports/hiv-surveillance.html. Accessed September 30, 2023.
2. Marcus JL, Leyden WA, Alexeeff SE, et al. Comparison of overall and comorbidity-free life expectancy between insured adults with and without HIV infection, 2000-2016. JAMA Netw Open 2020;3(6):e207954.
3. Xu J, Murphy SL, Kochanek KD, et al. Mortality in the United States, 2021. NCHS Data Brief 2022;(456):1–8.
4. Freiberg MS, Chang CC, Kuller LH, et al. HIV infection and the risk of acute myocardial infarction. JAMA Intern Med 2013;173(8):614–22.
5. Feinstein MJ, Hsue PY, Benjamin LA, et al. Characteristics, prevention, and management of cardiovascular disease in people living with HIV: A scientific statement from the American Heart Association. Circulation 9 2019;140(2):e98–124.
6. Benjamin EJ, Virani SS, Callaway CW, et al. Heart disease and stroke statistics-2018 update: A report from the American Heart Association. Circulation 2018; 137(12):e67–492.
7. Rojewski AM, Baldassarri S, Cooperman NA, et al. Exploring issues of comorbid conditions in people who smoke. Nicotine Tob Res 2016;18(8):1684–96.
8. Deeks SG. HIV infection, inflammation, immunosenescence, and aging. Annu Rev Med 2011;62:141–55.
9. Thiara DK, Liu CY, Raman F, et al. Abnormal myocardial function is related to myocardial steatosis and diffuse myocardial fibrosis in HIV-infected adults. J Infect Dis 2015;212(10):1544–51.
10. Alvaro-Meca A, Berenguer J, Díaz A, et al. Stroke in HIV-infected individuals with and without HCV coinfection in Spain in the combination antiretroviral therapy era. PLoS One 2017;12(6):e0179493.
11. Balcarek K, Venhoff N, Deveaud C, et al. Role of pyrimidine depletion in the mitochondrial cardiotoxicity of nucleoside analogue reverse transcriptase inhibitors. J Acquir Immune Defic Syndr 2010;55(5):550–7.
12. Sabin CA, Reiss P, Ryom L, et al. Is there continued evidence for an association between abacavir usage and myocardial infarction risk in individuals with HIV? A cohort collaboration. BMC Med 2016;14:61.
13. Marcus JL, Neugebauer RS, Leyden WA, et al. Use of abacavir and risk of cardiovascular disease among HIV-infected individuals. J Acquir Immune Defic Syndr 2016;71(4):413–9.
14. Friis-Møller N, Reiss P, Sabin CA, et al. Class of antiretroviral drugs and the risk of myocardial infarction. N Engl J Med 2007;356(17):1723–35.
15. Achhra AC, Lyass A, Borowsky L, et al. Assessing cardiovascular risk in people living with HIV: Current tools and limitations. Curr HIV AIDS Rep 2021;18(4): 271–9.
16. Thompson MA, Horberg MA, Agwu AL, et al. Primary care guidance for persons with human immunodeficiency virus: 2020 Update by the HIV Medicine Association of the Infectious Diseases Society of America. Clin Infect Dis 2021;73(11): e3572–605.

17. Panel on Antiretroviral Guidelines for Adults and Adolescents, U.S. Department of Health and Human Services. Guidelines for the Use of Antiretroviral Agents in Adults and Adolescents with HIV. https://clinicalinfo.hiv.gov/en/guidelines/adult-and-adolescent-arv Accessed September 30, 2023.

18. van Zoest RA, Law M, Sabin CA, et al. Predictive performance of cardiovascular disease risk prediction algorithms in people living with HIV. J Acquir Immune Defic Syndr 2019;81(5):562–71.

19. Grundy SM, Stone NJ, Bailey AL, et al. 2018 AHA/ACC/AACVPR/AAPA/ABC/ACPM/ADA/AGS/APhA/ASPC/NLA/PCNA Guideline on the management of blood cholesterol: A report of the American College of Cardiology/American Heart Association Task Force on Clinical Practice Guidelines. Circulation 2019;139(25):e1082–143.

20. Friis-Møller N, Ryom L, Smith C, et al. An updated prediction model of the global risk of cardiovascular disease in HIV-positive persons: The Data-collection on Adverse Effects of Anti-HIV Drugs (D:A:D) study. Eur J Prev Cardiol 2016;23(2):214–23.

21. Appel LJ, Moore TJ, Obarzanek E, et al. A clinical trial of the effects of dietary patterns on blood pressure. DASH Collaborative Research Group. N Engl J Med 1997;336(16):1117–24.

22. Martínez-González MA, Gea A, Ruiz-Canela M. The Mediterranean diet and cardiovascular health. Circ Res 2019;124(5):779–98.

23. Malik VS, Popkin BM, Bray GA, et al. Sugar-sweetened beverages and risk of metabolic syndrome and type 2 diabetes: A meta-analysis. Diabetes Care 2010;33(11):2477–83.

24. Moscou-Jackson G, Commodore-Mensah Y, Farley J, et al. Smoking-cessation interventions in people living with HIV infection: A systematic review. J Assoc Nurses AIDS Care Jan-Feb 2014;25(1):32–45.

25. Whelton PK, Carey RM, Aronow WS, et al. 2017 ACC/AHA/AAPA/ABC/ACPM/AGS/APhA/ASH/ASPC/NMA/PCNA Guideline for the prevention, detection, evaluation, and management of high blood pressure in adults: A report of the American College of Cardiology/American Heart Association Task Force on Clinical Practice Guidelines. Hypertension 2018;71(6):e13–115.

26. ElSayed NA, Aleppo G, Aroda VR, et al. 10. Cardiovascular disease and risk management: Standards of care in diabetes-2023. Diabetes Care 2023;46(Suppl 1):S158–s190.

27. Okeke NL, Webel AR, Bosworth HB, et al. Rationale and design of a nurse-led intervention to extend the HIV treatment cascade for cardiovascular disease prevention trial (EXTRA-CVD). Am Heart J 2019;216:91–101.

28. Musoke L, Bosworth HB, Dickson C, et al. A telehealth-delivered intervention to extend the veteran HIV treatment cascade for cardiovascular disease prevention: V-EXTRA-CVD study protocol for a randomized controlled trial. HIV Res Clin Pract 2023;24(1):2261747.

29. Hoek AG, van Oort S, Mukamal KJ, et al. Alcohol consumption and cardiovascular disease risk: Placing new data in context. Curr Atheroscler Rep 2022;24(1):51–9.

30. Kevil CG, Goeders NE, Woolard MD, et al. Methamphetamine use and cardiovascular disease. Arterioscler Thromb Vasc Biol 2019;39(9):1739–46.

31. Moszczynska A. Current and emerging treatments for methamphetamine use disorder. Curr Neuropharmacol 2021;19(12):2077–91.

32. Chou R, Cantor A, Dana T, et al. Statin use for the primary prevention of cardiovascular disease in adults: Updated evidence report and systematic review for the US Preventive Services Task Force. JAMA 2022;328(8):754–71.

33. Funderburg NT, Jiang Y, Debanne SM, et al. Rosuvastatin reduces vascular inflammation and T-cell and monocyte activation in HIV-infected subjects on antiretroviral therapy. J Acquir Immune Defic Syndr 2015;68(4):396–404.

34. Grinspoon SK, Fitch KV, Zanni MV, et al. Pitavastatin to prevent cardiovascular disease in HIV infection. N Engl J Med 2023;389(8):687–99.

35. Aberg JA, Sponseller CA, Ward DJ, et al. Pitavastatin versus pravastatin in adults with HIV-1 infection and dyslipidaemia (INTREPID): 12 week and 52 week results of a phase 4, multicentre, randomised, double-blind, superiority trial. Lancet HIV 2017;4(7):e284–94.

36. Ward NC, Watts GF, Eckel RH. Statin toxicity. Circ Res 2019;124(2):328–50.

37. Hoetelmans R, Lasure A, Koester A, et al. The effect of TMC114, a potent next-generation HIV protease inhibitor, with low-dose ritonavir on atorvastatin pharmacokinetics [poster no. H-865]. Washington, DC: Poster presented at: 44th Annual Interscience Conference on Antimicrobial Agents and Chemotherapy; 2004.

38. Natural Medicines (internet database). Available at: https://naturalmedicines.therapeuticresearch.com/. Accessed September 25, 2023.

39. Biktarvy [package insert]. Foster City, CA: Gilead Sciences, Inc.; 2022.

40. Cabenuva [package insert]. Middlesex, UK: ViiV Healthcare; 2023.

41. Isentress [package insert]. Lebanon, NJ: Merck & Co, Inc.; 2014-2022.

42. Stribild [package insert]. Foster City, CA: Gilead Sciences, Inc.; 2021.

43. Tivicay [package insert]. Middlesex, UK: ViiV Healthcare; 2022.

44. Jenkins DJA, Spence JD, Giovannucci EL, et al. Supplemental vitamins and minerals for cardiovascular disease prevention and treatment: JACC Focus Seminar. J Am Coll Cardiol 2021;77(4):423–36.

45. Cofer LB, Barrett TJ, Berger JS. Aspirin for the primary prevention of cardiovascular disease: Time for a platelet-guided approach. Arterioscler Thromb Vasc Biol 2022;42(10):1207–16.

46. Ajufo E, Ayers CR, Vigen R, et al. Value of coronary artery calcium scanning in association with the net benefit of aspirin in primary prevention of atherosclerotic cardiovascular disease. JAMA Cardiol 2021;6(2):179–87.

47. Sabin CA, Worm SW, Weber R, et al. Use of nucleoside reverse transcriptase inhibitors and risk of myocardial infarction in HIV-infected patients enrolled in the D:A:D study: a multi-cohort collaboration. Lancet 2008;371(9622):1417–26.

48. Worm SW, Sabin C, Weber R, et al. Risk of myocardial infarction in patients with HIV infection exposed to specific individual antiretroviral drugs from the 3 major drug classes: the data collection on adverse events of anti-HIV drugs (D:A:D) study. J Infect Dis 2010;201(3):318–30.

49. Eyawo O, Brockman G, Goldsmith CH, et al. Risk of myocardial infarction among people living with HIV: an updated systematic review and meta-analysis. BMJ Open 2019;9(9):e025874.

50. Vos AG, Venter WDF. Cardiovascular toxicity of contemporary antiretroviral therapy. Curr Opin HIV AIDS 2021;16(6):286–91.

51. Ryom L, Lundgren JD, El-Sadr W, et al. Cardiovascular disease and use of contemporary protease inhibitors: the D:A:D international prospective multicohort study. Lancet HIV 2018;5(6):e291–300.

52. Byonanebye DM, Polizzotto MN, Maltez F, et al. Impact of INSTI and TAF-related BMI changes and risk on hypertension and dyslipidemia in RESPOND. Brisbane, Australia: Abstract presented at: IAS 2023, the 12th IAS Conference on HIV; 2023. Abstract 5470.
53. Venter F, Sokhela S, Bosch B, et al. Risks of hypertension with first-line dolutegravir (DTG) and tenofovir alafenamide (TAF) in the NAMSAL and ADVANCE trials. Brisbane, Australia: Abstract presented at: IAS 2023, the 12th IAS Conference on HIV; 2023. Abstract 5640.

A Scoping Review of Approaches to Reduce Stigma and Discrimination Against People with HIV in Health-Care Settings in the United States: Few Recent Interventions Identified

Sarah E. Janek, BSN, RN, ACRN[a],*, Elizabeth T. Knippler, MPH[a],
Ali T. Saslafsky, BSN, RN, MSN, APRN, FNP-C[a],
Marta I. Mulawa, MHS, PhD[a,b]

KEYWORDS

- Scoping review • Stigma • HIV • Stigma reduction intervention

KEY POINTS

- Human immunodeficiency virus (HIV) stigma and discrimination is pervasive throughout the US health-care system and prevents people living with HIV from seeking and staying in treatment and care.
- Few intervention studies specific to HIV stigma reduction in the United States have been developed within the past 5 years, leaving a large gap for interventions.
- Existing interventions have involved health-care professional students and exemplify the importance of destigmatizing HIV care early in education, professional development, and training.
- A lack of standardized operationalization and measures of stigma pose a barrier to understanding and intervening on the HIV stigma in health-care settings.
- Future interventions are needed, especially those that counter intersectional stigma, allowing for stigma reduction not only for HIV but also other minoritized identities.

Funding: This work was supported by the National Institute on Minority Health and Health Disparities (mPIs: Bauermeister and Muessig, R01MD013623). *Funded by*: NIMHD. *Grant number(s)*: R01MD013623. S.E. Janek was supported by the Duke University School of Nursing.
[a] Duke University School of Nursing, 307 Trent Drive, Durham, NC 27710, USA; [b] Duke Global Health Institute, Duke University, Durham, NC, USA
* Corresponding author. Duke University School of Nursing, 307 Trent Drive, Box 3322, Durham, NC 27710.
E-mail address: sarah.janek@duke.edu

INTRODUCTION

Approximately 1.2 million people in the United States are living with human immunode-ficiency virus (HIV)[1] with only 57.8% of people with HIV estimated to be retained in care.[2] These outcomes are worse among minoritized populations, exacerbating sexual health inequities experienced by racial and ethnic minoritized groups and sexual and gender minoritized groups.[1,3] Although there are multiple and compounding factors that contribute to these inequities, such as structural racism, lack of health insurance, or dis-parities in access to quality care, stigma proves to be a large factor inhibiting persons from engaging in HIV prevention and treatment.[3,4] Stigma has been historically defined "as the co-occurrence of labeling, stereotyping, separation, status loss, and discrimina-tion in a context in which power is exercised."[5] During the origin of the HIV epidemic in the 1980s, a more specific form of stigma emerged, acquired immunodeficiency syn-drome (AIDS)-related stigma,[6] which is now known as HIV stigma. HIV stigma continues today through prejudice and social devaluation of those living with HIV,[7,8] or those engaging in HIV prevention, and can manifest as internalized, anticipated, and enacted stigma.[9] Only 43% of Americans state they feel comfortable interacting with someone who is living with HIV,[10] which heavily influences how people living with HIV experience stigma and discrimination. Additionally, almost 8 in 10 people living with HIV in the US report feeling internalized HIV stigma, resulting in thoughts of shame and low self-esteem.[11] Medical advancements in HIV prevention and treatment offer promising path-ways toward HIV stigma reduction across the nation but additional efforts are needed to realize this potential.

HIV can now be managed as a chronic condition[12] due to advancements in treatment options that have also revolutionized HIV prevention; the Undetectable = Untransmittable (U=U) message,[13] for example, communicates how a person living with HIV cannot trans-mit HIV through sex if they have an undetectable viral load due to consistent antiretroviral treatment.[14] However, although these advancements aid in reducing stigma and discrim-ination toward people living with HIV, knowledge about U=U and the current state of HIV prevention and treatment options is not universal. As a result, HIV stigma persists and often prevents patients from seeking or staying in care.[13] In health-care settings, HIV stigma can manifest in multiple ways, including denial of care, provision of substandard care, and differential treatment (eg, excessive use of personal protective equipment and increased wait times).[15,16] In a recent nationally representative survey of adults with HIV, approximately 25% of all adults who had an HIV care visit within the past year reported experiencing discrimination in a US health-care setting.[17] Literature has shown that there is a lower likelihood of care engagement and retention in care for people with HIV if they experience HIV stigma in a health-care setting and when they perceive that same stigma will occur in the future.[8] Not only does stigma affect care-seeking behaviors but also medication adherence because individuals with greater internalized stigma and recent stigmatizing experiences have poorer rates of medication adherence that result in poorer health outcomes.[9]

In recognition of the importance of stigma, the National HIV/AIDS Strategy[3] explic-itly calls for reducing HIV stigma and discrimination by ensuring that health-care pro-fessionals complete education and training on stigma, discrimination, and unrecognized bias toward people with HIV as well as those who experience height-ened risk for HIV. Thus, interventions focused on reducing stigma toward people with HIV in health-care settings are critical to addressing the current HIV epidemic, and the inequities experienced involving treatment.

The aim of this scoping review is to synthesize the recent literature on interventions to reduce stigma and discrimination against people with HIV in health-care settings across the United States, as well as uncover the current gaps in recently evaluated stigma reduction interventions in these settings. Due to the advancements in HIV care, past interventions may not be as relevant to the current stigma experiences of people with HIV, and thus, we are synthesizing the literature from the prior 5 years. Earlier reviews have focused mainly on interventions related to personal and internalized HIV stigma,[18] or both pre-exposure prophylaxis (PrEP) and HIV stigma reduction interventions in specific populations such as men who have sex with men.[13] Another review has synthesized current HIV stigma reduction interventions but is rooted in understanding reducing stigma internationally rather than specifically within the United States.[19] This scoping review seeks to understand the contemporary approaches that have been examined to mitigate stigma and may serve as a positive direction for future implementation in the context of the US health-care system.

METHODS
Search Strategy

The search was developed and conducted by expert medical librarians in consultation with the research team and included a mix of keywords and subject headings related to HIV, stigma, and health-care staff. A search hedge was used to narrow publications to those using study designs appropriate for establishing a cause-and-effect relationship between the intervention/approach and stigma/discrimination outcomes (eg, randomized controlled trials [RCTs] and quasi-experimental designs inclusive of nonequivalent group designs and one-group pretest-posttest designs).

We searched electronic databases including MEDLINE via PubMed, Scopus via Elsevier, and CINAHL Complete via EBSCOhost. The search was limited to the past 5 years and conducted on July 3, 2023. The complete reproducible search strategy, including date ranges and search filters, is detailed in the Appendix 1.

Eligibility Criteria

Studies were included if they met each of the following criteria: (1) evaluated an intervention or approach to reduce stigma and/or discrimination against people with HIV, (2) focused on the health-care setting or delivery of health care, (3) conducted in the United States, (4) measured a relevant discrimination or HIV stigma outcome, and (5) study design met criteria.

Our definition of health-care setting and delivery was intentionally broad to capture a variety of settings and experiences where stigma or discrimination could occur. These included interactions with clinical care providers in formal health-care settings, delivery of health care in other settings (eg, home-based care and community-based organizations), interactions with HIV-specific providers, interactions with providers for issues unrelated to HIV (eg, dental care and physical therapy), and other experiences in health-care settings outside of provider interactions (eg, interactions with front desk staff, clinic environment, language, or questions on medical forms). We also included studies of health professions students and trainees due to their interactions with patients during clinical training and future employment.

Relevant outcomes measuring discrimination or stigma included outcomes related to a provider or staff or outcomes reported by a person with HIV. This criterion allowed both provider beliefs and attitudes and patient experiences, such as discrimination at a clinic, to be included.

In order to focus on stigma and discrimination against people with HIV, we excluded studies that focused solely on discrimination related to HIV prevention services such as PrEP. Studies that addressed other stigmas or discrimination relevant to HIV care (eg, discrimination based on drug use, gender identity, sexual orientation, or race/ethnicity) but did not measure HIV stigma were excluded from this review.

We also excluded studies that (1) did not evaluate an intervention, (2) did not present quantitative data on a relevant outcome, (3) had a sample size less than 10, or (4) were not in English. Review articles were excluded from our review but were systematically flagged to check for any missed articles that should be included in our review; the references included in the flagged papers were reviewed and yielded no additional included studies.

Selection Process

After the initial search, all identified references were uploaded into Covidence, a software system for managing systematic reviews.[20] The software removed any duplicate references.

During title and abstract screening, each reference was reviewed independently by 2 authors. Studies were excluded if they did not clearly meet inclusion criteria based on the title and/or abstract. Any disagreements between the 2 independent reviewers were discussed among the larger team and resolved by consensus. During the next stage of review, the full text of each reference was carefully reviewed independently by all 4 reviewers. Each reference was discussed by the full team and a final decision on inclusion was made by consensus. This review's selection process is presented using the Preferred Reporting of Items for Systematic Reviews and Meta-Analyses (PRISMA) flowchart[21] in **Fig. 1**.

Data Extraction

Each citation meeting the inclusion criteria underwent data extraction by all 4 reviewers, with 1 reviewer assigned as the primary reviewer. Extracted items included information about the study sample and setting, intervention characteristics, research design characteristics, and outcomes. Extracted data were reviewed as a team and finalized by consensus.

RESULTS

A total of 1562 citations were identified from the database search (see **Fig. 1**). Following the removal of duplicates (n = 298), 1264 studies were screened in the title and abstract phase and 13 studies were screened in full text. Three studies[22–24] met the inclusion criteria for this review and their characteristics are detailed in **Table 1**.

Overview of Included Interventions

The studies represented geographic areas across the United States, including north central Florida,[24] southern California,[23] and the Mid-Atlantic region.[22] All studies included HCPs or trainees and ranged in sample sizes from 62 to 768 participants. Two studies focused on trainees including first-year and second-year health professional students[24] and third-year undergraduate nursing students.[22] The third study included a wide range of practicing HCPs in an academic medical institution.[23]

Both studies involving students used online stigma-reduction interventions that featured a virtual patient simulation and used a pretest and posttest design to measure stigma-related outcomes.[22,24] Raponi and colleagues[24] evaluated a 3-module, longitudinal case-based curriculum featuring a hypothetical patient, where teams of interprofessional health students worked together on assessments and learning activities, focusing on interdisciplinary teamwork skills. Altmiller and colleagues evaluated a student-focused intervention for third-year undergraduate nursing students that

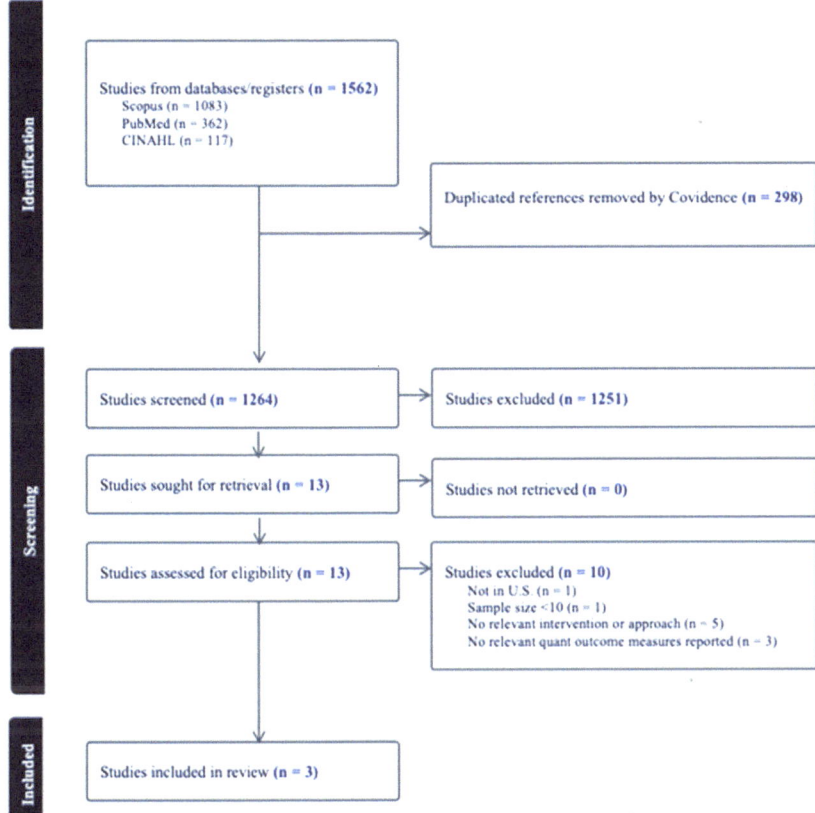

Fig. 1. Study selection process reported by PRISMA.

included a virtual patient diagnosed with HIV in the clinic setting.[22] All students completed a pretest followed by a lecture focusing on HIV/AIDS care. Students in the intervention arm worked on the virtual patient simulation section that week and completed a posttest after the assignment, whereas students in the control arm completed a posttest immediately after the lecture and later completed the virtual patient simulation assignment. Davtyan and colleagues evaluated a one-time, multipart intervention for practicing HCPs.[23] HCPs enrolled in the treatment arm participated in a lecture about HIV stigma in health-care settings, a Photovoice component presented by Stigma Trainers (women of color living with HIV), and an interactive workshop including various hypothetical scenarios. During the Photovoice component of the intervention, the Stigma Trainers shared stories and images they took to capture their personal experiences of living with HIV. Participants in the control arm only received an electronic version of the first lecture component.

Stigma/Discrimination Outcomes Measured

No single standardized measurement of stigma or discrimination was used throughout the 3 studies. Raponi and colleagues measured a stigma-related outcome through students' self-reported comfort caring for patients with HIV using a 5-point Likert scale.[24] Additionally, students were asked to provide an adjective to describe their attitudes that were formulated into pre-and-post-test word clouds. Altmiller and

Table 1
Characteristics of included studies

First Author and Year	Geography and Setting	Population	Intervention Description	Length of Assessment	Study Design	Sample Size	Results
Raponi et al,[24] 2022	University in north central Florida	First-year and second-year health professional students in audiology, dentistry, medicine, nursing, pharmacy, physical therapy, occupational therapy, public health, and speech language	Online, three-module, longitudinal case-based curriculum to facilitate interprofessional learning for students in interdisciplinary teams related to issues associated with HIV/AIDS in the United States	Approximately 6 weeks; student teams have 2 weeks to complete each module	Pre-post; no comparison group	N = 768	Students' level of comfort in providing care for a patient with HIV/AIDS were significantly higher after the third session compared with before the first session ($P \leq .001$). Significant difference was found in sentiment associated with students' adjectives about taking care of a patient with HIV at start of curriculum compared with conclusion of curriculum ($P < .01$).

| Davtyan et al,[23] 2020 | Academic medical institution in southern California | Health-care workers (Physicians [MD only], Nurses [LVN, NP, RN]), allied health-care workers (health-care providers [HCPs] who provide diagnostic and therapeutic patient care) | One time, 2-h training of HIV/AIDS stigma including Photovoice (3 parts: Overview of HIV stigma in Health-Care Settings (lead researcher led), Women of Color Reflect on HIV Stigma Through Photovoice (WOCLWH Stigma Trainers led), Let's Address Stigma Together (interactive workshop with Stigma Trainers) | Baseline (T1), within approximately 1 week after intervention/control (T2), and 3 months after intervention/control (T3) | RCT with individual-level randomization | N = 73 (n = 38 intervention, n = 35 control) | After controlling for educational level, knowledge of HIV/AIDS increased more for intervention vs control arm at T2 vs T1 ($\beta = 0.56$, $P < .01$). After controlling for educational level, attitudes toward people living with HIV improved more for intervention vs control arm at T2 vs T1 ($\beta = 0.58$, $P < .01$). No results that were significant between the control and intervention groups remained significant at the 3-month follow-up. |

(continued on next page)

Table 1
(continued)

First Author and Year	Geography and Setting	Population	Intervention Description	Length of Assessment	Study Design	Sample Size	Results
Altmiller et al,[22] 2022	University in mid-Atlantic region	Third-year undergraduate nursing students	A virtual patient simulation in which learners encountered a 52-year-old Vietnamese-American man being diagnosed with HIV in the clinic setting	Up to 2 weeks from pre-test	Non-randomized with comparison group: pre-post data	N = 62 (n = 30 intervention, n = 32 control)	No statistically significant effect on HPASS total posttest scores. Clinical significance present (HPASS scores decreased in both groups, and intervention group having greater decrease) across all 3 subscales.

Abbreviations: LVN, licensed vocational nurse; NP, nurse practitioner; RN, registered nurse; HPASS, health care provider HIV/AIDS stigma scale.

colleagues measured stigma using a validated instrument, the Health Care Provider HIV/AIDs Stigma Scale, in a pre-and-post-test fashion.[22] Davtyan and colleagues assessed knowledge of HIV/AIDS, attitudes toward people living with HIV, and observations of enacted stigma using 10-item scales with 4-point Likert scales. These measures were collected on 3 timepoints across 3 months.[23]

Intervention Results

Raponi and colleagues found that the 3-module curriculum resulted in a statistically significant increase in student comfort with providing care for patients with HIV, as well as improved sentiment toward this care, at the conclusion of their intervention.[24] Davtyan and colleagues also found significant results with their Photovoice intervention for practicing HCPs but found that the increases in knowledge and attitudes did not maintain significance 3 months after the intervention.[23] Altmiller and colleagues did not find any statistically significant effect on Health Care Provider HIV/AIDs Stigma Scale scores after their intervention for nursing students; however, they did find that these scores still decreased in both intervention and control, with the intervention group having a greater drop, indicating a potentially clinically significant reduction.[22]

DISCUSSION

Despite the commitment to reducing HIV stigma and discrimination within the National HIV/AIDS Strategy,[3] this scoping review of recent interventions to reduce stigma against people with HIV in US health-care settings found only 3 interventions that were evaluated within the past 5 years. This paucity of interventions may reflect complacency related to HIV and HIV stigma within the US health-care system and nation as a whole. Recent data, however, suggest that the United States is not on track to reaching the Ending the Epidemic 2030 targets, and one of the major barriers to progress continues to be health-care–related stigma and discrimination.[4] Interventions that effectively reduce HIV stigma and discrimination within the health-care system are urgently needed to improve health outcomes among people with HIV and to end the HIV epidemic in this country.

Our finding that there have been few recent HIV stigma reduction interventions in US health-care settings is consistent with other reviews on related topics. For example, Ferguson and colleagues found 19 global randomized and non-RCTs examining health-care stigma-reduction interventions, yet only one was conducted in the United States (in 2013).[19] Kutner and colleagues reviewed interventions to reduce stigma related to a broader range of factors in US health systems and found few studies that addressed HIV stigma or intersectional stigma; the most common stigma-related targets of interventions were related to alcohol or drug use or mental health.[25] Across these reviews, there has been a persistent gap in the evidence regarding the effectiveness of HIV-specific stigma reduction interventions in US health-care settings. Although lessons learned from interventions implemented in other countries may be valuable for application in the United States, it is important to note the unique history, context, and epidemiology of HIV under the complexities of the US health-care system.

This review highlights several additional advances in the interventions studied, including the intentional inclusion of interprofessional health-care providers, to mitigate stigma. These interventions are consistent with HIV being recognized as a chronic and manageable illness, with providers of all specialties needing training and stigma reduction approaches to care for people with HIV.[26] Additionally, 2 of the included studies evaluated interventions conducted with students.[22,24] These studies highlight the value of reducing stigma during formative training experiences, emphasizing the need for clinical training to go beyond the standardized teachings of pathophysiology and transmission of HIV.

Although incorporating stigma reduction into prelicensure education is crucial, educational interventions must be complemented by additional support and ongoing training for practicing clinicians and staff. This not only encourages continued reflection on potential bias but also allows for continued education on advances in HIV prevention and treatment that could influence attitudes and behaviors, such as U=U. Our review highlights the importance of integrating such ongoing trainings into expectations of employment; several studies reflected on the challenges of recruiting health-care workers into optional trainings. The Photovoice-informed HIV stigma training, for example, reported many challenges despite its use of various recruitment approaches.[23] It is also notable that one of these studies omitted from our review was excluded because they were only able to recruit 5 health-care workers, failing to meet their target of enrolling 15 health-care workers[27]; this study adapted and tested a bystander intervention to reduce HIV stigma among people living with HIV, friends and family members, and health-care workers. Thus, our results highlight the importance of the development of novel interventions for licensed health-care workers through required continuing education programs and trainings.

The findings of this review also speak to the novel approaches (eg, virtual patient simulations, Photovoice) that are being used in stigma-reduction interventions as well as the importance of using a participatory approach to intervention design. The Photovoice-informed HIV stigma training, for example, specifically included women of color living with HIV in leadership positions, working collaboratively with the academic researchers to design the training, develop content, and facilitate training delivery.[23] Photovoice, a photographic research technique, supports the participatory approach by prompting dialog and exploration of community and personal experiences.[28] This method has been particularly beneficial in women's health research[28] and served as an innovative approach in Davtyan and colleagues' study to support women of color living with HIV in sharing their experiences to train HCPs.[23]

Similar to other reviews on this topic, our review highlights the challenges of measuring HIV stigma when evaluating interventions conducted within health-care settings. These challenges develop due to the multifaceted and multilevel nature of stigma. The studies included in this review all used different stigma measures, and this heterogeneity in outcome measures explains the absence of meta-analyses on interventions to reduce HIV stigma and discrimination.[29] In our review, Altmiller and colleagues[22] measured stigma with the validated Health Care Provider HIV/AIDs Stigma Scale, although using this validated scale had significant limitations, including the irrelevance of several items to the virtual patient included in their intervention (eg, items focused on physical contact with patients or HIV related to injection drug use). Raponi and colleagues,[24] however, measured stigma using 2 nontraditional approaches. The first was a 1-item question about comfort providing care for a patient with HIV, with responses ranging on a 5-point Likert-type scale. This 1-item question was complemented by having students provide an adjective to describe their feelings about caring for people with HIV before the first session and after the third intervention module. These adjectives were analyzed using sentiment analysis and statistical analysis evaluated the extent to which sentiment changed because of the modules. Although all included studies captured the construct of stigma, this variation in measurement influences the ability to synthesize effects across studies, which is crucial for informing future intervention development and clinical care guidelines. Additionally, measures capturing provider attitudes or comfort may not fully capture the impact on care for people with HIV, including patient experiences of discrimination or quality of care. Thus, in order to move toward a destigmatized and nondiscriminatory approach to HIV care, we must consider the best ways to standardize the operationalization and measures of stigma and discrimination, while accounting for how these measures may need to adapt over time to adjust for changing sociopolitical context or scientific advances in treatment and care.

By highlighting approaches specifically designed to reduce stigma and discrimination against people with HIV in health-care settings, our review is intended to inform much-needed multilevel intersectional stigma reduction interventions. Because stigma operates on multiple levels of influence, intervening within those levels simultaneously is likely to enhance the impact of our efforts.[30] Given the unique impact of stigma and discrimination with the health-care setting, the synergistic potential of multilevel interventions will not be reached if they do not include effective approaches that intentionally focused on improving the health-care setting. Future research must also recognize that HIV stigma does not exist as a singular challenge but as the result of multiple oppressive structures in the United States, such as structural racism, sexism, and heterosexism, intersecting to exacerbate the HIV inequities experienced by minoritized groups.[31] HIV stigma, as well as stigma associated with minoritized identities, interlocks to create intersectional stigma that furthers underlying inequities[31] through the discrimination that prevents people living with HIV from seeking and receiving treatment. Multilevel interventions that engage health-care providers and health-care settings to reduce intersectional stigma are sorely needed. Specifically targeting and measuring HIV stigma in such studies will provide crucial insights as to the potential synergistic effects of these approaches.

SUMMARY

Our review adds a significant contribution to the extant literature through its synthesis of contemporary HIV stigma reduction interventions across US health-care settings. Our findings highlight the need for contemporary stigma-reduction interventions that address the persistence of stigma despite improved medical advancements, including treatment as prevention and PrEP. This review highlights critical gaps in HIV stigma measurement and interventions, laying a foundation for future research and clinical implications. By developing novel stigma-reduction interventions within health-care settings, the US health-care system can become less stigmatized toward patients with HIV and become more affirming and inclusive in its care approaches.

CLINICS CARE POINTS

- HIV stigma is a significant barrier to improved health outcomes for patients living with HIV in the United States, and stigma reduction interventions prove to be a promising path to creating a more affirmative health-care setting for patients.

- HIV stigma interventions and education are crucial during prelicensure education to create a learning environment focused on stigma reduction that translates into the workplace.

- Additional research and interventions are needed to reduce stigma in health-care workers specifically, calling for increased research participation from HCPs as well as interventions that are focused in the practicing health-care setting.

ACKNOWLEDGMENTS

The authors wish to thank Leila Ledbetter and Erin Simon at the Duke University Medical Center Library for their assistance developing and conducting the search.

DISCLOSURE

The authors declare that they do not have any financial conflicts of interest to report.

REFERENCES

1. U.S. Department of Health & Human Services. HIV & AIDS trends and U.S. statistics overview. HIV.gov. Published 2022 https://www.hiv.gov/hiv-basics/overview/data-and-trends/statistics. Accessed September 3, 2023.
2. Centers for Disease Control and Prevention. Monitoring selected national HIV prevention and care objectives by using HIV surveillance data United States and 6 dependent areas, 2019. Published May 25, 2021 https://www.cdc.gov/hiv/library/reports/hiv-surveillance/vol-26-no-2/index.html. Accessed September 3, 2023.
3. National HIV/AIDS Strategy for the United States 2022-2025. The White House; 2021 https://www.hiv.gov/federal-response/national-hiv-aids-strategy/national-hiv-aids-strategy-2022-2025. Accessed September 15, 2023.
4. Guilamo-Ramos V, Thimm-Kaiser M, Benzekri A. Is the USA on track to end the HIV epidemic? Lancet HIV 2023;10(8):e552–6. https://doi.org/10.1016/S2352-3018(23)00142-X.
5. Hatzenbuehler ML, Phelan JC, Link BG. Stigma as a fundamental cause of population health inequalities. Am J Publ Health 2013;103(5):813–21. https://doi.org/10.2105/AJPH.2012.301069.
6. Herek GM. AIDS and stigma. Am Behav Sci 1999;42:1106–16. https://doi.org/10.1177/00027649921954787.
7. Earnshaw VA, Chaudoir SR. From conceptualizing to measuring HIV stigma: A review of HIV stigma mechanism measures. AIDS Behav 2009;13(6):1160–77. https://doi.org/10.1007/s10461-009-9593-3.
8. Forney DJ, Sheehan DM, Dale SK, et al. The impact of HIV-related stigma on racial/ethnic disparities in retention in HIV care among adults living with HIV in Florida. J Racial Ethn Health Disparities 2023. https://doi.org/10.1007/s40615-023-01715-1.
9. Reif S, Wilson E, McAllaster C, et al. The relationship of HIV-related stigma and health care outcomes in the US Deep South. AIDS Behav 2019;23(3):242–50. https://doi.org/10.1007/s10461-019-02595-5.
10. 2022 state of HIV stigma. Published online 2022 https://s3.us-west-2.amazonaws.com/media.glaad.org/wp-content/uploads/2022/12/20055526/2022-State-of-HIV-Stigma-Report-Final-lores-9bd.pdf. Accessed September 30, 2023.
11. Internalized HIV-related stigma. 2018.
12. Bekker LG, Beyrer C, Mgodi N, et al. HIV infection. Nat Rev Dis Prim 2023;9(1):1–21. https://doi.org/10.1038/s41572-023-00452-3.
13. Ford OG, Rufurwadzo TG, Richman B, et al. Adopting U = U to end stigma and discrimination. J Int AIDS Soc 2022;25(3):e25891. https://doi.org/10.1002/jia2.25891.
14. Cohen MS, Chen YQ, McCauley M, et al. Antiretroviral therapy for the prevention of HIV-1 transmission. N Engl J Med 2016;375(9):830–9. https://doi.org/10.1056/NEJMoa1600693.

15. Nyblade L, Stockton MA, Giger K, et al. Stigma in health facilities: why it matters and how we can change it. BMC Med 2019;17(1):25. https://doi.org/10.1186/s12916-019-1256-2.

16. Centers for Disease Control and Prevention. Facts about HIV stigma 2022 https://www.cdc.gov/hiv/basics/hiv-stigma/index.html. Accessed September 3, 2023.

17. McCree DH, Beer L, Crim SM, et al. Intersectional discrimination in HIV health-care settings among persons with diagnosed HIV in the United States, Medical Monitoring Project, 2018-2019. AIDS Behav 2023. https://doi.org/10.1007/s10461-023-04076-2.

18. Ingram L, Stafford C, Deming ME, et al. A systematic mixed studies review of the intersections of social-ecological factors and HIV stigma in people living with HIV in the U.S. South. J Assoc Nurses AIDS Care JANAC 2019;30(3):330–43. https://doi.org/10.1097/JNC.0000000000000076.

19. Ferguson L, Gruskin S, Bolshakova M, et al. Systematic review and quantitative and qualitative comparative analysis of interventions to address HIV-related stigma and discrimination. AIDS Lond Engl 2023. https://doi.org/10.1097/QAD.0000000000003628.

20. Covidence systematic review software. 2022 https://www.covidence.org/. Accessed June 10, 2023.

21. Page MJ, McKenzie JE, Bossuyt PM, et al. The PRISMA 2020 statement: an updated guideline for reporting systematic reviews. BMJ 2021;372:n71. https://doi.org/10.1136/bmj.n71.

22. Altmiller G, Jimenez F, Wharton J, et al. HIV and contact tracing: Impact of a virtual patient simulation activity. Clin Simul Nurs 2022;64:58–66. https://doi.org/10.1016/j.ecns.2021.12.005.

23. Davtyan M, Bartell SM, Lakon CM. Assessing the efficacy of a PhotoVoice-informed HIV stigma training for health care workers. AIDS Behav 2020;24(1):65–80. https://doi.org/10.1007/s10461-019-02710-6.

24. Raponi JM, Blue AV, Janelle J, et al. A longitudinal interprofessional case based learning experience: The HIV/AIDS care continuum in the rural South. J Interprofessional Educ Pract 2022;29:100537. https://doi.org/10.1016/j.xjep.2022.100537.

25. Kutner BA, Vaughn MP, Giguere R, et al. A systematic review of intervention studies that address HIV-related stigmas among US healthcare workers and health systems: Applying a theory-based ontology to link intervention types, techniques, and mechanisms of action to potential effectiveness. Ann Behav Med 2023. https://doi.org/10.1093/abm/kaad022. kaad022.

26. Thompson MA, Horberg MA, Agwu AL, et al. Primary care guidance for persons with Human Immunodeficiency Virus: 2020 update by the HIV medicine association of the infectious diseases society of America. Clin Infect Dis Off Publ Infect Dis Soc Am 2021;73(11):e3572–605. https://doi.org/10.1093/cid/ciaa1391.

27. Bagchi AD, Thompson A, Damas K, et al. Step UP! To Stamp Out Stigma: Adapting and testing a bystander intervention to reduce HIV-related stigma. J Public Health 2022;30(1):185–93. https://doi.org/10.1007/s10389-020-01284-1.

28. Wang CC. Photovoice: a participatory action research strategy applied to women's health. J Womens Health 1999;8(2):185–92. https://doi.org/10.1089/jwh.1999.8.185.

29. Feyissa GT, Lockwood C, Woldie M, et al. Reducing HIV-related stigma and discrimination in healthcare settings: A systematic review of quantitative evidence. PLoS One 2019;14(1):e0211298. https://doi.org/10.1371/journal.pone.0211298.

30. Rao D, Elshafei A, Nguyen M, et al. A systematic review of multi-level stigma interventions: state of the science and future directions. BMC Med 2019;17(1):41. https://doi.org/10.1186/s12916-018-1244-y.
31. Bowleg L. The problem with intersectional stigma and HIV equity research. Am J Publ Health 2022;112(S4):S344–6. https://doi.org/10.2105/AJPH.2022.306729.

APPENDIX 1: SEARCH STRATEGIES

Librarian Searcher: Erin Simon, Duke University Medical Center Library.
Peer-Review: Leila Ledbetter, MLIS, AHIP, Duke University Medical Center Library.
Date: July 3, 2023.
Database: MEDLINE (PubMed), Inclusive Date Coverage: 2018-2023.

Set #	Search Strategy	Results
1 HIV	"HIV"[Mesh] OR "HIV Infections"[Mesh] OR "Acquired Immunodeficiency Syndrome"[Mesh] OR "HIV Seropositivity"[Mesh] OR "AIDS Serodiagnosis"[Mesh] OR "Anti-Retroviral Agents"[Mesh] OR "Acquired Immunodeficiency Syndrome"[tiab] OR aids[tiab] OR hiv[tiab] OR "human immunodeficiency virus"[tiab] OR antiretroviral [tiab] OR "Anti-Retroviral"[tiab] OR seropositive[tiab] or '"sero status"[tiab] OR seropositivity[tiab] OR Serodiagnosis[tiab] OR Serodiagnoses[tiab]	541,204
2 Stigma	"social stigma"[mesh] OR "Social Alienation"[Mesh] OR "Social Isolation"[Mesh] OR "shame"[mesh] OR "prejudice"[mesh] OR "social discrimination"[mesh] OR stigma[tiab] OR stigmas[tiab] OR stigmatize[tiab] OR stigmatise[tiab] OR stigmatized[tiab] OR stigmatized[tiab] OR shame[tiab] OR shameful[tiab] OR shaming[tiab] OR shames[tiab] OR shamed[tiab] OR blame[tiab] OR blames[tiab] OR blamed[tiab] OR blaming[tiab] OR prejudice[tiab] OR prejudiced[tiab] OR prejudicing[tiab] OR prejudices[tiab] OR discriminate[tiab] OR discriminates[tiab] OR discriminated[tiab] OR discrimination[tiab] OR discriminating [tiab] OR mistreat[tiab] OR mistreats[tiab] OR mistreated[tiab] OR mistreatment[tiab] OR mistreating[tiab] OR alienate[tiab] OR alienates[tiab] OR alienated[tiab] OR alienation[tiab] OR alienating[tiab]	367,348
3 Healthcare staff	"health personnel"[mesh] OR "allied health personnel"[mesh] OR "attitude of health personnel"[mesh] OR "health personnel"[tiab] OR (((health[tiab] AND care[tiab]) OR healthcare[tiab]) AND (provider*[tiab] OR worker*[tiab] OR professional*[tiab])) OR caregivers[tiab] OR "allied health personnel"[tiab] OR anatomists[tiab] OR anesthesiologist*[tiab] OR "nurse anesthetist*"[tiab] OR audiologist*[tiab] OR coroner*[tiab] OR "medical examiner*"[tiab] OR dentist*[tiab] OR "dental staff"[tiab] OR doula*[tiab] OR "emergency medical dispatcher*"[tiab] OR epidemiologist*[tiab] OR ((dental[tiab] OR medical[tiab] OR nursing[tiab]) AND faculty[tiab]) OR "health educator*"[tiab] OR (("health facility" OR hospital [tiab]) AND (personnel[tiab] OR administrator*[tiab])) OR "infection control practitioner*"[tiab] OR ((medical[tiab]) AND (chaperone*[tiab] OR "laboratory personnel"[tiab] OR staff [tiab])) OR nurse*[tiab] OR nursing[tiab] OR nutritionist*[tiab] OR ((occupational[tiab] OR physical[tiab]) AND therapist*[tiab]) OR physician*[tiab] OR doctor* OR psychotherapist*[tiab]	1,928,165

(continued on next page)

Set #	Search Strategy	Results
(continued)		
4	#1 AND #2 AND #3	4596
5 US	Europe[mesh] OR Africa[mesh] OR asia[mesh] OR "south America"[mesh] OR "central America"[mesh] OR "latin America"[mesh] OR Canada[mesh] OR mexico[mesh] OR Greenland[mesh]	3,199,526
6	#4 NOT #5	2560
7 Study design	"Single-Blind Method"[Mesh] OR "Double-Blind Method"[Mesh] OR "Cohort Studies"[Mesh] OR "Follow-Up Studies"[Mesh] OR "Longitudinal Studies"[Mesh] OR "Prospective Studies"[Mesh] OR "Retrospective Studies"[Mesh] OR "Case-Control Studies"[Mesh] OR "Cross-Sectional Studies"[Mesh] OR "Controlled Before-After Studies"[Mesh] OR "Interrupted Time Series Analysis"[Mesh] OR "Cross-Over Studies"[Mesh] OR "Randomized Controlled Trials as Topic"[Mesh] OR "Meta-analysis as topic"[Mesh] OR "Evaluation studies as topic"[Mesh] OR "Randomized Controlled Trial"[pt] OR "Controlled Clinical Trial"[pt] OR "Clinical Trial"[pt] OR "Observational Study"[pt] OR "Evaluation Study"[pt] OR "Comparative Study"[pt] OR "Meta-Analysis"[pt] OR "Systematic Review"[pt] OR systematic [subset] OR randomized[tiab] OR randomised[tiab] OR randomization[tiab] OR randomisation[tiab] OR placebo[tiab] OR randomly[tiab] OR trial[tiab] OR trials[tiab] OR groups[tiab] OR "single blind"[tiab] OR "single blinded"[tiab] OR "double blind"[tiab] OR "double blinded"[tiab] OR "evaluation study"[tiab] OR "evaluation studies"[tiab] OR "intervention study"[tiab] OR "intervention studies"[tiab] OR cohort[tiab] OR cohorts[tiab] OR longitudinal[tiab] OR longitudinally[tiab] OR prospective[tiab] OR prospectively[tiab] OR retrospective[tiab] OR retrospectively[tiab] OR follow-up[tiab] OR "follow up"[tiab] OR followup[tiab] OR case-control[tiab] OR "case control"[tiab] OR "case controlled"[tiab] OR case-controlled [tiab] OR cross-sectional[tiab] OR "cross sectional"[tiab] OR crossover[tiab] OR "cross over"[tiab] OR "comparative study"[tiab] OR "comparative studies"[tiab] OR meta-analysis [tiab] OR meta-analyses[tiab] OR "meta analysis"[tiab] OR "meta analyses"[tiab] OR metaanalysis[tiab] OR metaanalyses [tiab] OR meta-analytic[tiab] OR "meta analytical"[tiab] OR metaanalytic[tiab]	9,895,397
8	#6 AND #7	859
9	#8 AND ("2018/06/01"[Date - MeSH]: "3000"[Date - MeSH])	362

Database: CINAHL Plus with full text (EBSCOhost), Inclusive Date Coverage: 2018-2023.

Set #	Search Strategy	Results
1 HIV	(MH "Human Immunodeficiency Virus+") OR (MH "HIV Infections+") OR (MH "Acquired Immunodeficiency Syndrome") OR (MH "HIV Seropositivity") OR (MH "AIDS Serodiagnosis") OR (MH "Anti-Retroviral Agents+") OR TI(hiv OR "human immunodeficiency virus" OR hiv OR aids OR "acquired immunodeficiency syndrome" OR "hiv	156,925

(continued on next page)

	(continued)	
Set #	**Search Strategy**	**Results**
	seropositivity" OR "anti-retroviral agent*" OR "antiretroviral agent*" OR "anti retroviral agent*" OR seropositive OR seropositivity IR serodiagnosis OR serodiagnoses) OR AB(hiv OR "human immunodeficiency virus" OR hiv OR aids OR "acquired immunodeficiency syndrome" OR "hiv seropositivity" OR "anti-retroviral agent*" OR "antiretroviral agent*" OR "anti retroviral agent*" OR seropositive OR seropositivity IR serodiagnosis OR serodiagnoses)	
2 Stigma	(MH "Stigma") OR (MH "Prejudice+") OR (MH "Social Alienation") OR (MH "Social Isolation+") OR (MH "Shame+") OR (MH "Discrimination+") OR (MH "Perceived Discrimination") OR TI(stigma OR stigmas OR stigmatize OR stigmatise OR stigmatized OR prejudice* OR alienation OR isolation OR discriminat* OR shame OR shameful OR shaming OR shames OR shamed OR blame OR blames OR blamed OR blaming OR prejudice OR prejudiced OR prejudicing OR prejudices OR mistreat OR mistreats OR mistreated OR mistreatment OR alienate OR alienates OR alienated OR alienation OR alienating) OR AB(stigma OR stigmas OR stigmatize OR stigmatise OR stigmatized OR prejudice* OR alienation OR isolation OR discriminat* OR shame OR shameful OR shaming OR shames OR shamed OR blame OR blames OR blamed OR blaming OR prejudice OR prejudiced OR prejudicing OR prejudices OR mistreat OR mistreats OR mistreated OR mistreatment OR alienate OR alienates OR alienated OR alienation OR alienating)	168,434
3 Healthcare staff	(MH "Health Personnel+") OR (MH "Health Personnel, Unlicensed") OR (MH "Personnel, Health Facility+") OR (MH "Rural Health Personnel") OR (MH "Health Personnel, Infected") OR (MH "Alternative Health Personnel+") OR (MH "Health Personnel, Minority+") OR (MH "Health Information Management Personnel+") OR (MH "Occupational Health Services+") OR (MH "Mental Health Personnel+") OR (MH "Allied Health Personnel+") OR (MH "Multiskilled Health Practitioners") OR (MH "Health Professionals with Disabilities+") OR (MH "Military Health") OR (MH "Attitude of Health Personnel+") OR (MH "Employee Attitudes") OR TI(provider* OR caregiver* OR anatomist* OR anesthesiologist* OR audiologist* OR coroner* OR "medical examiner*" OR dentist* OR "dental staff" OR doula* OR "emergency medical dispatcher*" OR epidemiologist* OR nurse* OR nursing OR "health educator*" OR "infection control practitioner*" OR nutritionist* OR therapist* OR physician* OR psychotherapist*) OR AB(provider* OR caregiver* OR anatomist* OR anesthesiologist* OR audiologist* OR coroner* OR "medical examiner*" OR dentist* OR "dental staff" OR doula* OR "emergency medical dispatcher*" OR epidemiologist* OR nurse* OR nursing OR "health educator*" OR "infection control practitioner*" OR	1,436,257

(continued on next page)

(continued)		
Set #	**Search Strategy**	**Results**
	nutritionist* OR therapist* OR physician* OR doctor* OR psychotherapist*)	
4	S1 AND S2 AND S3	2929
5 US	(MH "Europe+") OR (MH "Africa+") OR (MH "Asia+") OR (MH "South America+") OR (MH "Central America+") OR (MH "Mexico") OR (MH "Greenland") OR (MH "Canada+")	1,264,011
6	S4 NOT S5	1577
7 Study design	(ZT "randomized controlled trial") OR (MH "Randomized Controlled Trials") OR TI ("randomized controlled trial" OR "controlled clinical trial" OR randomized OR randomised OR randomization OR randomisation OR placebo OR randomly OR trial OR trials OR groups OR "single blind" OR "single blinded" OR "double blind" OR "double-blinded) OR AB ("randomized controlled trial" OR "controlled clinical trial" OR randomized OR randomised OR randomization OR randomisation OR placebo OR randomly OR trial OR trials OR groups OR "single blind" OR "single blinded" OR "double blind" OR "double-blinded) OR (MH "Retrospective Design") OR (MH "Empirical Research") OR (MH "Nonexperimental Studies+") OR TI ("evaluation study" OR "evaluation studies" OR "intervention study" OR "intervention studies" OR "case-control" OR cohort OR cohorts OR longitudinal OR longitudinally OR prospective OR prospectively OR retrospective OR retrospectively OR "comparative study" OR crossover OR "cross over") OR AB ("evaluation study" OR "evaluation studies" OR "intervention study" OR "intervention studies" OR "case-control" OR cohort OR cohorts OR longitudinal OR longitudinally OR prospective OR prospectively OR retrospective OR retrospectively OR "comparative study" OR crossover OR "cross over") OR MH "Systematic Review" OR MH "Meta Analysis" OR TI ("systematic review" OR "systematic reviews" OR "meta-analysis" OR "meta-analyses") OR AB ("systematic review" OR "systematic reviews" OR "meta-analysis" OR "meta-analyses")	1,833,440
8	S6 AND S7	289
9	Limiters - Published Date: 20180101-	117

Database: Scopus (Elsevier), Inclusive Date Coverage: 2018-2023.

Set #	**Search Strategy**	**Results**
1 HIV	TITLE-ABS ({HIV Infections} OR {Acquired Immunodeficiency Syndrome} OR {HIV Seropositivity} OR {AIDS Serodiagnosis} OR {Anti-Retroviral Agents} OR {Acquired Immunodeficiency Syndrome} OR aids OR hiv OR {human immunodeficiency virus} OR antiretroviral OR anti-retroviral OR seropositive OR {sero status} OR seropositivity OR serodiagnosis OR serodiagnoses)	629,050
2 Stigma	TITLE-ABS ({social stigma} OR {Social Alienation} OR {Social Isolation} OR shame OR prejudice OR {social discrimination}	679,232

(continued on next page)

Set #	Search Strategy	Results
(continued)		
	OR stigma OR stigmas OR stigmatize OR stigmatise OR stigmatized OR stigmatized OR shame OR shameful OR shaming OR shames OR shamed OR blame OR blames OR blamed OR blaming OR prejudice OR prejudiced OR prejudicing OR prejudices OR discriminate OR discriminates OR discriminated OR discrimination OR discriminating OR mistreat OR mistreats OR mistreated OR mistreatment OR mistreating OR alienate OR alienates OR alienated OR alienation OR alienating)	
3 Healthcare staff	TITLE-ABS ({health personnel} OR {attitude of health personnel} OR {health personnel} OR (((health AND care) OR healthcare) AND (provider* OR worker* OR professional*)) OR caregivers OR {allied health personnel} OR anatomists OR anesthesiologist* OR {nurse anesthetist*} OR audiologist* OR coroner* OR {medical examiner*} OR dentist* OR {dental staff} OR doula* OR {emergency medical dispatcher*} OR epidemiologist* OR ((dental OR medical OR nursing) AND faculty) OR {health educator*} OR (({health facility} OR hospital) AND (personnel OR administrator*)) OR {infection control practitioner*} OR ((medical) AND (chaperone* OR {laboratory personnel} OR staff)) OR nurse* OR nursing OR nutritionist* OR ((occupational OR physical) AND therapist*) OR physician* OR doctor* OR psychotherapist*)	2,019,781
4	#1 AND #2 AND #3	3771
5 US	TITLE-ABS (europe OR africa OR asia OR {south America} OR {central America} OR canada OR mexico OR greenland)	1,685,146
6	#4 AND NOT #5	3100
7 Study design	TITLE-ABS (randomized OR randomised OR randomization OR randomisation OR placebo OR randomly OR trial OR trials OR study OR studies OR groups OR group OR {case-control} OR cohort OR cohorts OR longitudinal OR longitudinally OR prospective OR prospectively OR retrospective OR retrospectively OR observational OR {follow up} OR {meta-analysis} OR program OR intervention OR evaluation OR comparative OR {systematic review} OR {meta-synthesis} OR nonrandom OR {non-random} OR nonrandomized OR {non-randomized} OR nonrandomised OR {non-randomised} OR quasi-experiment OR quasiexperiment OR quasirandom OR quasi-random OR quasi-control OR quasicontrol OR {quazi-experiment} OR quaziexperiment OR quazirandom OR {quazi-random} OR {quazi-control} OR quazicontrol OR {pre-post} OR {posttest} OR {post-test} OR pretest OR pre-test OR {time series} OR {time points} OR {before and after} OR {before and during} OR interview OR questionnaire OR {focus group} OR qualitative OR ethnography OR fieldwork OR {field work} OR {key informant} OR {methodological study} OR {methodology study} OR {method study} OR {methods study})	35,588,494
8	#6 AND #7	2626
9	#8 AND PUBYEAR > 2017 AND PUBYEAR < 2024	1083

The Intersection of Mental Health and Sexual and Gender Minority Identities for Older Adults Living with Human Immunodeficiency Virus

A Narrative Review

David Agor, DNP, PMHNP-BC, HIVPCP[a,b,*], Brandon A. Knettel, PhD[c,d,e], Kenneth Daici[f], Steven Meanley, MPH, PhD[b,g]

KEYWORDS

- Sexual and gender minorities (SGM, OR LGBTQIA+) • Older adults • HIV
- Depression • Psilocybin • Syndemics

KEY POINTS

- More than 50% of people living with HIV are aged 50 years and older.
- Sexual/gender minority (SGM) older adults bear a higher burden of HIV incidence and prevalence compared with their heterosexual counterparts.
- SGM older adults living with HIV (OALWH) are disproportionately affected by mental illness, especially depression.
- There are limited evidenced based, culturally congruent mental health interventions for SGM OALWH.
- Culturally congruent intervention models hold promise for improving health outcomes and quality of life for this priority population.

[a] Department of Family and Community Health, University of Pennsylvania, School of Nursing, 418 Curie Boulevard, 218L E, Philadelphia, PA 19104, USA; [b] University of Pennsylvania Eidos Center, Philadelphia, PA, USA; [c] Duke School of Nursing, 307 Trent Drive, Durham, NC 27710, USA; [d] Duke Global Health Institute, Duke University, Durham, NC, USA; [e] Duke Global Mental Health Program, Duke University, Durham, NC, USA; [f] Brown University, 69 Brown Street, Box 9734, Providence, RI 02912, USA; [g] University of Pennsylvania School of Nursing, 418 Curie Boulevard, 231L, Philadelphia, PA 19104, USA
* Corresponding author.
E-mail address: dagor@upenn.edu

Nurs Clin N Am 59 (2024) 253–271
https://doi.org/10.1016/j.cnur.2024.01.005
0029-6465/24/© 2024 Elsevier Inc. All rights reserved.

INTRODUCTION

During the early years of the HIV epidemic, life expectancy postdiagnosis was merely 1 to 2 years, leading to a predominant scientific focus on developing effective therapies to improve survival. However, the advancement of life-saving therapeutics and the resulting transition of HIV to a chronic illness have highlighted the need to attend to social determinants of health, HIV care engagement, and comorbid health challenges. This includes increased attention to comorbid mental health challenges experienced by people living with HIV (PLWH) across the life span. According to the National Institute of Mental Health, rates of depression among PLWH range between 9% and 32%, or more than double the rates in the general population.[1,2] PLWH also face disproportionate risks of a variety of other health challenges, including substance use disorders, death by suicide, diabetes, and high blood pressure.[3,4]

The burden of HIV disproportionately affects racial/ethnic minoritized groups and among sexual and gender minority (SGM) populations, particularly among men who have sex with men (MSM) and transwomen.[5,6] MSM alone accounted for 70% of new HIV infections in the United States in 2021.[7–10] HIV infections are also increasing among older adults, with 17% of new HIV cases in 2018 diagnosed in individuals aged 50 years and older.[11] This may be due to factors such as inconsistent condom use, low rates of biomedical prevention uptake (eg, preexposure prophylaxis and postexposure prophylaxis) in this population, and a lack of targeted prevention and intervention programs tailored specifically to older adults.[7,12]

Stigma and discrimination have been identified as major barriers that deter SGM older adults from seeking timely HIV preventative care and prevent SGM older adults living with HIV (OALWH) from seeking necessary ancillary services (eg, mental health treatment).[13,14] SGM individuals currently in older adulthood came of age when homosexuality was psychopathologized in the Diagnostic and Statistical Manual of Mental Disorders, and terms such as GRID (gay-related immune deficiency) were commonly used to describe HIV by organizations such as the Centers for Disease Control and the National Institutes of Health.[8,15,16] Structural stigma and homonegativity, both in the general public and in the health-care system, commonly contribute to discriminatory and other nonaffirming experiences for SGM OALWH.[17–19] Such experiences cultivate mistrust in the health-care system, which contributes to delayed access to critical services and concealing one's sexual orientation and/or gender identity to providers.[18,20,21]

By the end of 2030, it is projected that 70% of PLWH in the United States will be 50 years of age or older.[22] Depression poses a significant concern among SGM OALWH, often referred to as the "new epidemic" due to the high burden of depressive disorders and symptomology among SGM individuals.[23,24]

The introduction of highly effective antiretroviral drugs has transformed HIV from a terminal condition to a manageable chronic illness, greatly increasing the life expectancy of PLWH to levels similar to HIV-seronegative individuals. Extended life expectancies have given rise to a prioritized focus on the unique biopsychosocial needs of OALWH, particularly SGM individuals who remain disproportionately affected by the HIV epidemic and negative mental health conditions in the United States. In response, the National Institutes of Health's Office of AIDS Research developed an HIV and Aging Working Group to promote the holistic study of the unique health challenges experienced by OALWH and to encourage age and culturally congruent interventions for this population.[25] To aid these efforts, it is critical to review the body of research on mental health interventions for OALWH, and how they address the intersecting social lived experiences of SGM individuals.

Moreover, experiences of marginalization among OALWH from multiple minoritized communities may lead to allostatic stress overload and increased susceptibility to mental health challenges such as depression, loneliness, stigma, and stress-induced psychopathology. Despite these challenges, there remains a dearth of empirical studies exploring effective mental health interventions for SGM OALWH. Identifying effective mental health interventions for this population is critical for supporting HIV disease management and quality of life. This review's main objectives are to review published mental health interventions conducted among SGM OALWH studies and to develop recommendations for future research and practice in this area.

METHODS

We followed Moher and colleagues' (2009) recommendations of the Preferred Reporting Items for Systematic Reviews and Meta-Analysis (PRISMA) search strategy and screening process in this review.[26] Two electronic databases (PubMed and APA PsycINFO) were queried in April 2023 for titles and abstracts from 2013 to 2023 using varied search keywords and MeSH terms. The search keywords used across the databases were Mood disorders, social isolation, HIV, HIV infections, HIV Long-Term Survivors, sexual and gender minorities, bisexuality, health services for transgender persons, limited to articles published in English excluding Adolescent or child, infant. Details of the search strategy for each database are presented in Appendix 1. We used Covidence, a screening and data extraction software, to conduct screening and data extraction for this review.

In April 2023, we conducted a systematic search on the PubMed and APA PsycINFO databases, yielding 740 articles. After 181 duplicate citations were removed, we had 559 abstracts for initial screening. The inclusion criteria included studies in SGM individuals aged 50 years and older, conducted in the United States, written in English, published within the past decade (2013–2023), and describing an intervention focused on addressing mood disorders and/or associated symptoms (including affective disorders, major depressive disorder, loneliness, social isolation, and stigma) in the context of HIV. We implemented double reviewers to maintain the rigor and quality along each stage of the review process. We used discussion, consensus, and third reviewer to resolve conflicts. This approach ensured that biases were minimized and disagreements in the screening process were resolved through consensus.

We excluded 26 studies in the full-text screening stage for not meeting the predefined sample population (no SGM, PLWHIV, or older adults), methodology (intervention group), and data quality, all of which were essential to maintain the rigor and quality of our review. Two articles are included in the review (**Fig. 1**).

RESULTS
General Characteristics of Intervention Studies

Populations with many intersectional social disadvantages such as SGM OALWH may benefit from interventions that consider how their social, behavioral, and health experiences are situated at the intersections of their social identities, such as heterosexist stigma and dealing with discriminatory laws.[13,27–29] There is a dearth of research on the development of mental health interventions for SGM OALWH—We identified only 2 studies that were exclusively mental health interventions for SGM OALWH.[14,27]

Anderson and colleagues (2020)[14,] conducted a single-site, open-label pilot study that examined the feasibility, relative safety, and potential efficacy of psilocybin-assisted group therapy for demoralization in older long-term AIDS survivors (OLTAS). The study included 18 self-identified gay men aged 50 years or older and OLTAS with

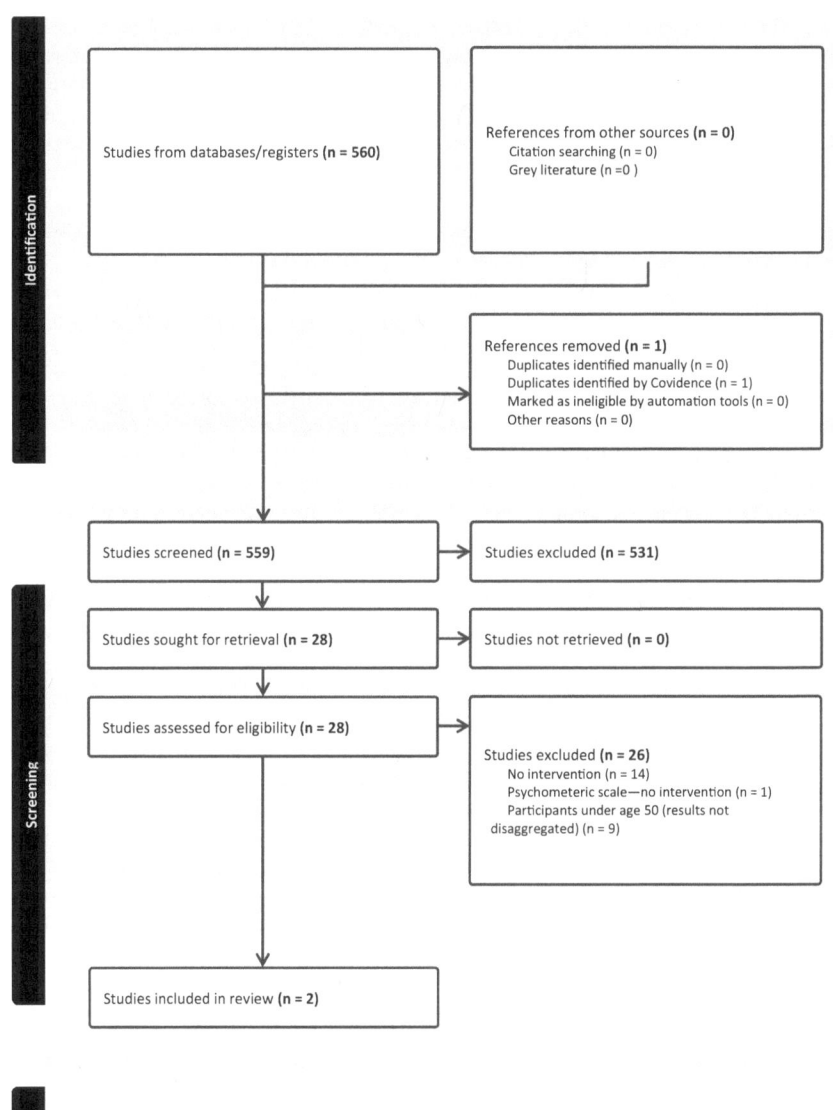

Fig. 1. PRISMA diagram outlining search strategy.

moderate-to-severe demoralization. The sample consisted of 77% White, 5.6% Hispanic, and 5.6% African American individuals. The intervention involved Brief Supportive Expressive Group Therapy (SEGT), modified for psilocybin administration. Crystalline psilocybin was administered at 0.3 mg/kg po for Cohort 1 and 0.36 mg/kg po for Cohorts 2 and 3. Individual therapy proceeded with psilocybin administration, then group therapy. The study found that psilocybin-assisted group therapy was feasible, relatively safe, and potentially reduced demoralization in OLTAS.

Heckman and colleagues (2014)[27] conducted a 3-arm randomized controlled trial (RCT) with 4-month and 8-month follow-ups: examining the effectiveness of 2 teletherapy interventions for depressive symptoms in older adults living with HIV/AIDS. The sample consisted of 361 individuals, including MSM and heterosexual individuals aged 50 years and older, who self-reported HIV status and scored positive on the geriatric depression scale. The sample was 59% African American, 23% White, 11% Latino/Latina, and 7% and 56% have progress to AIDS. Participants were randomized to 1 of 3 groups: standard of care (SOC), telephone coping effectiveness training (tele-CET), or telephone supportive-expressive group therapy (tele-SEGT). The study found that tele-SEGT was more effective than SOC at reducing depressive symptoms at postintervention and 8-month follow-up. Tele-SEGT was also more effective than tele-CET at reducing depressive symptoms postintervention.

Both studies implemented several intervention strategies to address the mental health in SGM OALWH. We describe these strategies below.

Culturally and Age Adapted Therapies

Cognitive behavioral therapy (CBT) is an effective and widely used therapy across many mental health challenges.[30–32] However, the central tenet of CBT on reframing cognitive distortion does not explicitly address SGM minority stress, HIV-related biopsychosocial needs, and differing levels of stigma.[5,33,34] Critiques have characterized CBT as Eurocentric, that a focus on personal accountability for change may not reflect the experiences of marginalized communities, and that some core components of CBT might be culturally incongruent for racial and ethnic minorities and SGM OALWH.[13,28,35] The challenges that face SGM OALWH demand an adapted CBT sensitive to their unique lived experience, and early evidence suggests that culturally adapted CBT is efficacious in minoritized communities.[32] Both studies included in this review used adapted CBT in their intervention.[14,27]

Both studies adapted therapies for their intervention. Heckman and Colleagues adapted CBT with emphasis modeled after Lazarus and Folkman's Transactional Model of stress and coping for their tele-CET intervention—encouraging optimization of coping through social support. SGM OALWH had a higher attendance (7.25) rate in tele-CET compared with their heterosexual counterparts (5.79). However, the adapted CBT was less efficacious than their adapted tele-SEGT in reducing depressive symptoms for SGM OALWH (**Table 1** for study characteristics).

Heckman and colleagues[27] used tele-SEGT for their group intervention, whereas Anderson and colleagues[14] adapted SEGT for their individual and group session interventions emphasizing the practice of mindfulness. SEGT is an adapted palliative therapy modeled from humanistic psychology. SEGT encouraged SGM OALWH to foster empathy and positive regard, maintaining a present-moment focus and exploring their feelings about the challenges associated: with aging, HIV seropositive status, and living with HIV/AIDS. Tele-SEGT was more efficacious for improving depressive symptomology for SGM OALWH compared with SOC (B = -2.39, $P = .03$) and tele-CET (B = -1.95, $P = .07$). However, Anderson and colleagues did not measure therapy outcomes (see **Table 1** for study characteristics).

Mindfulness and Meditation-Based Stress Reduction

Mindfulness and meditation-based stress reduction (MMBSR) holds promise for improving stress-induced mental health psychopathologic conditions.[28,36] MMBSR has also shown promise among minoritized individuals.[37,38] The core psychotherapeutic principals of MMBSR accentuate present-moment awareness with openness, curiosity, and acceptance; nonjudgmental thoughts, emotion, and sensations; cultivating

Table 1
Summary of studies

Author, Year	Geography and Setting	Population and Sample Size	Intervention	Length of Assessment	Study Design	Results
Anderson, et al,[14] 2020	San Francisco, California	Self-identified gay men ≥50 y, OLTAS with moderate-to-severe demoralization N = 18 Mean age 59.2 y. Three sequential group therapy cohorts (n = 6)	Psilocybin-assisted group therapy: 0.3 mg/kg po for Cohort 1 and 0.36 mg/kg po for Cohorts 2 and 3 Individual therapy: one 90-min prepsilocybin and one session 2 h postpsilocybin. Group therapy: 90 min twice per week for 3 wk using Brief SEGT	Preintervention, postintervention, 3 mo follow-up	Single-site open-label pilot study for 7 wk	95% group therapy attendance Posttreatment and 3-mo follow-up, respectively, 88.9% and 66.7% of participants demonstrated at least a 2-point reduction in demoralization The study demonstrated the feasibility, relative safety, and potential efficacy of psilocybin-assisted group therapy for demoralization in OLTAS

| Heckman, et al,[27] 2014 | AIDS service organizations in 24 states | ≥50 y old living with HIV/AIDS, Geriatric depression score ≥10 N = 361 | Three interventions arms: • SOC • tele-CET group (tele-CET; Twelve 90-min therapy sessions using Lazarus and Folkman's Transactional Model of Stress and Coping using cognitive behavioral (CBT) principles • Telephone SEGT + SOC. Therapy: humanistic psychology: emphasis on fostering empathy, positive regard, therapist transparency, and maintaining a present-moment focus, exploring feelings on: difficulties associated with normal aging, being HIV-positive, and living with HIV/AIDS as an older adult | Preintervention, postintervention, 4-mo and 8-mo follow-ups | RCT | MSM in tele-SEGT reported fewer depressive symptoms postintervention compared with MSM in SOC (B = −2.39, $P = .03.009$, d = 0.44). Tele-SEGT participants reported fewer depressive symptoms at postintervention compared with tele-CET participants (B = 1.95, $P = .07$) tele-SEGT reduced depressive symptoms vs standard care through 8 mo for heterosexuals Tele-SEGT reduced depressive symptoms vs standard care at postintervention for MSM |

mindful awareness through practices such as meditation, body scans, and yoga; radical self-compassion; patience; and equanimity.

Both studies in this review used some variation of mindfulness in their interventions to address SGM minority stress and stigma for OALWH.[14,27] Researchers emphasized positive regard, self-empathy, personal trigger identification, and deep breathing exercises.[14,27] For example, Heckman and colleagues' study accentuated fostering empathy and positive regard, maintaining a present-moment, emotional exploration of challenges with aging, and living with HIV as an older adult.[27] Equally, Anderson and colleagues provided psychoeducation on the "here and now" processing and detoxifying death for SGM OALWH.[14] Because MMBSR was not treated as a stand-alone therapy but rather an adaptation to treatment, there was no outcome measure for MMBSR in both studies.

Group Therapy

Group therapy leverages the power of group dynamics for healing. Group therapy is a time and cost-effective psychotherapeutic intervention to address unique bio-psychosocial stressors affecting SGM OALWH.[14,27,28,35] Group therapy is apt for SGM OALWH because it helps to alleviate common challenges such as isolation and loneliness by talking and relating with others who may hold shared identities. Group therapy allowed SGM OALWH to validate each other, fostering shared identity and lived experience. There is a paucity of SGM-affirming spaces for OALWH. Culturally congruent group therapy for SGM, racial and ethnic minorities, and OALWH are efficacious and hold promise for addressing social isolation, sharing resources, and improving mental health outcomes.[13,14,27]

Anderson and colleagues[14] recruited a homogenous group to improve trust, safety, and peer validation for SGM OALWH, using breathing exercises, guided meditation, and mindfulness to emotionally ground the group. Anderson and colleagues[14] report that group therapy was cathartic for SGM OALWH because they found age-appropriate space, affirming their intersecting shared lived experience—SGM OALWH group therapy attendance rate was 95%, which was the primary outcome for group therapy. Equally, Heckman and colleagues[27] found that SGM OALWH had a higher group therapy attendance (8.11 session SEGT) than their heterosexual counterparts (6.95 SEGT sessions)—They report that the conjunction of group therapy and digital mental health might have increased privacy and anonymity that increased group therapy attendance.

Group therapy was effective in addressing HIV-related stigma and minority stress and improving loneliness by connecting SGM OALWH.[14,27] The outcome of group therapy was assessed by the therapeutic model (SEGT, adapted CBT, or psilocybin administration).

Digital Mental Health

Digital mental health (DMH) interventions use technologies (telephones, mobile applications, and computers) to deliver and support mental well-being and promote mental health awareness.[27] DMH interventions provide unique opportunities for SGM OALWH to receive mental health care by maintaining a sense of anonymity and reducing the stigma associated with physical HIV and mental health clinics. DMH interventions also reduce logistical barriers, such as transportation challenges or issues with mobility that may increase with age.[27]

Heckman and colleagues (2014)[27] used DMH and found it was feasible for SGM OALWH—Although only the SGM OALWH SEGT arm had a statistically significant reduction in depression (B = −1.95, P = .7). Heckman and colleagues[27] randomized participants to 3 arms, the 2 DMH (tele-CERT) and tele-SEGT. The session consisted of 90 minutes per session for 12 sessions. Research assistants called participants a day before to remind them of the session and other necessary research protocols. The therapist facilitated mutual support for SGM OALWH, improved social and family support, and positive emotional expression.

DMH interventions improved mental health outcomes, reduced stigma, and increased adherence to antiretroviral therapy (ART)for SGM OALWH. Further, group therapy with DMH helps alleviate a sense of isolation and loneliness for participants.[14,27] DMH was clinically significant in reducing isolation and depressive symptoms among SGM OALWH.

Pharmacological-Assisted Psychotherapeutic Interventions

Anderson and colleagues (2020) [14] were unique in their mental health intervention; they provided psilocybin-assisted individual and group therapy. Psilocybin-assisted group therapy has an emerging evidence base among people living with chronic illness. This study demonstrated effectiveness in improving depressive symptoms (assessed by demoralization) among SGM OALWH: with a 95% attendance and demoralization pre-post (mean difference -6.67 [SD 6.51]) and 3-month follow-up (mean difference -5.78 [SD 6.01]). Psilocybin-assisted group therapy also holds promise for addressing stigma, shame, and social isolation prevalent among SGM OALWH. The authors reported zero serious medication side effects, although self-limiting anxiety existed. It is noteworthy that most participants were not naive to psilocybin.

DISCUSSION

This narrative review sought to identify, compile, and synthesize current research on mental health interventions for SGM OALWH. Several critical implications emerge from the 2 studies included in the review (see **Table 1**). There is a notable paucity of research focused on mental health intervention specifically for SGM OALWH—the dearth of mental health interventions for this population suggests that mental health is not being equitably prioritized for SGM OALWH. Equally, this shortage of mental health intervention studies is critical given the fifth annual state of HIV care released in November 2023 cited mental health (61%), aging with HIV (60.4%), and stigma and discrimination (57.8%) as the highest care priorities for PLWH.

Current adapted therapies show promise in improving mental health and behavioral outcomes for SGM OALWH, such as depression, coping, and accessing social support systems. This aligns with critiques that traditional CBT may not fully address minority stress. However, the interventions predominantly featured CBT and SEGT modalities. Meanwhile, Anderson and colleagues' psilocybin-assisted therapy pilot showed feasibility and safety in this population. Although an emerging area needing more research, psilocybin-assisted therapy could uniquely address existential distress regarding aging/HIV. More research is warranted on the potential benefits of other treatment modalities for this population. Given the higher tendency for loneliness and isolation among SGM OALWH, it is imperative to consider group therapy (face-to-face or DMH) as a vital intervention to help ameliorate the harmful effects of isolation in this population. DMH might be well suited to overcoming barriers and improving access for this group.

Addressing Intersectional Stigma, Discrimination, and Trauma

The community of SGM OALWH is not a monolith and includes a wide array of intersecting social identities and experiences that need to be considered when designing and delivering interventions. For example, some older adults may value privacy and anonymity when it comes to speaking about their HIV diagnosis, making a digital intervention preferable to in-person or group therapy.[13,27,39] This may be due to their exposure to HIV stigma, as older adults lived through the early years of the HIV epidemic of the 1980s, as well as the associated wave of prejudice that targeted people living with HIV and SGM individuals. In this regard, mental health interventions targeting SGM OALWH must use cultural humility, which involves accounting for people's beliefs and values due to their personal, historical, or cultural contexts.[18]

Intersectionality describes how various social identities interact to produce a unique, compounded experience and identity defined by the individual.[25,40,41] SGM OALWH are a prime example because they have at least 3 marginalized identities that can contribute to a triple stigma: SGM identity, older age, and living with HIV.[8,25,36] SGM from racial and ethnic minority backgrounds face further stigma and marginalization, as do SGM OALWH who are experiencing mental health challenges.[5,36,42] Because of intersectional stigma and discrimination, SGM OALWH may have smaller social networks compared with their younger peers.[5,36,42] OALWH have a significantly higher chance of living alone and higher rates of morbidity and mortality.[20] Due to the social isolation faced by such a stigmatized community, interventions should focus on social connection and the processing of experiences of others with shared identities.[14,27]

Intersectionality also extends to social lived experiences across gender, disability status, religiosity, and socioeconomic status. According to Chen and colleagues, racial and ethnic minoritized SGM older adults, especially those from Black and Hispanic backgrounds, report higher levels of racism, face greater discrimination, and lack safe spaces to meet other people with similar intersectional identities due to the youth-centric and majority White SGM community spaces.[21] Foreign-born SGM adults face similar issues, with decreased health care access in their area and more unfair treatment from health-care providers.[21] These social stressors often translate into poor mental health outcomes.[21] Intersectional stigma is a driving force for mental health disparities and demands a prioritized need for interventions to support people from multiple minoritized backgrounds.[5,13]

Interventions must also be trauma-informed by considering the traumatic experiences SGM OALWH may have gone through, as well as the ways they manifest into varying mental health conditions such as depression. Many of the mental health concerns of people living with HIV have been found to be linked in some way to trauma, further suggesting that interventions must address trauma.[19] Enhance Sexual Health Intervention for Men, a stress reduction intervention designed for HIV-positive bisexual African Americans with histories of childhood sexual assault, was found to significantly improve depression symptoms when compared with a general health promotion program.[14,27,35] Addressing trauma is critical to obtaining a compressive picture of someone's mental health situation, allowing providers to establish trust, integrate knowledge about trauma into their interventions, and improve outcomes for conditions such as depression.

Tailored Interventions for Gender-Diverse Older Adults Living with Human Immunodeficiency Virus

Although grouped with sexual minorities under the SGM umbrella, gender minorities (people who are transgender, nonbinary, gender fluid, genderqueer, and so forth) have specific needs and challenges that may require specifically tailored interventions. According to a systematic review describing the health care needs of gender-diverse older people, transgender older adults have significantly higher rates of various health conditions, including depression and anxiety.[23] Hunter-Jones and colleagues found that DMH mindfulness-based adapted cognitive therapy holds promise for improving self-reported quality of life for gender minority participants.[13,27,28]

The unique biopsychosocial needs of gender minoritized populations are not adequately captured in intervention studies focused on HIV and aging focus, which is predominantly sexual minority men and MSM. This highlights a significant research gap, given the unique health disparities and psychosocial challenges experienced at the intersection of advanced age, HIV status, and gender/sexual minority status. There is an urgent need for studies exploring the specific needs of SGM older adult gender minority individuals living with HIV.

Syndemic Interventions to Address Coexisting Psychosocial Barriers and Support Human Immunodeficiency Virus Disease Management Among Older Adults Living with Human Immunodeficiency Virus

Despite medical breakthroughs in recent decades, not all OALWH receive consistent ART treatment and support that make living with HIV a manageable, chronic disease. Earlier studies suggest that PLWH experiences a syndemic of psychosocial and

---

Box 1
Biopsychosocial sexual/gender minority older adults living with HIV data

Mental health and HIV
- More than 50% of all PLWHs are aged 50 years or older[50]
- In 2019, racial and ethnic minority older adults accounted for 42% of HIV cases among older adults aged 50 years and older[51]
- OALWH presenting with advanced HIV are 14 times more likely to die within a year compared with earlier counterparts[52]
- More than 50% of SGM older adults are sexually active, suggesting a need for comprehensive sexual health care[52,53]
- Health-care providers often report discomfort discussing sexual well-being with SGM older adults[52]
- Racial and ethnic minorities (REM) SGM OALWH experience higher HIV deterioration and death than their White older SGM[51,52]
- More than 15% of older PLWH identify as bisexual[52]
- Older lesbian and bisexual women's primary HIV risk factor was injection drug use US center for disease, prevention and control (CDC)
- Around 3% of transgender adults are living with HIV; transgender women have a higher HIV prevalence rate of approximately 22%, with higher rates among racial and ethnic minority transwomen[52]
- Most older transgender adults living with HIV are transwomen[52]

Data from Refs.[50–53]

Mental health and risk factors among sexual and gender minority older adults
- Mental health disorder is highest among transgender older adults than other older sexual minorities: 16% had attempted suicide at least once in their lifetime[54]
- SGM older adults are 4 times less likely to have children compared with their heterosexual counterparts[52]
- Higher SGM in group discrimination for SGM OALWH[52]
- SGM culture has a negative view of aging because of its youth-centeredness: overreliance on physical appearance and youthfulness.[52]
- SGM older adults are twice as likely to live alone, less likely to have a significant other, or have close family to assist with care or health-care decisions.[52]
- About 65% of older transgender believe there would be limited access to care as they aged[52]
- About 70% of SGM older adults may "recloset" themselves when seeking elder housing[52]

Data from Refs.[52,54]

Table 2	
SGM OALWH mental health resources for providers and patients	
Resources (Alphabetical)	**Description**
Human Rights Campaign: *Long-Term Care Equality Index*[55]	Benchmarks long-term care facilities for SGM-inclusive policies and practices
Movement Advancement Project (MAP)[56]	SGM state-level resource hub: providing research, advocacy, and analysis to promote equality
Pride counseling[57]	Provides online SGM culturally congruent counseling
Services & Advocacy for SGM Elders (*Sage*)[58]	National advocacy organization dedicated to improving the lives of SGM older adults and SGM OALWH

structural social conditions that compound one another in elevating individuals' risk for health-compromising behaviors and subsequent deleterious health outcomes.[43–45] For example, limited access to HIV medical care often manifests from a combination of financial, geographic/physical, sociocultural, and mental health barriers. Notably, there is substantial evidence that depression and a sense of hopelessness are comorbid psychosocial challenges often faced by OALWH that are interconnected with other individual, interpersonal, and structural barriers that negatively impact HIV disease management.[22] Not receiving ART may also elicit and exacerbate syndemic issues, including comorbid mental health conditions, because it decreases immune functioning. Because depression positively correlates with nonadherence to ART, interventions supporting HIV disease management among SGM OALWH must also address the multilevel barriers linked to mental health challenges. Unfortunately, none of the studies in this review addressed syndemic conditions.

Syndemic interventions for PLWH, especially for PLWH in older adulthood, are poorly conceptualized.[46] Earlier studies have acknowledged challenges with designing and evaluating syndemic interventions, including focusing on individual-level factors, such as eliciting common barriers to desired behavioral outcomes (eg, consistent condom use) and constructing action opportunities and plans tailored to the individual, including service referrals. Syndemic experts suggest a critical need to consider social determinants and systems-level approaches (ie, "syndemic care system") in addition to individual-level tailoring to maximize the effectiveness of syndemic interventions.[47,48] In the context of SGM OALWH, syndemic interventions should identify common salient barriers to HIV treatment and mental health, the social structures that perpetuate these barriers, and intervene across these ecological levels, considering policy solutions, scale-up of community and clinical service provision, and tailoring to intersectional, individual-level lived social experiences.[49]

SUMMARY

Overwhelming evidence suggests a critical need to address mental health disparities that disproportionately affect SGM OALWH in the United States. Yet, there remains a dearth of mental health-focused interventions tailored to SGM OALWH. The development and evaluation of randomized trials containing large and diverse sample sizes of SGM OALWHs are urgently needed. In **Box 1**, we outline recent statistics highlighting the intersections of HIV, mental health, aging SGM status, and race/ethnicity.

Ultimately, providers must practice cultural humility and sensitivity to SGM OALWH. Given the high rates of trauma exposure in this population, trauma-informed care must be the SOC and address co-occurring mental health conditions that limit engagement in HIV medical care. Clinicians having a repertoire of affirming local, regional, and national SGM OALWH resources to refer patients to is an invaluable resource that can improve health outcomes for this priority population. National-level resources may provide a launching point for identifying locally tailored services (**Table 2**).

Furthermore, knowing that many SGM older adults will never disclose their SGM identity, therefore, creating an affirming clinical environment for all patients without making heterosexual assumptions is critical for improving health outcomes. Clinicians can boost the resilience of this population with culturally congruent and trauma-informed care. Finally, policymakers urgently need to prioritize funding interventions that address the salient social determinants that hinder HIV and mental health-care engagement among SGM OALWH.

CLINICS CARE POINTS

- SGM OALWH are a higher risk for depression and loneliness
- Clinicians should use evidence-based, culturally congruent psychometrics to assess for mental illness among SGM OALWH
- Use culturally congruent adapted psychotherapy for SGM OALWH
- Provide SGM OALWH access to OALWH-specific national and local resources

DISCLOSURE

Funding for this review was made possible (in part) by Grant Number 5H79SM080386-05 from SAMHSA. The views expressed neither reflect the official policies of the Department of Health and Human Services nor does mention of trade names, commercial practices, or organizations imply endorsement by the US Government.

REFERENCES

1. NIMH » HIV and AIDS and Mental Health. Available at: https://www.nimh.nih.gov/health/topics/hiv-aids. [Accessed 30 November 2023].
2. Leibowitz AA, Desmond KA. The impact of mental health conditions on public insurance costs of treating HIV/AIDS. AIDS Behav 2020;24(6):1621–31.
3. Ma Y, Xiang Q, Yan C, et al. Relationship between chronic diseases and depression: the mediating effect of pain. BMC Psychiatr 2021;21(1):436.
4. Fattouh N, Hallit S, Salameh P, et al. Prevalence and factors affecting the level of depression, anxiety, and stress in hospitalized patients with a chronic disease. Perspect Psychiatr Care 2019;55(4):592–9.
5. Pachankis JE, McConocha EM, Reynolds JS, et al. Project ESTEEM protocol: a randomized controlled trial of an LGBTQ-affirmative treatment for young adult sexual minority men's mental and sexual health. BMC Publ Health 2019;19(1):1086.
6. Parsons JT, Rendina HJ, Moody RL, et al. Feasibility of an emotion regulation intervention to improve mental health and reduce hiv transmission risk behaviors for HIV-positive gay and bisexual men with sexual compulsivity. AIDS Behav 2017;21(6):1540–9.
7. HIV incidence | HIV and gay and bisexual men | HIV by group | HIV/AIDS | CDC. Available at: https://www.cdc.gov/hiv/group/msm/msm-content/incidence.html. [Accessed 18 December 2021].
8. De Jesus M, Ware D, Brown AL, et al. Social-environmental resiliencies protect against loneliness among HIV-Positive and HIV- negative older men who have

sex with men: Results from the Multicenter AIDS Cohort Study (MACS). Soc Sci Med 2021;272:113711.

9. Arscott J, Humphreys J, Merwin E, et al. "That guy is gay and black. that's a red flag." how HIV stigma and racism affect perception of risk among young black men who have sex with men. AIDS Behav 2020;24(1):173–84.

10. CROI press release: lifetime HIV risk | CDC. 2016. Available at: https://www.cdc.gov/nchhstp/newsroom/2016/croi-press-release-risk.html. [Accessed 15 April 2021].

11. Antibiotic resistant gonorrhea - STD information from CDC. Available at: https://www.cdc.gov/std/gonorrhea/arg/default.htm. [Accessed 5 March 2022].

12. HIV surveillance | reports| resource library | HIV/AIDS | CDC. Available at: https://www.cdc.gov/hiv/library/reports/hiv-surveillance.html. [Accessed 26 July 2023].

13. English D, Smith JC, Scott-Walker L, et al. Feasibility, acceptability, and preliminary HIV care and psychological health effects of iTHRIVE 365 for black same gender loving men. J Acquir Immune Defic Syndr 2023;93(1):55–63.

14. Anderson BT, Danforth A, Daroff PR, et al. Psilocybin-assisted group therapy for demoralized older long-term AIDS survivor men: An open-label safety and feasibility pilot study. EClinicalMedicine 2020;27:100538.

15. National Academies of Sciences. In: White J, Sepúlveda M-J, Patterson CJ, editors. Engineering, and medicine; division of behavioral and social sciences and education; committee on population; committee on understanding the well-being of sexual and gender diverse populations. Understanding the well-being of LGBTQI+ populations. National Academies Press (US); 2020. https://doi.org/10.17226/25877.

16. Emlet CA, O'Brien KK, Fredriksen Goldsen K. The global impact of HIV on sexual and gender minority older adults: challenges, progress, and future directions. Int J Aging Hum Dev 2019;89(1):108–26.

17. Hatzenbuehler ML. Structural stigma: Research evidence and implications for psychological science. Am Psychol 2016;71(8):742–51.

18. Pachankis JE, Bränström R. How many sexual minorities are hidden? projecting the size of the global closet with implications for policy and public health. PLoS One 2019;14(6):e0218084.

19. Mazonson P, Berko J, Loo T, et al. Loneliness among older adults living with HIV: the "older old" may be less lonely than the "younger old". AIDS Care 2021;33(3):375–82.

20. Casey LS, Reisner SL, Findling MG, et al. Discrimination in the united states: experiences of lesbian, gay, bisexual, transgender, and queer americans. Health Serv Res 2019;54(Suppl 2):1454–66.

21. Yu H, Bauermeister JA, Flores DD. LGBTQ+ health education interventions for nursing students: A systematic review. Nurse Educ Today 2023;121:105661.

22. HIV by Age | HIV by Group | HIV/AIDS | CDC. Available at: https://www.cdc.gov/hiv/group/age/index.html?CDC_AA_refVal=https%3A%2F%2Fwww.cdc.gov%2Fhiv%2Fgroup%2Fage%2Folderamericans%2Findex.html. [Accessed 26 July 2023].

23. Bromberg DJ, Paltiel AD, Busch SH, et al. Has depression surpassed HIV as a burden to gay and bisexual men's health in the United States? A comparative modeling study. Soc Psychiatry Psychiatr Epidemiol 2021;56(2):273–82.

24. Bernard C, Dabis F, de Rekeneire N. Prevalence and factors associated with depression in people living with HIV in sub-Saharan Africa: A systematic review and meta-analysis. PLoS One 2017;12(8):e0181960.

25. High KP, Brennan-Ing M, Clifford DB, et al. HIV and aging: state of knowledge and areas of critical need for research. A report to the NIH Office of AIDS

Research by the HIV and Aging Working Group. J Acquir Immune Defic Syndr 2012;60(Suppl 1):S1–18.

26. Moher D, Liberati A, Tetzlaff J, et al, PRISMA Group. Preferred reporting items for systematic reviews and meta-analyses: The PRISMA statement. PLoS Med 2009; 6(7):e1000097.

27. Heckman BD, Lovejoy TI, Heckman TG, et al. The moderating role of sexual identity in group teletherapy for adults aging with HIV. Behav Med 2014;40(3):134–42.

28. Hunter-Jones J, Gilliam S, Davis C, et al. Process and outcome evaluation of a mindfulness-based cognitive therapy intervention for cisgender and transgender african american women living with HIV/AIDS. AIDS Behav 2021;25(2):592–603.

29. English D, Carter JA, Bowleg L, et al. Intersectional social control: The roles of incarceration and police discrimination in psychological and HIV-related outcomes for Black sexual minority men. Soc Sci Med 2020;258:113121.

30. Cuijpers P, Miguel C, Harrer M, et al. Cognitive behavior therapy vs. control conditions, other psychotherapies, pharmacotherapies and combined treatment for depression: a comprehensive meta-analysis including 409 trials with 52,702 patients. World Psychiatr 2023;22(1):105–15.

31. O'Cleirigh C, Safren SA, Taylor SW, et al. Cognitive behavioral therapy for trauma and self-care (CBT-TSC) in men who have sex with men with a history of childhood sexual abuse: a randomized controlled trial. AIDS Behav 2019;23(9): 2421–31.

32. Pachankis JE, Harkness A, Maciejewski KR, et al. LGBQ-affirmative cognitive-behavioral therapy for young gay and bisexual men's mental and sexual health: A three-arm randomized controlled trial. J Consult Clin Psychol 2022. https://doi.org/10.1037/ccp0000724.

33. Blashill AJ, Safren SA, Wilhelm S, et al. Cognitive behavioral therapy for body image and self-care (CBT-BISC) in sexual minority men living with HIV: A randomized controlled trial. Health Psychol 2017;36(10):937–46.

34. Pachankis JE, Hatzenbuehler ML, Rendina HJ, et al. LGB-affirmative cognitive-behavioral therapy for young adult gay and bisexual men: A randomized controlled trial of a transdiagnostic minority stress approach. J Consult Clin Psychol 2015;83(5):875–89.

35. Williams JK, Glover DA, Wyatt GE, et al. A sexual risk and stress reduction intervention designed for HIV-positive bisexual African American men with childhood sexual abuse histories. Am J Public Health 2013;103(8):1476–84.

36. Hunter-Jones JJ, Gilliam SM, Carswell AL, et al. Assessing the acceptability of a mindfulness-based cognitive therapy intervention for african-american women living with HIV/AIDS. J Racial Ethn Health Disparities 2019;6(6):1157–66.

37. Woods-Giscombé C, Black AR. Mind-body interventions to reduce risk for health disparities related to stress and strength among african american women: the potential of mindfulness-based stress reduction, loving-kindness, and the NTU therapeutic framework. Complement Health Pract Rev 2010;15(3):115–31.

38. Sun S, Nardi W, Loucks EB, et al. Mindfulness-based interventions for sexual and gender minorities: a systematic review and evidence evaluation. Mindfulness (N Y) 2021;12(10):2439–59.

39. Root E, Caskie G. eMental health literacy and the relationship to barriers to mental health care. Innov Aging 2020;4(Supplement_1):305.

40. Joudeh L, Harris OO, Johnstone E, et al. "Little red flags": barriers to accessing health care as a sexual or gender minority individual in the rural southern united states-a qualitative intersectional approach. J Assoc Nurses AIDS Care 2021; 32(4):467–80.

41. Hong C, Ochoa AM, Wilson BDM, et al. The associations between HIV stigma and mental health symptoms, life satisfaction, and quality of life among Black sexual minority men with HIV. Qual Life Res 2023. https://doi.org/10.1007/s11136-023-03342-z.

42. English D, Hickson DA, Callander D, et al. Racial discrimination, sexual partner race/ethnicity, and depressive symptoms among black sexual minority men. Arch Sex Behav 2020;49(5):1799–809.

43. Achterbergh RCA, van der Helm JJ, van den Brink W, et al. Design of a syndemic based intervention to facilitate care for men who have sex with men with high risk behaviour: the syn.bas.in randomized controlled trial. BMC Infect Dis 2017; 17(1):398.

44. Shiau S, Krause KD, Valera P, et al. The burden of COVID-19 in people living with HIV: A syndemic perspective. AIDS Behav 2020;24(8):2244–9.

45. Tsuyuki K, Pitpitan EV, Levi-Minzi MA, et al. Substance use disorders, violence, mental health, and HIV: differentiating a syndemic factor by gender and sexuality. AIDS Behav 2017;21(8):2270–82.

46. Chakrapani V, Kaur M, Tsai AC, et al. The impact of a syndemic theory-based intervention on HIV transmission risk behaviour among men who have sex with men in India: Pretest-posttest non-equivalent comparison group trial. Soc Sci Med 2022;295:112817.

47. Gilbert L, Stoicescu C, Goddard-Eckrich D, et al. Intervening on the Intersecting Issues of Intimate Partner Violence, Substance Use, and HIV: A Review of Social Intervention Group's (SIG) Syndemic-Focused Interventions for Women. Res Soc Work Pract 2023;33(2):178–92.

48. Graham TS, Thornicroft G. The syndemic approach in relation to clinical practice and research in psychiatry. Consortium Psychiatricum 2020;1(2):3–6.

49. Rod MH, Rod NH, Russo F, et al. Promoting the health of vulnerable populations: Three steps towards a systems-based re-orientation of public health intervention research. Health Place 2023;80:102984.

50. Wing EJ. The Aging Population with HIV Infection. Trans Am Clin Climatol Assoc 2017;128:131–44.

51. Services US Department of Health and Human. What is the impact of HIV on racial and ethnic minorities in the US. 2020. Available at: https://www.hiv.gov/hiv-basics/overview/data-and-trends/impact-on-racial-and-ethnic-minorities/.

52. Simone M, Meyer H, Eskildsen M, Appelbaum J. In: The Fenway Guide to Lesbian, Gay, Bisexual, and Transgender Health, 133-136, 2nd edition. Philadelphia, PA: American College of Physicians; 2015. p. 141–6.

53. National Institute on Aging. Improving the health and well-being of sexual and gender minority older adult. Available at:. National Institute on Aging; 2023 https://www.nia.nih.gov/news/improving-health-and-well-being-sexual-and-gender-minority-older-adults. [Accessed 4 October 2023].

54. Grant JM, Tanis JM. Injustice at every turn. A report of the National; 2011.

55. The LEI. Available at: https://thelei.org/. [Accessed 19 October 2023].

56. Movement advancement project | organizations working to improve the lives of LGBT Americans. Available at: https://www.lgbtmap.org/resource-page. [Accessed 19 October 2023].

57. Rhodes EC, Damio G, LaPlant HW, et al. Promoting equity in breastfeeding through peer counseling: the US Breastfeeding Heritage and Pride program. Int J Equity Health 2021;20(1):128.

58. Your Rights & Resources. SAGE. Available at: https://www.sageusa.org/your-rights-resources/. [Accessed 19 October 2023].

APPENDIX 1: SEARCH STRATEGY REPORT: DATE: 4/6/2023

Total # of References: 740
# of Duplicates Removed: 181
Total # of References to Screen: 559
Database: PubMed

Set #		Results
1	"Mood Disorders"[Mesh] OR "Social Isolation"[Mesh] OR "Loneliness"[Mesh] OR "mood disorder"[tiab] OR "mood disorders"[tiab] OR "affective disorder"[tiab] OR "affective disorders"[tiab] OR depression [tiab] OR depressive[tiab] OR loneliness[tiab] OR lonely[tiab] OR "social isolation"[tiab] OR "social exclusion"[tiab]	
2	HIV[mesh] OR "HIV infections"[mesh] OR "HIV Long-Term Survivors"[Mesh] OR "Anti-HIV Agents"[Mesh] OR "Acquired Immunodeficiency Syndrome"[mesh] OR HIV[tiab] OR "human immunodeficiency virus"[tiab] OR AIDS[tiab] OR "Acquired Immunodeficiency Syndrome"[tiab]	
3	"sexual and gender minorities"[Mesh] OR "Bisexuality"[Mesh] OR "health services for transgender persons"[Mesh] OR homosexuality[Mesh] OR "homosexuality, female"[Mesh] OR "homosexuality, male"[Mesh] OR "transgender persons"[Mesh] OR LGBT[tiab] OR LGBTI[tiab] OR LGBTQ* [tiab] OR GLBT[tiab] OR GLBTQ[tiab] OR bisexual[tiab] OR bisexuals[tiab] OR bisexuality[tiab] OR homosexual[tiab] OR homosexuals[tiab] OR homosexuality[tiab] OR gay[tiab] OR gays[tiab] OR intersex[tiab] OR lesbian[tiab] OR lesbianism[tiab] OR lesbians[tiab] OR "men having sex with men"[tiab] OR "men who have sex with men"[tiab] OR "men who have sex with other men"[tiab] OR pansexual[tiab] OR polysexual[tiab] OR queer[tiab] OR "sexual minorities"[tiab] OR "sexual minority"[tiab] OR "sexual and gender minority"[tiab] OR "sexual and gender minorities"[tiab] OR transgender*[tiab] OR transsexual*[tiab] OR transman[tiab] OR "trans man"[tiab] OR "trans men"[tiab] OR transmen [tiab] OR transsexualism[tiab] OR transwoman[tiab] OR "trans woman"[tiab] OR "trans women"[tiab] OR transwomen[tiab] OR "two spirit"[tiab] OR two-spirit[tiab] OR "women who have sex with women"[tiab] OR asexual[tiab] OR asexuals[tiab] OR asexuality[tiab] OR nonbinary[tiab] OR agender[tiab] OR Bigender[tiab] OR Genderqueer [tiab] OR Gender-diverse[tiab] OR "gender diverse"[tiab] OR Gender-expansive[tiab] OR "gender expansive"[tiab] OR Same-gender-loving [tiab] OR "same gender loving"[tiab]	
4	#1 AND #2 AND #3	1373
5	#4 NOT (("Adolescent"[Mesh] OR "Child"[Mesh] OR "Infant"[Mesh]) NOT "Adult"[Mesh])	1338
6	#5 AND ("randomized controlled trial"[ptyp] OR "controlled clinical trial"[ptyp] OR randomized[tiab] OR randomised[tiab] OR randomization [tiab] OR randomisation[tiab] OR placebo[tiab] OR randomly[tiab] OR trial [tiab] OR groups[tiab] OR "Comparative Study"[ptyp] OR "clinical trial"[pt] OR "clinical trial"[tiab] OR "clinical trials"[tiab] OR "evaluation studies"[ptyp] OR "evaluation studies as topic"[MeSH] OR "evaluation study"[tiab] OR "evaluation studies"[tiab] OR drug therapy[sh] OR "intervention study"[tiab] OR "intervention studies"[tiab] OR "case-control studies"[MeSH] OR "case-control"[tiab] OR "cohort studies"[MeSH] OR cohort[tiab] OR "longitudinal studies"[MeSH] OR longitudinal[tiab] OR longitudinally[tiab] OR prospective[tiab] OR prospectively[tiab] OR "retrospective studies"[MeSH] OR retrospective [tiab] OR "follow up"[tiab] OR "comparative study"[pt] OR "comparative	678

(continued on next page)

(continued)

Set #		Results
	studies"[tiab] OR nonrandom[tiab] OR "non-random"[tiab] OR nonrandomized[tiab] OR "non-randomized"[tiab] OR nonrandomised [tiab] OR "non-randomised"[tiab] OR quasi-experiment*[tiab] OR quasiexperiment*[tiab] OR quasirandom*[tiab] OR quasi-random*[tiab] OR quasi-control*[tiab] OR quasicontrol*[tiab] OR (controlled[tiab] AND (trial[tiab] OR study[tiab])) OR "pre-post"[tiab] OR "posttest"[tiab] OR "post-test"[tiab] OR pretest[tiab] OR pre-test[tiab] OR ("time series"[tiab] AND interrupt[tiab]) OR ("time points"[tiab] AND (multiple[tiab] OR one [tiab] OR two[tiab] OR three[tiab] OR four[tiab] OR five[tiab] OR six[tiab] OR seven[tiab] OR eight[tiab] OR nine[tiab] OR ten[tiab] OR month[tiab] OR monthly[tiab] OR day[tiab] OR daily[tiab] OR week[tiab] OR weekly [tiab] OR hour[tiab] OR hourly[tiab])) OR (before[tiab] AND after[tiab]) OR (before[tiab] AND during[tiab])) NOT (Editorial[ptyp] OR Letter[ptyp] OR Comment[ptyp] OR "Review" [ptyp] OR "Systematic Review"[ptyp]) NOT (animals[mh] NOT humans[mh])	
7	#6 AND English[lang]	662
8	#7 AND (("2013"[Date - Publication]: "3000"[Date - Publication]))	390

Database: APA PsycInfo

Set #		Results
1	DE "Affective Disorders" OR DE "Disruptive Mood Dysregulation Disorder" OR DE "Major Depression" OR DE "Persistent Depressive Disorder" OR DE "Premenstrual Dysphoric Disorder" OR DE "Seasonal Affective Disorder" OR DE "Social Isolation" OR DE "Patient Seclusion" OR DE "Loneliness" OR TI ("mood disorder" OR "mood disorders" OR "affective disorder" OR "affective disorders" OR depression OR depressive OR loneliness OR lonely OR "social isolation" OR "social exclusion") OR AB ("mood disorder" OR "mood disorders" OR "affective disorder" OR "affective disorders" OR depression OR depressive OR loneliness OR lonely OR "social isolation" OR "social exclusion")	
2	DE "HIV" OR DE "AIDS" OR TI (HIV OR "human immunodeficiency virus" OR AIDS OR "Acquired Immunodeficiency Syndrome") OR AB (HIV OR "human immunodeficiency virus" OR AIDS OR "Acquired Immunodeficiency Syndrome")	
3	DE "Sexual Minority Groups" OR DE "LGBTQ" OR DE "Asexuality" OR DE "Bisexuality" OR DE "Homosexuality" OR DE "Intersex" OR DE "Transgender" OR DE "Transsexualism" OR TI (LGBT OR LGBTI OR LGBTQ* OR GLBT OR GLBTQ OR bisexual OR bisexuals OR bisexuality OR homosexual OR homosexuals OR homosexuality OR gay OR gays OR intersex OR lesbian OR lesbianism OR lesbians OR "men having sex with men" OR "men who have sex with men" OR "men who have sex with other men" OR pansexual OR polysexual OR queer OR "sexual minorities" OR "sexual minority" OR "sexual and gender minority" OR "sexual and gender minorities" OR transgender* OR transsexual* OR transman OR "trans man" OR "trans men" OR transmen OR transsexualism OR transwoman OR "trans woman" OR "trans women" OR transwomen OR "two spirit" OR two-spirit OR "women who have sex with women" OR asexual OR asexuals OR asexuality OR nonbinary OR agender OR Bigender OR Genderqueer OR Gender-diverse OR "gender diverse" OR Gender-expansive OR "gender expansive" OR Same-gender-loving OR "same gender loving") OR AB (LGBT OR LGBTI OR LGBTQ* OR GLBT OR GLBTQ OR	

(continued on next page)

Set #		Results
(continued)		
	bisexual OR bisexuals OR bisexuality OR homosexual OR homosexuals OR homosexuality OR gay OR gays OR intersex OR lesbian OR lesbianism OR lesbians OR "men having sex with men" OR "men who have sex with men" OR "men who have sex with other men" OR pansexual OR polysexual OR queer OR "sexual minorities" OR "sexual minority" OR "sexual and gender minority" OR "sexual and gender minorities" OR transgender* OR transsexual* OR transman OR "trans man" OR "trans men" OR transmen OR transsexualism OR transwoman OR "trans woman" OR "trans women" OR transwomen OR "two spirit" OR two-spirit OR "women who have sex with women" OR asexual OR asexuals OR asexuality OR nonbinary OR agender OR Bigender OR Genderqueer OR Gender-diverse OR "gender diverse" OR Gender-expansive OR "gender expansive" OR Same-gender-loving OR "same gender loving")	
4	#1 AND #2 AND #3	1158
5	#4 NOT (TI (Adolescent OR Child OR Children OR Pediatric* OR Infant) NOT TI (Adult OR Adults))	1145
6	#5 AND (DE "Clinical Trials" OR DE "Cohort Analysis" OR DE "Followup Studies" OR DE "Longitudinal Studies" OR DE "Prospective Studies" OR TI (randomized OR randomised OR randomization OR randomisation OR placebo OR randomly OR trial OR groups OR "clinical trial" OR "clinical trials" OR "evaluation study" OR "evaluation studies" OR intervention OR interventions OR case-control OR cohort OR longitudinal OR longitudinally OR prospective OR prospectively OR retrospective OR "follow up" OR "comparative studies" OR nonrandom OR "non-random" OR nonrandomized OR "non-randomized" OR nonrandomised OR "non-randomised" OR quasi-experiment* OR quasiexperiment* OR quasirandom* OR quasi-random* OR quasi-control* OR quasicontrol* OR (controlled AND (trial OR study)) OR "pre-post" OR "posttest" OR "post-test" OR pretest OR pre-test OR ("time series" AND interrupt) OR ("time points" AND (multiple OR one OR two OR three OR four OR five OR six OR seven OR eight OR nine OR ten OR month OR monthly OR day OR daily OR week OR weekly OR hour OR hourly)) OR (before AND after) OR (before AND during) OR AB (randomized OR randomised OR randomization OR randomisation OR placebo OR randomly OR trial OR groups OR "clinical trial" OR "clinical trials" OR "evaluation study" OR "evaluation studies" OR intervention OR interventions OR case-control OR cohort OR longitudinal OR longitudinally OR prospective OR prospectively OR retrospective OR "follow up" OR "comparative studies" OR nonrandom OR "non-random" OR nonrandomized OR "non-randomized" OR nonrandomised OR "non-randomised" OR quasi-experiment* OR quasiexperiment* OR quasirandom* OR quasi-random* OR quasi-control* OR quasicontrol* OR (controlled AND (trial OR study)) OR "pre-post" OR "posttest" OR "post-test" OR pretest OR pre-test OR ("time series" AND interrupt) OR ("time points" AND (multiple OR one OR two OR three OR four OR five OR six OR seven OR eight OR nine OR ten OR month OR monthly OR day OR daily OR week OR weekly OR hour OR hourly)) OR (before AND after) OR (before AND during)) NOT (DE "Literature Review" OR DE "Meta Analysis" OR TI ("meta-analysis" OR "meta-analyses" OR "systematic review" OR "systematic reviews" OR editorial))	797
7	#6 AND Narrow by Language: - english	788
8	#7 AND Limiters - Publication Year: 2013–2023	423
9	#8 AND Source Types: Academic Journals	350

Cancer Prevention and Screening for People Living with Human Immunodeficiency Virus

Melody Wilkinson, DNP, APRN, FNP-C*,
Karen McCrea, DNP, APRN, FNP-C, Amy Culbertson, DNP, APRN, FNP-BC

KEYWORDS

- Human immunodeficiency virus • Cancer • Prevention • Screening • Guidelines

KEY POINTS

- Due to improvements in treatment for human immunodeficiency virus (HIV), people living with HIV (PLWH) now have an improved life expectancy and increased risks of developing cancer.
- Effective management of HIV decreases the risk of developing some cancers.
- Cancer screening and prevention in PLWH improves health outcomes.
- Multiple cancer screening guidelines for the general population and a lack of HIV-specific cancer screening guidelines can complicate clinical decision-making.
- Health care providers must remain aware of current cancer screening recommendations for PLWH.

INTRODUCTION

People living with human immunodeficiency virus (HIV) (PLWH) have near-normal life expectancies and now experience more non-HIV–related comorbidities and deaths due to advances in antiretroviral therapy (ART) which has become more effective and less toxic.[1–3] Due to the increase in life expectancy, HIV is now considered a chronic disease. It is essential that health care providers effectively promote well-being, prevent future disease, and manage comorbidities across the lifespan in order to optimize the health and longevity of this population.[1,4]

Cancer is the leading cause of death worldwide.[5] PLWH are diagnosed with cancer more often and experience worse cancer-related health outcomes than the general population.[2] They are at increased risk of developing both HIV/acquired immunodeficiency syndrome (AIDS)–defining cancers (ADCs) as well as non-HIV/AIDS-defining cancers

School of Nursing, Georgetown University, 3700 Reservoir Road, Washington, DC 20057, USA
* Corresponding author.
E-mail address: mrw83@georgetown.edu

(NADCs).[6] Cancer prevention and screening in PLWH is essential and leads to earlier diagnosis and treatment, resulting in improved health outcomes and increases long-term survival.[1,7,8]

BACKGROUND

There are approximately 38.4 million PLWH worldwide and the numbers increase annually with 1.5 million people newly diagnosed with HIV in 2021.[9] Of those living with HIV, 1.6 million reside in North America. This number includes the estimated 13% of PLWH who are not yet diagnosed.[9–11]

Identifying the precise incidence of cancer among PLWH is difficult due to incomplete cancer and HIV data registries. However, multiple population-based studies are consistent in their findings. These large cohort studies demonstrate year-over-year declines in cancer rates among PLWH while also finding that PLWH continue to experience higher rates of cancer than the general population.[1,2,8,12] Since advances in ART have led to increased life expectancies in individuals with HIV, the types of cancers seen in PLWH are more closely aligned with the general population.[1,2,12]

While treatment with ART results in a decreased incidence of ADC, the incidence of ADC remains higher in PLWH than the general population. According to the American Cancer Society (ACS),[13] PLWH are 500 times more likely to be diagnosed with Kaposi's sarcoma (KS), 12 times more likely to be diagnosed with non-Hodgkins lymphoma, and 3 times more likely to be diagnosed with cervical cancer. As PLWH live longer, they are also at an increased risk of developing NADC. They develop anal, liver, lung, and oral/pharynx cancer as well as Hodgkin lymphoma at higher rates than the general population.[1,8,13] In addition to experiencing an increased risk of developing cancer, PLWH are also more likely to experience treatment complications, disease relapse, and death.[7,13,14]

HUMAN IMMUNODEFICIENCY VIRUS AND CANCER

Replicating HIV virus impacts nearly every system in the body. It causes (1) decreased cell-mediated immunity, (2) direct tissue damage, and (3) systemic indirect tissue damage.[15] This leads to the development of end-organ damage, opportunistic infections, and malignancy. These risk factors can be mitigated by early and effective ART.[2]

Independent risk factors for PLWH developing cancer include male gender, older age, low CD4 count, previous NADCs, no ART, and early ART treatment initiated in the year 2000 or prior.[7] The risks of developing ADCs are associated with late-stage HIV diagnosis, CD4 count less than 200 cells/m^3 after 6 months on ART, low CD4 count nadir, and long periods of having a low CD4 count.[7] All risk factors for PLWH significantly increase with age.[15] PLWH are twice as likely as the general population to develop NADCs, even when they are taking appropriate and effective ART. In large part, this is due to the increased risks associated with developing malignancies related to oncogenic viruses, which occur 5 times more frequently in PLWH than in the general population.[2,12]

In addition to biological factors, social determinants of health and lifestyle behaviors also contribute to cancer risks. Social determinants of health such as access to health care, insurance status, income levels, and education are associated with utilization of appropriate health screenings and improved HIV disease management.[14] PLWH have increased barriers in accessing health care services and are disproportionately impacted by health inequity. Diet, physical inactivity, tobacco use, and alcohol consumption increase the risk of developing cancer in all people.[5] PLWH have higher rates of tobacco and alcohol use, further increasing their risk of cancer.[1,2]

ACQUIRED IMMUNODEFICIENCY SYNDROME–DEFINING CANCERS

KS, B-cell non-Hodgkin lymphoma, and invasive cervical cell carcinoma are classified as ADCs.[9,11] KS and B-cell non-Hodgkin lymphoma are diagnosed solely on clinical presentation. While screening guidelines do not exist for these cancers, they are available for cervical cancer.[3,11] It is imperative that providers caring for PLWH understand how to assess for and diagnose ADC. These cancers occur at a much higher rate in PLWH (**Fig. 1**).[14]

As HIV progresses, the immune system deteriorates, and once latent, viruses can lead to illness and the development of cancers. While all 3 of the ADCs are oncogenic in nature, some NADCs are also caused by the reactivation of viruses (**Table 1**).[2,9,11,12,15] The symbiotic nature of HIV and other viruses underscores the importance of early HIV diagnosis and effective ART to suppress HIV.

NON-ACQUIRED IMMUNODEFICIENCY SYNDROME–DEFINING CANCERS

NADCs are a mixture of oncogenic and solid-organ tumors. The most common NADCs in PLWH are lung, anal, head and neck, liver, prostate, kidney, and lymphatic system.[7] Lung and anal cancer represent close to half of NADCs in this population. Interestingly, stomach, colorectal, kidney, uterus, prostate, breast, brain, and thyroid cancers have lower incidences in PLWH than the general population.[12] This phenomenon is not fully understood and is not solely explained by potential increased screening that may exist for patients engaged in HIV treatment. Researchers speculate that this may be due to potential antineoplastic properties of ART or from the virus itself (see **Fig. 1**).[12]

While PLWH experience increased incidence of cancer, there are very few specific screening or treatment guidelines for this population. PLWH are often excluded from clinical trials, limiting HIV-specific cancer screening, prevention, and treatment

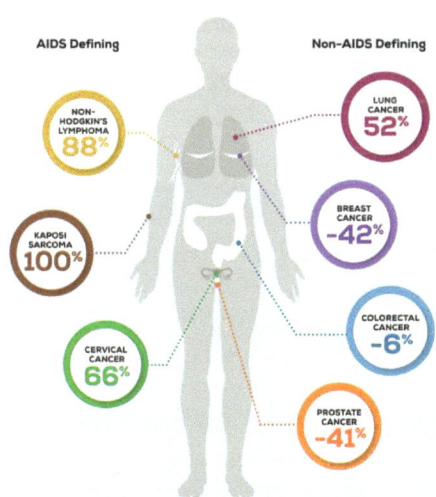

Fig. 1. Excess risk of cancers among people living with human immunodeficiency virus (PLWH) in the United States. Corrigan, K.L., Wall, K.C., Bartlett, J.A. and Suneja, G. (2019), Cancer disparities in people with HIV: A systematic review of screening for non-AIDS–defining malignancies. Cancer, 125: 843-853. https://doi.org/10.1002/cncr.31838.

Table 1
Oncogenic cancers

Cancer	Virus	Definition
Kaposi's sarcoma	Human herpesvirus-8	ADC
B-cell non-Hodgkin lymphoma	Epstein-Barr virus	ADC
Cervical cell carcinoma	Human papillomavirus 16 & 18	ADC
Squamous cell carcinoma	Human papillomavirus 16 & 18	NADC
Anal cell carcinoma	Human papillomavirus 16 & 18	NADC
Liver adenocarcinoma	Hepatitis B virus, hepatitis C virus	NADC
Smooth muscle tumor	Epstein-Barr virus	NADC
Oropharyngeal	Human papillomavirus 16 & 18	NADC
Colorectal cancer	JC virus	NADC

Abbreviations: ADC, acquired immunodeficiency syndrome–defining cancer; JC virus, John Cunningham virus; NADC, non-acquired immunodeficiency syndrome–defining cancer.

recommendations.[12] It is imperative that providers understand best practices in cancer prevention and screening and apply standard of care when caring for PLWH.

CANCER PREVENTION AND SCREENING FOR PEOPLE LIVING WITH HUMAN IMMUNODEFICIENCY VIRUS

Public health efforts focus on decreasing the incidence of cancer as well as mitigating the burden that cancer causes for individuals, families, and communities. These efforts are reflected in comprehensive population-health strategies that include primary, secondary, and tertiary cancer prevention measures (**Fig. 2**). Primary prevention focuses on preventing cancer, secondary prevention focuses on screening and early identification of pre-cancer and cancer, while tertiary strategies focus on improving quality of life and mitigating long-term impacts of cancer.[9,16–18]

For PLWH, good adherence with ART and effective management of HIV disease are paramount. Other primary cancer prevention strategies mirror those of the general population and focus on behavioral, lifestyle, and environmental risk reduction and

Primary Prevention	Secondary	Tertiary Prevention
Tobacco free living	Cancer Screening	Cancer symptom management
Limit alcohol	Early cancer identification	Palliative Care
Improve nutrition & exercise	Early cancer treatment	
Maintain healthy weight	Early treatment of HBV and HCV	
Decrease UV light exposure		
Minimize ionized		

Fig. 2. Cancer prevention strategies. HBV, hepatitis B virus; HCV, hepatitis C virus; UV, ultraviolet.

protective therapeutics.[9,17–19] These are strategies that all health care providers should routinely integrate into health promotion and disease prevention approaches when caring for PLWH. Behavior modification can be challenging for patients and implementing strategies such as motivational interviewing can be effective for helping individuals identify why change is important and to invest in the process. While lifestyle changes can help decrease the development of cancer, they will not stop the development of all cancers.[19]

After exposure to carcinogens, cancer may take years to develop which creates opportunities for early detection of pre-cancer and cancer.[17] Routine cancer screening can identify abnormalities that suggest specific pre-cancer or cancer in individuals not yet experiencing symptoms.[5] This allows for prompt diagnosis and treatment. Early intervention may offer opportunities to stagnate the cancer, inhibit or reverse carcinogens, or remove cancerous lesions. However, it is also important to recognize that there are potential harms associated with implementing population-based screening recommendations, such as false-positive screening results, unnecessary biopsy, and overdiagnosis.[18]

Screening guidelines are typically developed by international and national organizations or governmental agencies. HIV-specific cancer screening guidelines exist for cervical and HIV-specific recommendations exist for anal cancer.[3] However, most other cancer screening recommendations apply to the general population and do not address specific considerations for PLWH. In the absence of HIV-specific guidelines, primary care providers should follow evidence-based screening recommendations for the general population. In addition to cervical cancer, the most commonly screened for cancers in the primary care setting include breast, colorectal, lung, and prostate cancers.[16] Some cancers do not have screening guidelines for the general population but it is necessary to consider potential implications for PLWH due to their heightened risk.[3] A thorough literature review did not demonstrate a comprehensive set of cancer screening recommendations for PLWH. A detailed summary of evidence-based US, Canadian, and global cancer screening guidelines is included in **Table 2** and synthesized in the following sections.

CERVICAL CANCER

Cervical cancer ranks as the fourth most common cancer worldwide.[20–22] Invasive cervical cancer is an ADC and PLWH are up to 6 times more likely to be afflicted versus individuals without HIV.[21] The majority of cervical cancers are caused by the human papillomavirus (HPV) which is more prevalent in PLWH. HPV is more likely to persist and progress more rapidly to cervical cancer in the presence of HIV.[21,23]

Within the United States, 2 sets of guidelines exist to assist practitioners with clinical decision-making regarding cervical cancer screening in PLWH. These include the US Department of Health and Human Services (HHS) guidelines[21] and the Infectious Disease Society of America (IDSA) guidelines.[3] Both recommend screening at the time of HIV diagnosis and testing intervals vary depending on age and screening methodology of Pap/cytology versus HPV DNA. The 2 differ slightly with regards to the onset of screening and frequency of screening intervals. Both recommend screening cessation for patients who have undergone hysterectomy with cervix removal for noncancer related reasons.[20,23]

Guidelines differ globally. Canada lacks a national cervical cancer screening standard for PLWH. However, Cancer Care Ontario suggests immunocompromised persons receive Pap/cytology screening annually.[24–26] The World Health Organization (WHO)[22] offers more nuanced guidelines and recommends the starting age for screening occur later than what is recommended in the United States.

Table 2
Cancer screening recommendations for people living with human immunodeficiency virus

Cervical Cancer Screening for People Living with Human immunodeficiency virus

HHS (USA)	Initial screening
	  Age 21
	Screening at diagnosis
	  Ages 21–29: Annually with Pap/cytology testing until 3 consecutive negative tests, then every 3 y
	  Ages 30 and over: Annually with Pap/cytology alone OR Pap/cytology with HPV DNA test until 3 negative tests, then every 3 y
	Screening after diagnosis
	  Ages 21–29: Pap/cytology only—every 3 y (HPV/DNA not recommended in this age group).
	  Ages 30 and over: Pap/cytology only—every 3 y OR Pap/cytology and HPV DNA—every 3 y.
	When to stop screening
	  Stop with hysterectomy for benign reasons.
	  If no hysterectomy, continue screening throughout the woman's lifetime with consideration of factors such as life expectancy.

IDSA (USA)	Initial screening
	  Onset of sexual activity; no later than age 21
	Screening at diagnosis:
	  Ages 21–29: Annually with Pap/cytology testing until 3 consecutive negative tests, then every 3 y
	  Ages 30 and over: Annually with Pap/cytology alone until 3 negative tests, then every 3 y.
	  If Pap/cytology and HPV DNA and receive a negative result once, can go to every 3 y.
	Screening after diagnosis
	  Ages 21–29: Pap/cytology only—every 3 y (HPV/DNA—no recommendation in this age group).
	  Ages 30 and over: Pap/cytology only OR Pap/cytology and HPV DNA—every 3 y
	When to stop screening
	  Stop with hysterectomy for benign reasons.
	  No recommended age to stop screening.

CCO (Canada)	Screening with Pap/cytology yearly

WHO (Global)	Initial screening
	  Age 25
	Screening at diagnosis
	  No recommendations
	Screening after diagnosis
	  Ages 25–49 (should be given priority for screening): Pap/cytology or VIA alone—every 3 y OR Pap/cytology and HPV DNA—every 3–5 y.
	  Ages 50–65 without cervical cancer screening history: Pap/cytology or VIA alone—every 3 y until 2 consecutive negative results OR Pap/cytology and HPV DNA—every 3–5 y until 2 consecutive negative results.
	When to stop screening
	  Over age 50 with 2 consecutive negative results

(continued on next page)

Table 2 (continued)	
Anal cancer screening for PLWH	
IDSA (USA)	DARE annually Can use anal cytology for those who practice receptive anal sex, but only if access to follow-up care and HRA if abnormalities found. No periodicity is given for anal cytology.
HHS (USA)	DARE annually Can use anal cytology for those who practice receptive anal sex, but only if access to follow-up care and HRA if abnormalities found. No periodicity is given for anal cytology.
NYSDHAI (USA)	Under age 35: DARE if complain of symptoms. Age 35 or older: Ask about symptoms, perform a visual inspection and DARE (annually and if symptoms present) May perform cytology annually in those ages 35 and older May stop screening if limited life expectancy (<10 y) and/or if there are 2 consecutive negative cytology screens in those who are not sexually active.
EACS (European)	Digital rectal examination every 1–3 y with or without cytology in HIV positive MSM (high-risk PLWH)
IANS (Global)	DARE for high-risk PLWH individuals annually
Breast cancer screening via mammography for PLWH	
USPSTF (USA)	Ages 40–74: Every 2 y
ACS (USA)	Ages 40–44: Risk/benefit discussion Ages 45–54: Annually Ages 55+: Every 2 y Continue as long as the woman is in good health and expected to live 10 y or longer.
CTFPH (Canada)	Ages 40–49: Not routinely recommended/shared decision-making Ages 50–74: Every 2–3 y (Ages 70–74 can be shared decision-making)
CCS (Canada)	Ages 40–49: Risk/benefit discussion Ages 50–74: Every 2 y Ages 75 and older: Risk/benefit discussion
WHO (Global)	Well-resourced areas: Ages 40–49: Only through shared decision-making in the context of rigorous research program Ages 50–69: Every 2 y Ages 70–75: Only through shared decision-making in the context of rigorous research program Limited-resourced areas: Ages 50–69 only: Every 2 y Limited-resourced areas and weak health care: Prioritize symptomatic women Consider clinical breast examination
Colorectal cancer screening for the general population at average risk	
USPSTF (USA)	Ages 45–75 Choose one option through shared-decision making: gFOBT—Yearly FIT—Yearly sDNA-FIT—Every 1–3 y Flexible sigmoidoscopy—Every 5 y CT colonography—Every 5 y Colonoscopy—Every 10 y

(continued on next page)

Table 2 (continued)	
ACS (USA)	Ages 45–75 Choose one option through shared-decision making: gFOBT—Yearly FIT— Yearly sDNA-FIT—Every 1–3 y Flexible sigmoidoscopy—Every 5 y CT colonography—Every 5 y Colonoscopy—Every 10 y
CCS (Canada)	Average risk: Ages 50–74 Choose one option through shared decision-making: gFOBT—Every 2 y FIT—Every 2 y
CTFPHC (Canada)	Average risk: Ages 50–74 Choose one option through shared decision-making: gFOBT—Every 2 y FIT—Every 2 y Flexible sigmoidoscopy—Every 10 y
WHO (Global)	Recommends screening—no specific parameters
Lung cancer screening for the general population	
USPSTF (USA)	Annual screening for ages 50–80 with at least a 20 pack-year history who currently smoke or have quit in the past 15 y. Screening stops at age 81 or when the patient has stopped smoking for 15 y.
ACS (USA)	Annual screening for ages 55–74 with at least a 30 pack-year history who currently smoke or have quit in the last 15 y. Screening stops at age 75 or when the patient has stopped smoking for 15 y.
CPTFHC (Canada)	Screen at least 3 consecutive times ages 55–74 with at least a 30 pack-year history who currently smoke or have quit in the last 15 y. Screening stops at age 75 or when the patient has stopped smoking for 15 y.
CCS (Canada)	Recommend following CPTFHC
Prostate cancer screening for the general population	
USPSTF (USA)	Men at average risk: Ages 55–69 y may have PSA screening if they express a desire with a risk/benefit discussion. No periodicity recommendations
ACS (USA)	Men at average risk: Ages 50 and older who are expected to live at least 10 years can screen with PSA or DRE with a risk/benefit discussion Follow-up depends upon PSA level: <2.5 ng/mL, retest every 2 y More than 2.5 mg/mL, retest annually
CTFPHC (Canada)	Recommends against screening.
CCS (Canada)	Men at average risk: Age 50 or older can consider PSA testing with risk/benefit discussion Follow-up testing depends upon results individualized based on results
WHO (Global)	No recommendations
Liver cancer screening for PLWH	
AASLD (USA)	Screen high-risk every 6 mo with both u/s and AFP

(continued on next page)

Table 2 (continued)	
CASL/AMMI (Canada)	Screen hepatitis B patients coinfected with HIV every 6 mo with u/s. Does not recommend AFP levels
Other global recommendations	Screen high-risk patients every 6 mo with u/s

Abbreviations: AASLD, American Association for the Study of Liver Diseases; ACS, American Cancer Society; AFP, alpha-fetoprotein; CASL/AMMI, Canadian Association for the Study of the Liver and Association of Medical Microbiology and Infectious Disease; CCO, Cancer Care Ontario; CCS, Canadian Cancer Society; CT, computed tomography; CTFPH, Canadian Task Force on Preventive Health; CTFPHC, Canadian Task Force on Preventive Health Care; DARE, digital anal rectal exam; DNA, deoxyribonucleic acid; DRE, digital rectal exam; EACS, European AIDS Clinical Society; FIT, fecal immunochemical test; gFOBT, guaiac fecal occult blood test; HHS, US Department of Health and Human Services; HIV, human immunodeficiency virus; HPV, human papillomavirus; HRA, high-resolution anoscopy; IANS, International Anal Neoplasia Society; IDSA, Infectious Diseases Society of America; NYSDHAI, New York State Department of Health AIDS Institute; PLWH, people living with human immunodeficiency virus; PSA, prostate-specific antigen; sDNA-FIT, multitarget stool DNA test with fecal immunochemical test; U/S, ultrasound; USPSTF, US Preventive Services Task Force; VIA, visual inspection with acetic acid; WHO, World Health Organization.

ANAL CANCER

Anal cancer is also often caused by HPV and is one of the most common NADCs in PLWH.[7,21,27–30] HIV-positive men who have sex with men (MSM) are at a 37-fold increased risk when compared to the general population.[31] While HIV-positive MSM have the highest risk of anal cancer, all PLWH are at an increased risk, especially those who practice receptive anal sex, have abnormal cervical Pap results, or have anogenital warts.[32]

There is no national consensus regarding anal cancer screening in PLWH in the United States or Canada; however, several organizations have created clinical practice recommendations. Although not standardized, these typically include digital anal rectal exam (DARE) and the use of cytology for individuals at high risk but only if high resolution anoscopy is available for follow-up. Identifying and treating anal high-grade squamous intraepithelial lesions has been proven to reduce the risk of progression to anal cancer by up to 57% when compared to active monitoring.[33] While the screening recommendations are inconsistent, the research is compelling and highlights the importance of screening and early intervention.

The IDSA and HHS screening recommendations for PLWH are nearly identical with both recommending DARE for all PLWH annually.[3,20] The New York State Department of Health AIDS Institute guidelines are more detailed and include age parameters.[34] Additional recommendations are available from the Canadian Agency for Drugs and Technology in Health,[29] European AIDS Clinical Society,[35] and the International Anal Neoplasia Society.[36] The WHO offers a risk-based scale that practitioners can use when assessing patient risk.[28]

BREAST CANCER

Breast cancer is an NADC, and PLWH are more likely to experience abnormal presentations, be diagnosed at advanced stages, and experience poorer outcomes, relapse or death compared to people without HIV.[2,3,27,37] Despite the difference in disease presentation and progression, the actual incidence of breast cancer rates in PLWH is lower when compared to the general population.[2,14,27,37–39] Some estimate that

PLWH experience lower breast cancer rates, at approximately 40% to 50% of the population of people without HIV.[14,38] While it is unclear why this phenomenon occurs, it is speculated that ART may play a role in decreasing the development of some cancers.[12] The breast cancer screening recommendations for PLWH are the same as for the general population.[3]

In the United States, there are several national guidelines, which differ slightly but generally recommend that screening with mammogram begin at the age of 40 and conclude at age 74.[13,40] There are also multiple screening guidelines internationally that recommend screening begin at age 50. The Canadian Task Force on Preventive Health[41] and the Canadian Cancer Society (CCS)[42] both recommend breast cancer screening for women aged 50 to 74. As per the WHO,[43] global screening should be directed based on locally available resources, with priority given to screening women aged 50 to 69 every 2 years.

COLORECTAL CANCER

Colorectal cancer (CRC) is the third most common cancer worldwide.[44] Despite its common occurrence in the general population, as with breast cancer, this NADC has been found to occur at lower rates in PLWH.[2,38,45] These rates are predicted to stay the same or to further decrease in the United States by 2030.[2] Therefore, the CRC screening recommendations for PLWH are the same as for the general population.[3,14,28,38,44]

Within the United States, the US Preventive Services Task Force (USPSTF)[46] and ACS[47] both provide recommendations for CRC screening. For those at average risk of colon cancer, screening should start at age 45. The intervals of screening are dependent on the type of testing utilized. Both recommend routine screening end at age 75. Canadian recommendations from CCS[48] and Canadian Task Force on Preventive Health Care[49] suggest that screening begin at a later age. Of note, they do not recommend colonoscopy as a routine screening test. The WHO[50] recommends screening via stool samples but lacks specific guidance regarding periodicity.

LUNG CANCER

Of all the NADCs, lung cancer ranks as the most common and causes the most deaths in PLWH.[2,27,51,52] People with HIV are more likely to smoke which is considered a leading risk factor for developing lung cancer. However, when studies are controlled for smoking in PLWH, there is still a higher incidence of lung cancer.[7] Despite the increased incidence of lung cancer in this population, no national screening guidelines exist specifically for PLWH.

Organizations with primary care guidelines for the treatment of PLWH, such as IDSA, recommend following the USPSTF or the ACS guidelines.[3] Both organizations endorse using low-dose computed tomography and outline their recommendations based upon age, number of pack-years, years since quitting smoking, and end-screening age. Canadian guidelines align closely with the US guidelines but differ in the frequency of screening intervals.[53,54] There are no global guidelines; however, some individual countries have created their own.[55]

PROSTATE CANCER

Similar to colon and breast cancer, prostate cancer is an NADC that occurs at lower rates in PLWH versus the general population.[2,14,27,38,56] The lower incidence persists even after researchers account for decrease in testosterone levels and decreased prostate cancer screenings in PLWH.[38,56] As with other cancers in PLWH, prostate cancer is associated with increased morbidity and mortality than in the general population.[27] It is projected to be one of the most common cancers in PLWH by 2030.[2] There are no HIV-specific screening guidelines for prostate cancer.[3]

US guidelines recommend screening based on risk and patient preference with some differences in age of initiation and screening frequency.[57,58] Canadian guidelines vary from suggesting not screening to screening based on risks versus benefits.[59,60] While several additional countries have individual prostate screening guidelines, there are no global recommendations.

LIVER CANCER

Liver cancer is an NADC affecting PLWH in greater numbers than the general population. It is predicted to be the third most common cancer in PLWH by 2030.[2] PLWH have a higher incidence of hepatitis B and C virus infection which predispose patients to cirrhosis.[3,27] It is estimated that 85% to 95% of patients with cirrhosis of the liver will develop hepatocellular cancer (HCC).[61] Additionally, PLWH are more likely to use tobacco which has also been linked to the development of HCC.[27]

It is essential that providers screen all PLWH for viral hepatitis coinfection and offer treatment if indicated. This identifies patients who may benefit from preventive hepatitis B vaccination. For patients living with hepatitis B and C, they may benefit from additional screening tests for HCC. Recommendations in the United States and abroad call for screening every 6 months with ultrasound. They vary regarding the use of alpha-fetoprotein tests.[3,62,63] Early and consistent treatment of HIV and concurrent treatment of viral hepatitis, if present, results in a decreased risk for cancer development and better health outcomes.[27,61]

OROPHARYNGEAL CANCER

Risk factors for developing head and neck cancers in PLWH mimic those of the general population, but the incidence of developing head and neck cancer is elevated.[64] Risk factors include tobacco use, alcohol consumption, and exposure to HPV.[7,64] Currently, there are no national or international guidelines or general consensus related to oropharyngeal cancer screening. PLWH who present with symptoms concerning for oropharyngeal cancer should be referred promptly for evaluation.

IMPLICATIONS FOR PRACTICE

PLWH face increased risk of developing some cancers and associated morbidities and mortalities.[2] High-quality primary and specialty care can help to prevent and mitigate cancer risks and outcomes. It is imperative to identify and screen patients appropriately for HIV. Early diagnosis, referral, and treatment initiation for HIV result in improved health outcomes and decreased risk of developing cancer. Care providers should emphasize primary health promotion and disease prevention education which include discussions about the role of diet, exercise, smoking cessation, alcohol intake, condomless sex and vaccinations in cancer prevention and overall well-being. Key vaccinations that decrease cancer risk include HPV and hepatitis B.[3]

Once a positive HIV status is confirmed, every effort should be made to collaborate between primary and specialty care to optimize health outcomes and decrease complications. All barriers to care access should be explored and addressed in an effort to retain PLWH in active disease treatment and management. PLWH have significantly increased life expectancies due to improved ART. This longevity contributes to increased cancer risk. Primary and specialty care providers need to communicate effectively to ensure that all PLWH receive up-to-date, evidence-based cancer screenings, determining which individuals should be screened, how they should be screened, and at what intervals can be daunting. Multiple guidelines from various national and international organizations differ in their recommendations, potentially causing confusion for both the provider and patient.

Following evidence-based guidelines with earlier screening initiation and increased screening intervals may be one way to improve cancer detection. Conversely, earlier and more frequent screenings may lead to increased stress related to testing anxiety, false-positive findings, and increased financial burden. Ultimately, the decision of when and how often to screen for various cancers in PLWH should be determined through mutual goal-setting. This requires a relationship of mutual respect and trust between the patient and provider and necessitates that the provider be familiar with and conversant about differing recommendations and guidelines.

Guidelines are constantly being revised and updated based on new and evolving evidence. In order to provide high-quality care to PLWH, it is the responsibility of the provider to remain updated with the latest recommendations. This can be accomplished by reading evidence-based journals, attending conferences, subscribing to newsletters and email feeds, and routinely visiting organizational Web sites. Every clinic should have a system in place to disseminate new and relevant information related to optimal patient care.

SUMMARY

Early identification and effective treatment of HIV is the most important factor in improving cancer-related outcomes for PLWH. Primary and secondary prevention are tools to enhance health, decrease cancer risks, and detect cancer in earlier stages and should be implemented routinely. While there are variations among the cancer-screening recommendations, providers should partner with patients in a model of shared decision-making to improve health outcomes and implement appropriate cancer screenings.

CLINICS CARE POINTS

- Screen all individuals for HIV as per recommended guidelines.
- Refer all PLWH to specialty care for early initiation of HIV treatment.
- Treat underlying health conditions that increase the risk of cancer for PLWH.
- Facilitate communication between primary care and specialty care.
- Remain up-to-date on cancer screening recommendations and guidelines for PLWH.
- Through shared decision-making, screen all PLWH for cancers as appropriate.

DISCLOSURE

The authors declare that they have no commercial or financial interests that relate to the content in this article.

REFERENCES

1. Lee SO, Lee JE, Lee S, et al. Nationwide population-based incidence of cancer among patients with HIV/AIDS in South® Korea. Sci Rep 2022;12. https://doi.org/10.1038/s41598-022-14170-5.
2. Shiels MS, Islam JY, Rosenberg PS, et al. Projected cancer incidence rates and burden on incident cancer cases in HIV-infected adults in the United States through 2030. Ann Intern Med 2018;168(12). https://doi.org/10.7326/M17-2499.
3. Thompson AM, Horberg MA, Agwu AL, et al. Primary care guidance for persons with Human Immunodeficiency Virus: 2020 update by the HIV Medicine Association of the Infectious Diseases Society of America. Clin Infect Dis 2021;73(11): e3572–605.
4. Wilkinson M, Biernacki P, Knestrick J. HIV in primary care: Case study of common chronic comorbidities. J Nurse Pract 2022;18:525–8.
5. World Health Organization (WHO). Cancer. https://www.who.int/health-topics/cancer . Updated 2023. Accessed August 22, 2023.
6. National Cancer Institute (NCI). Cancer. US Department of Health and Human Services National Institutes of Health. http://www.cancer.gov . Accessed August 22, 2023.
7. Chiu CG, Smith D, Salters KA, et al. Overview of cancer incidence and mortality among people living with HIV/AIDS in British Columbia, Canada: Implications for HAART use and NADM development. BMC Cancer 2017;17(270). https://doi.org/10.1186/s12885-017-3229-1.
8. Hernandez-Ramirez RU, Shiels MS, Dubrow R, et al. Spectrum of cancer risk among HIV-infected people in the United States during the modern antiretroviral therapy era: a population-based registry linkage study. Lancet HIV 2017;4(11): e495–504.
9. World Health Organization (WHO). HIV. https://www.who.int/health-topics/hiv-aids . Updated 2023. Accessed August 22, 2023.
10. Government of Canada. HIV and AIDS. https://www.canada.ca/en/public-health/services/diseases/hiv-aids.html . Accessed August 22, 2023.
11. Centers for Disease Control and Prevention (CDC). Evidence of HIV treatment and viral suppression in preventing the sexual transmission of HIV. Centers for Disease Control and Prevention; 2022. Available at: https://www.cdc.gov/hiv/risk/art/evidence-of-hiv-treatment.html. Accessed August 22, 2023.
12. Shmakova A, Gemini D, Vassetzky Y. HIV-1, HAART and cancer: a complex relationship. Int J Cancer 2019;146:2666–79.
13. American Cancer Society (ACS). HIV infection and cancer. https://www.cancer.org/cancer/risk-prevention/infections/hiv-infection-aids.html. Updated 2023. Accessed August 22, 2023.
14. Corrigan KL, Wall KC, Bartlett JA, et al. Cancer disparities in people with HIV: a systematic review of screening for non-AIDS-defining malignancies. Cancer 2019;125(6):843–53.
15. Lucas S, Nelson AM. HIV and the spectrum of human disease. J Pathol 2015;235: 229–41.
16. National Comprehensive Cancer Control Program (NCCCP). https://www.cdc.gov/cancer/ncccp/index.htm . Centers for Disease Control and Prevention (CDC). Updated July 12, 2023. Accessed August 22, 2023.
17. Looman-Kroop HA, Umar A. CAncer prevention and screening: the next step in the era of precision medicine. npj Precis Oncol 2019;3:3.

18. Nagai K, Saito AM, Saito TI, et al. Reporting quality of randomized controlled trials in patients with HIV on antiretroviral therapy: a systematic review. Trials 2017; 18:625.

19. Rock CL, Thompson C, Gansler T, et al. American Cancer Society guideline for diet and physical activity for cancer prevention. CA:A Journal for Clinicians 2020;70(4):245–71.

20. United States Health and Human Services (HHS). Guidelines for the prevention and treatment of opportunistic infections in adults and adolescents with HIV. https://clinicalinfo.hiv.gov/en/guidelines/hiv-clinical-guidelines-adult-and-adolescent-opportunistic-infections/human-0 . Accessed August 22, 2023.

21. World Health Organization (WHO). New WHO recommendations on screening and treatment to prevent cervical cancer among women living with HIV. 2021. https://www.who.int/publications/i/item/9789240030961 . Accessed August 22, 2023.

22. Sung H, Ferlay J, Siegel R, et al. Global cancer statistics 2020: GLOBOCAN estimates of incidence and mortality worldwide for 36 cancers in 185 countries. CA Cancer J Clin 2021;71(3):209–49.

23. Chapman CL, Harris AL. Cervical cancer screening for women living with HIV. Nurs Womens Health 2016;20(4):392–8.

24. Cancer Care of Ontario (CCO). Cervical cancer FAQs for healthcare providers. https://www.cancercareontario.ca/en/guidelines-advice/cancer-continuum/screening/resources-healthcare-providers/cervical-screening-faqs#ui-accordion-9-header-0 . Accessed August 28, 2023.

25. Hosein, SR. Delays in cervical cancer screening among some HIV-positive Canadian women. 2019. Canadian AIDS Treatment Information Exchange. https://www.catie.ca/catie-news/delays-in-cervical-cancer-screening-among-some-hiv-positive-canadian-women. Accessed August 28, 2023.

26. De Pokomandy A, Burchell AN, Salters K, et al. Cervical cancer screening among women living with HIV: a cross-sectional study using the baseline questionnaire data from the Canadian HIV Women's Sexual and Reproductive Health Cohort Study (CHIWOS). CMAJ Open 2019;7(2):E217–26.

27. Chiao EY, Coghill A, Kizub D, et al. The effect of non-AIDS-defining cancers on people living with HIV. Lancet Oncol 2021;22(6):e240–53.

28. Clifford GM, Georges D, Shiels MS, et al. A meta-analysis of anal cancer incidence by risk group: towards a unified anal cancer risk scale. Int J Cancer 2020;148(1):38–47.

29. Canadian Agency for Drugs and Technology in Health (CADTH). Anal cancer screening in high-risk populations; a review of the clinical utility, diagnostic accuracy, cost-effectiveness, and guidelines. Ottawa, CA: CADTH Rapid Response Report: Summary With Critical Appraisal; 2019. p. 1922–8147 (online).

30. American Cancer Society. Risk factors for anal cancer. https://www.cancer.org/cancer/types/anal-cancer/causes-risks-prevention/risk-factors.html . Published 2020. Accessed August 28, 2023.

31. Colon-Lopez V, Shiels MS, Machin M, et al. Anal cancer risk among people with HIV infection in the United States. J Clin Oncol 2018;36(1):68–75.

32. Albuquerque A, Rios E, Schmitt F. Recommendations favoring anal cytology as a method for anal cancer screening: a systematic review. Cancers 2019;11(12):1942.

33. Palefsky JM, Lee JY, Jay N, et al. Treatment of anal high-grade squamous intraepithelial lesions to prevent anal cancer. N Engl J Med 2022;386(24):2273–82.

34. New York State Department of Health AIDS Institute (NYSDHAI). Screening for anal disease. https://www.hivguidelines.org/guideline/hiv-anal-cancer/?mycollection=hpv-care#tab_3 Reviewed 9 Aug 2022. Accessed August 28, 2023.

35. European AIDS Clinical Society (EACS). EACS guidelines 2022 version 11.1. https://www.eacsociety.org/guidelines/eacs-guidelines/Published 2022. Accessed August 28, 2023.

36. Hillman RJ, Berry-Lawhorn JM, Ong JJ, et al. International Anal Neoplasia Society (IANS) guidelines for the practice of digital anal rectal examination. J Lower Gennital Tract Dis 2019;23(2):138–46.

37. D'Andrea F, Ceccarelli M, Facciolà A, et al. Breast cancer in women living with HIV. Eur Rev Med Pharmacol Sci 2019;23(3):1158–64.

38. Coghill AE, Engels EA, Schymura MJ, et al. Risk of breast, prostate, and colorectal cancer diagnoses among HIV-infected individuals in the United States. J Natl Cancer Inst 2018;110(9):959–66.

39. Coburn SB, Shiels MS, Silverberg MJ, et al. Secular trends in breast cancer risk among women with HIV initiating ART in North America. J Acquir Immune Defic Syndr 2021;87(1):663–70.

40. United States Preventive Services Task Force (USPSTF). Breast cancer: screening. https://www.uspreventiveservicestaskforce.org/uspstf/draft-recommendation/breast-cancer-screening-adults . Updated May 9, 2023. Accessed August 28, 2023.

41. Canadian Task Force on Preventive Health Care (CTFPH). Breast cancer update (2018). https://canadiantaskforce.ca/guidelines/published-guidelines/breast-cancer-update/Updated 2018. Accessed August 28, 2023.

42. Canadian Cancer Society (CCS). Screening for breast cancer. https://cancer.ca/en/cancer-information/cancer-types/breast/screening#:~:text=If%20you%20are%2050%20to,mammogram%20is%20right%20for%20you Updated 2023. Accessed August 28, 2023.

43. World Health Organization (WHO). WHO position paper on mammography screening. https://www.who.int/publications/i/item/who-position-paper-on-mammography-screening Published Feb 16, 2014, Accessed August 28, 2023.

44. Xi Y, Xu P. Global colorectal cancer burden in 2020 and projections to 2040. Transl Oncol 2021;14(10). https://doi.org/10.1016/j.tranon.2021.101174.

45. Goedert JJ, Hosgood HD, Biggar RJ, et al. Screening for cancer in persons living with HIV infection. Trends Cancer 2016;2(8):416–28.

46. United States Preventive Services Task Force (USPSTF). Colorectal cancer: screening. https://www.uspreventiveservicestaskforce.org/uspstf/recommendation/colorectal-cancer-screening Updated May 18, 2021. Accessed August 28, 2023.

47. American Cancer Society (ACS). Colorectal cancer screening guidelines. https://www.cancer.org/health-care-professionals/american-cancer-society-prevention-early-detection-guidelines/colorectal-cancer-screening-guidelines.html Updated 2018. Accessed August 28, 2023.

48. Canadian Cancer Society (CCS). Screening for colorectal cancer. https://cancer.ca/en/cancer-information/cancer-types/colorectal/screening Updated 2023. Accessed August 28, 2023.

49. Canadian Task Force on Preventive Health Care (CTFPHC). Colorectal cancer-clinician recommendation table. https://canadiantaskforce.ca/tools-resources/colorectal-cancer-clinician-recommendation-table/Updated 2023. Accessed August 28, 2023.

50. World Health Organization (WHO). Colorectal cancer. https://www.who.int/news-room/fact-sheets/detail/colorectal-cancer Updated July 11, 2023. Accessed August 28, 2023.
51. Kong CY, Sigel K, Criss SD, et al. Benefits and harms of lung cancer screening in HIV-infected individuals with CD4+ cell count at least 500 cells/μl. AIDS 2018; 32(10):1333–42.
52. National Comprehensive Cancer Network (NCCN). NCCN clinical practice guidelines in oncology (NCCN Guidelines®) cancer in people with HIV. Version 1.2023. https://www.nccn.org/Accessed August 28, 2023.
53. Canadian Cancer Society (CCS). Lung cancer. https://cancer.ca/en/cancer-information/cancer-types/lung Reviewed May 2020. Accessed August 28, 2023.
54. Canadian Task Force on Preventive Health Care (CTFPHC). Lung cancer (2016). https://canadiantaskforce.ca/guidelines/published-guidelines/lung-cancer/ Reviewed 2023. Accessed August 28, 2023.
55. Pinsky P. Lung cancer screening with low-dose CT: a world-wide view. Transl Lung Cancer Res 2018;7(3):234–42.
56. Sun D, Cao M, Li H, et al. Risk of prostate cancer in men with HIV/AIDS: a systematic review and meta-analysis. Prostate Cancer Prostatic Dis 2021;24:24–34.
57. United States Preventive Services Task Force (USPSTF). Prostate cancer: screening. https://www.uspreventiveservicestaskforce.org/uspstf/recommendation/prostate-cancer-screening Updated May 8, 2018. Accessed August 28, 2023.
58. American Cancer Society (ACS). American Cancer Society recommendations for prostate cancer early detection. https://www.cancer.org/cancer/types/prostate-cancer/detection-diagnosis-staging/acs-recommendations.html Rvised Feb. 24, 2023. Accessed August 28, 2023.
59. Canadian Cancer Society. Prostate-specific antigen (PSA) test. https://cancer.ca/en/treatments/tests-and-procedures/prostate-specific-antigen-psa-test#:~:text=If%20you%20are%20at%20average,to%20be%20at%20high%20risk Reviewed 2023. Accessed August 28, 2023.
60. Canadian Task Force on Preventive Health Care (CTFPHC). Prostate cancer (2014). https://canadiantaskforce.ca/guidelines/published-guidelines/prostate-cancer/Reviewed 2023. Accessed August 28, 2023.
61. Yilmaz N, Yilmaz UE, Suer K, et al. Screening for hepatocellular carcinoma: summary of current guidelines up to 2018. Hepatoma Res 2018;4:46.
62. Singal AG, Llovet JM, Yarchoan M, et al. AASLD practice guidance on prevention, diagnosis and treatment of hepatocellular carcinoma. Hepatology 2023. https://doi.org/10.1097/HEP.0000000000000466.
63. Coffin CS, Fung SK, Alvarez A, et al. Management of Hepatitis B Virus (HBV) Infection: Executive Summary: 2018 Guidelines from the Canadian Association for the Study of the Liver (CASL) and Association of Medical Microbiology and Infectious Disease (AMMI) Canada. Can Liver J 2018;1(4):156–217.
64. D'Souza G, Carey TE, William WN Jr, et al. Epidemiology of head and neck squamous cell cancer among HIV-infected patients. J Acquir Immune Defic Syndr 2014;65(5):603–10.

Biomedical Approaches and Disparities in HIV Prevention

Jared Carter-Davis, AGNP-C, MSN, AAHIVS[a],*,
Ellen Seymour, AGNP-C, MSN, MPH, AAHIVS, DNP Candidate[b,1]

KEYWORDS

- Pre-exposure prophylaxis (PrEP) • PrEP disparities • HIV prevention • PrEP outlook
- PrEP initiation and management

KEY POINTS

- New human immunodeficiency virus (HIV) infections continue to occur in the United States, with certain groups disproportionately impacted.
- Oral and injectable pre-exposure prophylaxis (PrEP) is highly effective in preventing HIV and offers individuals at risk of acquiring HIV an opportunity to prevent infection.
- Significant disparities remain in PrEP access and uptake.
- Strategies to address this disparity must occur at the individual, provider, and system levels.

INTRODUCTION

Despite advances in human immunodeficiency virus (HIV) treatment since the start of the epidemic, HIV remains a public concern. HIV pre-exposure prophylaxis (PrEP) was first approved by the Food and Drug Administration (FDA) in 2012 and is highly efficacious in preventing HIV infection. Since its approval, uptake has steadily increased and directly contributed to decreased rates of new infections; however, blatant disparities remain. According to the US Centers for Disease Control and Prevention (CDC), the populations with the highest risk of HIV acquisition and highest rates of new infections have the lowest rates of PrEP use.[1] It is clear that the inequitable distribution of PrEP must be addressed. Nurses play a key role in increasing PrEP education, access, and uptake in these disparate populations, and have a meaningful impact on population outcomes. Therefore, it is imperative nurses are thoroughly educated on PrEP for HIV prevention. To that end, the objectives of this article are to describe the current

[a] Division of Infectious Diseases, East Carolina University, ECU Adult Specialty Care, 2390 Hemby Lane, Greenville, NC 27834, USA; [b] Access Community Health Network, 5401 South Wentworth Avenue, Chicago, IL 60609, USA
[1] Present address: 4135 DuBois Boulevard, Brookfield, IL 60513.
* Corresponding author. 2303 B Sweet Bay Drive, Greenville, NC 27834.
E-mail address: carterdavisj23@ecu.edu

Nurs Clin N Am 59 (2024) 289–296
https://doi.org/10.1016/j.cnur.2024.03.001
0029-6465/24/© 2024 Elsevier Inc. All rights reserved.

state of HIV and HIV prevention in the United States, identify people who could benefit from PrEP, discuss currently approved PrEP modalities and their guidelines, highlight current disparities in PrEP access and uptake, and discuss strategies for achieving equity in HIV prevention.

BACKGROUND

According to the CDC, there are approximately 1.2 million people living with HIV in the United States with 36,136 new infections in 2021.[2] Furthermore, it is estimated that 13% of people living with HIV are undiagnosed. Rates of new HIV infections remain disproportionately high in black men who have sex with men (MSM) (BMSM), LatinX MSM, and black women. BMSM remain the group with the highest rates of new HIV infections.[2]

HIV is a virus that is transmitted from 1 individual to another through blood, semen, vaginal secretions, anal secretions, and breast milk. In the earliest decades of the HIV epidemic, those who acquired HIV had few, if any, treatment options. Highly active antiretroviral therapy was first introduced in the late 1980s and the initial antiretroviral treatment regimens were introduced in the mid-1990s. Since then, HIV treatment regimens have continued to advance. However, HIV prevention options remained limited until 2010 when the Pre-exposure Prophylaxis Initiative clinical trial showed that when taken daily, the antiretroviral drug Truvada (tenofovir disoproxil fumarate/emtricitabine [TDF/FTC]) was effective in reducing risk of HIV acquisition in HIV-negative MSM.[3] Following this study, several other large-scale randomized controlled trials demonstrated that Truvada was also effective in reducing HIV acquisition in heterosexual men and women, people who inject drugs, and in serodiscordant couples, in which 1 partner is HIV positive and the other is HIV negative. This evidence led the FDA to approve oral Truvada for use as PrEP for HIV prevention in 2012. Subsequently, oral Descovy (tenofovir alafenamide [TAF/FTC]) was approved for use as PrEP in 2019, and most recently, injectable Apretude (cabotegravir [CAB-LA]) was approved in 2021.[3]

Since PrEP was first approved, awareness, access, and uptake of this HIV prevention method has steadily and significantly increased. The CDC estimates that in 2021, of the 1.2 million people who could benefit from PrEP use, approximately 30% have received a PrEP prescription compared to only 13% in 2017.[4] However, PrEP distribution remains uneven, with significant variability by race/ethnicity, sex, age, and geographic location.[4] In 2021, it was estimated that less than one-quarter of the black and LatinX people who were eligible for PrEP received a prescription compared to three-quarters of white people.[4] In addition, PrEP uptake is estimated to be 3 times higher in males than in females.[4] These inequities must be addressed to effectively end the HIV epidemic in the United States.

BIOMEDICAL APPROACHES TO HUMAN IMMUNODEFICIENCY VIRUS PREVENTION

Nurses play a vital role in identifying patients who could benefit from PrEP, in addition to ensuring continuity of care, care coordination, and retention and reengagement in comprehensive PrEP services. Therefore, it is important that nurses know PrEP eligibility indications, the appropriate screening prior to PrEP initiation, and the needed monitoring while on PrEP.

As of 2021, the US Public Service guidelines recommended that all sexually active people be educated about PrEP, and all who are sexually active or report injection drug use that places them at increased risk of HIV acquisition be offered a PrEP prescription.[1] It is important to complete a thorough, nonjudgmental sexual and substance use history to assess for practices that may increase risk of HIV acquisition to determine if a person could benefit from PrEP use. Indications for PrEP use may include, but are not limited to, having sexual partners with HIV, 1 or more sexual partners with unknown HIV status, 1 or more bacterial sexually transmitted infections (STIs) in the past 6 months, substance use, use of substances prior to sex, alcohol use prior to sex, and inconsistent condom use. It is also important to note that any patient requesting PrEP should be offered and prescribed an appropriate PrEP regimen.[1]

There are currently 3 FDA-approved medications for use as PrEP for HIV prevention, 2 oral, and 1 long-acting injectable.[1] The oral options include Truvada and Descovy, both single tablets taken once daily. Apretude is a long-acting injectable medication, administered in a clinical setting, every 2 months. There are differing guidelines for each route (or modalities) of administration. Truvada (TDF/FTC 200 mg/300 mg) is a daily oral option for PrEP that is approved for all individuals weighing at least 35 kg, whereas Descovy (TAF/FTC 200 mg/25 mg) is a daily oral option that is currently only approved for cisgender men and transgender women.[1] Descovy is not currently approved and should not be prescribed for cisgender women or transgender men.[1] Both oral PrEP regimens have an overall efficacy of approximately 99% when taken as prescribed.[5] Prior to oral PrEP initiation, patients should have no signs or symptoms of acute HIV infection, and should be screened for HIV, hepatitis B, and other STIs. It is also important to check kidney function to determine that creatinine clearance is higher than 60 mL/min for Truvada initiation and higher than 30 mL/min for Descovy initiation. Lastly, patients of reproductive potential should be screened for pregnancy.[1] It is important to properly educate patients on adherence to PrEP, potential side effects, and potential drug interactions. The most common side effects of oral PrEP medications are fatigue, headache, nausea, vomiting, and diarrhea.[1] Furthermore, patients will need to follow up every 3 months for HIV screening to ensure they remain HIV negative, and for routine STI screening. In addition, kidney function should be monitored every 6 to 12 months and lipids monitored at least annually.[1]

Long-acting CAB-LA, brand name Apretude, was approved by the FDA in 2021, and is the first long-acting injectable PrEP regimen for all individuals weighing at least 35 kg. CAB-LA (600 mg/3 mL) is appropriate for those with significant renal disease that has rendered them ineligible for oral PrEP regimens, those with difficulty adhering to daily oral PrEP, and those who prefer every 2-month injection dosing instead of daily oral dosing. However, it has not yet been approved as an HIV prevention modality for injection drug use transmission risk, as this has not yet been studied.[1] Overall, CAB-LA has demonstrated a 79% reduction in HIV risk and was found to be highly efficacious in HIV prevention with minimal safety concerns.[6] Prior to initiation, patients should have no signs or symptoms of acute HIV infection and must be screened for HIV and STIs including syphilis, gonorrhea, and chlamydia. Laboratory testing for hepatitis B serology, creatinine clearance, lipids, and liver function are not indicated prior to initiation, or as ongoing monitoring with CAB-LA.[1] At the initial injection appointment, patients should be educated on potential side effects, management of injection site reactions, the importance of following up every 2 months for HIV screening with both antigen/antibody and HIV ribonucleic acid tests, and the need for routine STI screening. In addition, anyone receiving CAB-LA for PrEP should be educated about the "long tail" of CAB-LA and its risks. CAB-LA is associated with slowly declining drug concentrations, which can increase risk for HIV-associated drug resistance if a person acquires HIV during the "tail" period. Assuring people using CAB-LA understand this nuance is important in assuring the best long-term outcomes once someone stops using CAB-LA. A follow-up injection is recommended 1 month after the initial injection, and then every 2 months thereafter.[1]

DISPARITIES IN HUMAN IMMUNODEFICIENCY VIRUS INCIDENCE AND PRE-EXPOSURE PROPHYLAXIS UPTAKE
New Human Immunodeficiency Virus Infections

To understand the implications associated with disparities in PrEP uptake, it is first necessary to examine the disparate rates of new HIV infections in the United States. The incidence of HIV varies widely by race, gender, transmission risk factors, and geographic location. In 2021, black people had the highest incidence of HIV infections, representing 40% of new diagnoses, as compared with LatinX and white communities which represented 29% and 25%, respectively[2] (**Fig. 1**).

In addition, HIV incidence in 2021 was markedly higher among males, whose rate of new infections was 4 times that of females. Data examining sex and race, together, indicated that black males have a lifetime risk of acquiring HIV that is 6 times that of white males, and black females have almost 12 times the lifetime risk of white females.[7] Most infections among males were attributed to MSM sexual contact (81%), while among females, 82% of new infections were attributed to heterosexual sexual contact. BMSM had the highest incidence of HIV of all groups, followed by LatinX MSM and white MSM[8] (**Fig. 2**).[2]

Pre-exposure Prophylaxis Uptake

According to the CDC, in 2021, 78% of white people who were eligible for PrEP coverage were prescribed it, while only 11% of eligible black people and 21% of eligible LatinX people received PrEP prescriptions[9] (**Fig. 3**). In addition, there were 3 black and 6 LatinX PrEP users for every new HIV diagnosis within those groups, compared with 26 white PrEP users for every new HIV diagnosis among white people.[10]

PrEP coverage is also unevenly distributed by sex, with 34% of eligible males covered, compared with 12% of females. Among transgender women, in 7 major US cities, HIV prevalence was 40% in 2021, and while 92% were aware of PrEP, only 32% reported using it.[4] Concerning disparities in PrEP coverage were also evident across HIV transmission categories. While 78% of HIV-negative BMSM were aware of PrEP, only 19% had used it.[11]

There are myriad factors that impact rates of PrEP uptake among the populations most at risk for HIV infection. Commonly cited influences among BMSM include lack of general awareness of PrEP and the stigma associated with taking these medications. Two main facets of PrEP-related stigma have been identified: one related to stigma associated with homosexuality and the sexual behaviors of BMSM and the other associated with HIV itself.[12] Another factor impacting PrEP uptake among BMSM is the need to discuss their sexual practices with a care provider, which is

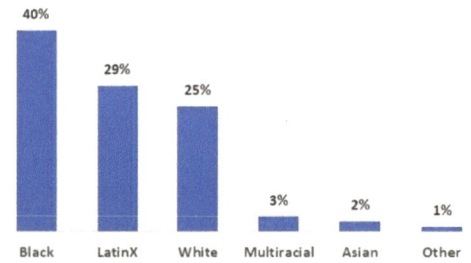

Fig. 1. US human immunodeficiency virus incidence by race, 2021. (*From* https://www.cdc.gov/hiv/basics/statistics.html.)

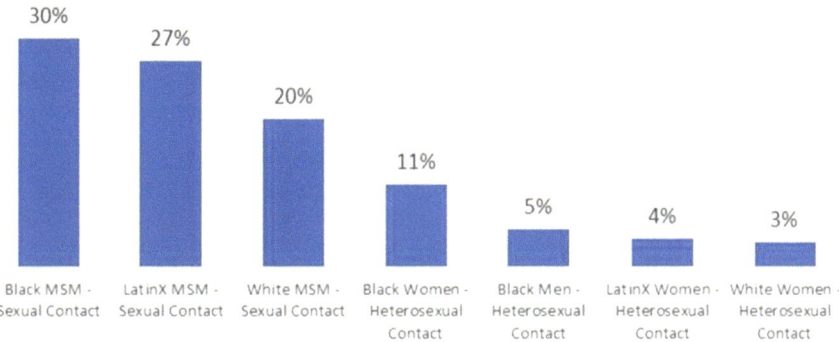

Fig. 2. Human immunodeficiency virus incidence by transmission category, 2021. (*From* https://www.cdc.gov/hiv/basics/statistics.html.)

adversely impacted by level of comfort with providers and medical mistrust secondary to experiences of racism in care settings.[13] Creating environments that allow open communication with one's provider is an essential part of the PrEP process, as the vast majority of those currently benefitting from PrEP initially gained awareness during visits with their care providers.[12]

Importantly, even if patients are willing to discuss their sexual practices with a provider, this does not ensure that their providers will possess the knowledge or willingness to conduct risk assessments or provide PrEP education and prescriptions. While every provider with prescriptive authority can prescribe PrEP medications, concerns about patient adherence, medication toxicities, drug resistances, and patients' ability to afford PrEP medications serve as barriers to prescribing PrEP.[14] Primary care providers' likelihood of prescribing PrEP, particularly in rural and suburban settings, is associated with their level of training, attitudes about PrEP effectiveness, stigma, perceptions about patients' risk behaviors, and the belief that PrEP should be prescribed by infectious disease specialists.[15,16] These provider-related barriers highlight the need for clinical nurses to ensure patients receive culturally competent screening for PrEP eligibility and provide assistance with accessing a provider who is willing to prescribe PrEP.

NEXT STEPS FOR PRE-EXPOSURE PROPHYLAXIS

Despite persistent disparities in PrEP uptake, there has been significant progress in overall use of PrEP for HIV prevention. In 2017, only about 13% of people who could benefit from PrEP were prescribed it, compared with about 30% in 2021.[4] The

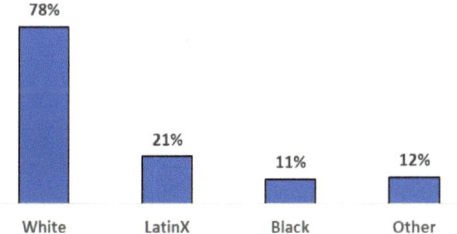

Fig. 3. Pre-exposure prophylaxis uptake by race/ethnicity, 2021. (*From* https://www.cdc.gov/hiv/group/racialethnic/other-races/prep-coverage.html.)

increase in PrEP use and improvements in testing and treatment have contributed to lower rates of new HIV infections, which declined 12% among MSM aged 13 to 24 years, from 2017 to 2021.[4] Nonetheless, as a central part of the national Ending the HIV Epidemic in the United States strategy, it is vital for additional resources to be dedicated to reducing barriers to PrEP uptake.

The White House has demonstrated dedication to eliminating disparities in PrEP uptake, including requests for substantial increases in government funding dedicated to increasing knowledge of PrEP, improving access to providers who prescribe PrEP, and assisting with medication and clinical care costs. Unfortunately, congress has been slow to provide much of this funding. Despite this, the CDC reports that financial barriers to PrEP uptake have declined by nearly half, primarily due to Medicaid expansion and coverage for PrEP medications and services under the Affordable Care Act.[4]

While a national strategy is necessary to confront PrEP uptake disparities comprehensively, numerous strategies have been implemented at the state and local levels with promising results. Efforts to increase consumer awareness of PrEP include targeted promotional campaigns that incorporate the use of radio and television advertising, social media campaigns, and the engagement of community partners and peers to increase credibility and trust among those who are eligible for PrEP therapy. To improve provider knowledge and buy-in, clinical resources and decision-making support have been provided by the CDC, in addition to testing and risk-assessment resources. Linkage facilitators, such as the PrEP Clinic Locator (https://preplocator. org/), allow individuals to find PrEP providers who offer HIV prevention services, regardless of insurance status and ability to pay for PrEP medications.[17]

The White House's fiscal year 2024 budget proposal included $850 million in funding to be distributed among the CDC, Resources and Services Administration, Indian Service, and National Institutes of in support of the national Ending the HIV Epidemic in the United States initiative, reducing HIV incidence, increasing PrEP access, and increasing the availability of services for individuals with HIV. The proposal is currently being evaluated by congress and represents an increased focus on confronting disparities in PrEP accessibility and uptake.[17]

SUMMARY

After approximately 4 decades, HIV remains a central public concern that requires continued focus, innovative interventions, and increased resources. PrEP is integral tool in the national initiative toward ending the HIV epidemic. There are 2 oral, and 1 injectable regimen that are all highly effective at preventing new HIV infections. Unfortunately, there are blatant disparities in access and uptake of PrEP, with the highest risk groups most impacted. It is vital for nurses to remain educated on the state of PrEP, increasing screening for eligibility and improving linkage to PrEP providers. There are numerous promising interventions designed to address disparities in both PrEP uptake and HIV incidence, ultimately contributing to the work of ending the HIV epidemic.

CLINICS CARE POINTS

- All sexually active individuals should be informed about and assessed for indications for PrEP.
- There are both oral and injectable forms of PrEP. Oral Truvada is approved for all individuals, oral Descovy is approved for cisgender men and transgender women and should not be given to cisgender women and transgender men.

- Injectable Apretude is approved for all individuals; however, it is not yet approved for HIV prevention in those who engage in injection drug use.
- Patients on PrEP must be screened for HIV every 3 months to ensure they are still HIV negative or to be linked to HIV care if test results are positive.
- Ongoing adherence education is important for those taking oral PrEP.
- Consistent care coordination and continuity of care by the care team is vital to ensuring positive outcomes

DISCLOSURES

The authors have nothing to disclose.

REFERENCES

1. Centers for Disease Control and Prevention. US Public Service Pre-exposure Prophylaxis for the prevention of HIV infection in the United States -2021 update A clinical practice guideline. 2021. Available at: https://www.cdc.gov/hiv/pdf/risk/prep/cdc-hiv-prep-guidelines-2021.pdf. [Accessed 1 February 2024].
2. Centers for Disease Control and Prevention. Basic Statistics. 2023. Available at: https://www.cdc.gov/hiv/basics/statistics.html. [Accessed 2 January 2024].
3. National Institute of National Institute of Allergy and Infectious Disease. Pre-exposure prophylaxis (PrEP) to reduce hiv risk. 2020. Available at: https://www.niaid.nih.gov/diseases-conditions/pre-exposure-prophylaxis-prep. [Accessed 2 February 2024].
4. PrEP for HIV prevention in the U.S. Centers for Disease Control and Prevention. 2023. Available at: https://www.cdc.gov/nchhstp/newsroom/fact-sheets/hiv/PrEP-for-hiv-prevention-in-the-US-factsheet.html. [Accessed 21 January 2024].
5. Centers for Disease Control and Prevention. PrEP effectiveness. 2022. Available at: https://www.cdc.gov/hiv/basics/prep/prep-effectiveness.html#:~:text=PrEP%20reduces%20the%20risk%20of,99%25%20when%20taken%20as%20prescribed. [Accessed 21 January 2024].
6. Fonner V, Ridgeway K, van der Straten A, et al. Safety and efficacy of long-acting injectable cabotegravir as preexposure prophylaxis to prevent HIV acquisition. AIDS 2023;37:957–66.
7. Overall lifetime risk of being diagnosed with HIV in the US decreases by 11%, but stark racial and geographical disparities persist. aidsmap.com. 2022. Available at: https://www.aidsmap.com/news/feb-2022/overall-lifetime-risk-being-diagnosed-hiv-us-decreases-11-stark-racial-and. [Accessed 8 January 2024].
8. HIV & AIDS trends and U.S. Statistics Overview. HIV.gov. December 7. 2023. Available at: https://www.hiv.gov/hiv-basics/overview/data-and-trends/statistics/. [Accessed 2 February 2024].
9. Prep coverage. Centers for Disease Control and Prevention. 2023. https://www.cdc.gov/hiv/group/racialethnic/other-races/prep-coverage.html. [Accessed 1 February 2024].
10. Interactive map. AIDSVu. 2022. Available at: https://aidsvu.org/prep-use-race-ethnicity-launch-22/. [Accessed 12 January 2024].
11. HIV prevention. Centers for Disease Control and Prevention. 2022. Available at: https://www.cdc.gov/hiv/group/bmsm/hiv-prevention.html. [Accessed 21 January 2024].

12. Lelutiu-Weinberger C, Golub SA. Enhancing prep access for black and Latino men who have sex with men. JAIDS Journal of Acquired Immune Deficiency Syndromes 2016;73(5):547–55.

13. Hsueh L, Layland EK, Kipke MD, et al. Linking racism and homonegativity to care system distrust among young men of color who have sex with men: Evidence from the y Young Men's (HYM) study. Soc Sci Med 2021;284:114219.

14. Siegler AJ, Bratcher A, Weiss KM, et al. Location Location Location: An exploration of disparities in access to publicly listed pre-exposure prophylaxis clinics in the United States. Ann Epidemiol 2018. Available at: https://www.sciencedirect.com/science/article/pii/S1047279717310475. [Accessed 23 January 2024].

15. Sell J, Chen R, Huber C, et al. Primary care provider HIV prep knowledge, attitudes, and prescribing habits: A cross-sectional survey of late adopters in rural and suburban practice. Journal of primary care & community 2023;. https://www.ncbi.nlm.nih.gov/pmc/articles/PMC9834790/. [Accessed 3 February 2024].

16. HIV pre-exposure prophylaxis (prep) care system. Centers for Disease Control and Prevention; 2023. Available at: https://www.cdc.gov/hiv/effective-interventions/prevent/prep/index.html. [Accessed 1 February 2024].

17. Ending the HIV epidemic funding. HIV.gov. 2024. Available at: https://www.hiv.gov/federal-response/ending-the-hiv-epidemic/funding. [Accessed 3 February 2024].

Overview of the US National HIV Strategy and Ending the HIV Epidemic Initiative

Kara S. McGee, DMS, MSPH, PA-C, AAHIVS

KEYWORDS

- HIV • Nurse-led interventions • Ending HIV epidemic

KEY POINTS

- Ending the HIV Epidemic in the United States is possible and the National HIV/AIDS Strategy for the United States 2022 to 2025 provides guidance on achieving this goal.
- Preventing new HIV infections by increasing access to HIV prevention services such as pre-exposure prophylaxis is an important strategy to decreasing new HIV infections in the United States.
- Nurses can play an important role in improving HIV-related health outcomes by increasing access to programs such as rapid HIV treatment and working with people with HIV to retain them in care.

INTRODUCTION

The US National HIV/AIDS Strategy (NHAS) is a comprehensive plan that outlines the nation's approach to addressing the HIV epidemic. The current NHAS, published in 2021, is the nation's third national HIV strategy and builds on the previous strategies published in 1993 and 2010. The NHAS sets specific goals for Ending the HIV Epidemic in the United States (EHE) by 2025. Along with the goals, the NHAS includes specific strategies to prevent new HIV infections, improve health outcomes for people with HIV, and address HIV-related health disparities. The overall vision of the NHAS is in **Fig. 1**.[1]

Closely aligned with the NHAS is the EHE plan. The EHE plan was published in 2019 by the US Department of Health and Human Services (DHHS) and focuses on realizing the NHAS goals in specific communities where HIV transmission rates are highest. The US DHHS partners with multiple sectors in the 57 priority jurisdictions to implement four key strategies to end of the HIV epidemic in the United States. The priority jurisdictions of the EHE plan are the 48 counties in the United States with the most new HIV cases plus San Juan, Puerto Rico, Washington, DC, and seven states with a large

MSN Program, Division of Infectious Diseases, Duke University School of Nursing, Duke University School of Medicine, 307 Trent Drive, Box 3322, Durham, NC 27710, USA
E-mail address: Kara.mcgee@duke.edu

Nurs Clin N Am 59 (2024) 297–308
https://doi.org/10.1016/j.cnur.2023.12.003
0029-6465/24/© 2024 Elsevier Inc. All rights reserved.

nursing.theclinics.com

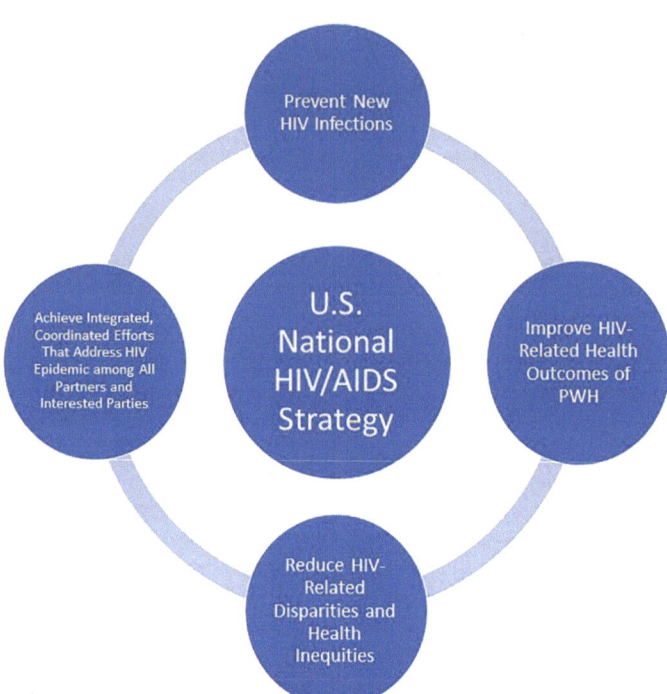

Fig. 1. The goals of the 2022 to 2025 NHAS.

number of HIV diagnoses in rural areas.[2] The EHE plan priority jurisdictions are listed in **Table 1**.

This article provides an overview of the NHAS and EHE and provides examples of programs and strategies that can be used to end the HIV epidemic in the United States.

HISTORY

The US NHAS has gone through several iterations since the onset of the HIV epidemic in the 1980s. The early federal response in the 1980s to 1990s was fragmented and lacked a cohesive strategy. In 1986, the US surgeon general C Everett Koop issued the "Surgeon General's Report on AIDS."[3] This report aimed to provide evidence-based information about the transmission, prevention, and the social and medical aspects of HIV/AIDS. Closely following the surgeon general's report, the US Centers for Disease Control and Prevention (CDC) started a national campaign, "America Responds to AIDS (ARTA)." The goal of ARTA was to increase awareness and provide education about HIV/AIDS and provides resources for people to obtain additional information.[4] During this time, activist groups and health care providers played a crucial role in raising awareness and advocating for resources and research.

In 1990, the US Congress passed the Ryan White Comprehensive AIDS Resources Emergency (CARE) Act. The CARE Act is named after Ryan White, a teenager who contracted HIV through a blood transfusion and provided federal funding for HIV/AIDS care and treatment services. It marked one of the early legislative responses to the epidemic and helped support HIV/AIDS care for those without adequate

Table 1
Ending the HIV epidemic in the United States plan priority jurisdictions

State	County(ies)	Territories	States
Arizona	Maricopa County	Puerto Rico,	Alabama
California	Alameda County	San Juan	Arkansas
	Los Angeles County	Municipio	Kentucky
	Orange County		Mississippi
	Riverside County		Missouri
	Sacramento County		Oklahoma
	San Bernardino County		South Carolina
	San Diego County		
	San Francisco County		
Florida	Broward County		
	Duval County		
	Hillsborough County		
	Miami-Dade County		
	Orange County		
	Palm Beach County		
	Pinellas County		
Georgia	Cobb County		
	DeKalb County		
	Fulton County		
	Gwinnett County		
Illinois	Cook County		
Indiana	Marion County		
Louisiana	East Baton Rouge Parish		
	Orleans Parish		
Maryland	Baltimore City		
	Montgomery County		
	Prince George's County		
Massachusetts	Suffolk County		
Michigan	Wayne County		
Nevada	Clark County		
New Jersey	Essex County		
	Hudson County		
New York	Bronx County		
	Kings County		
	New York County		
	Queens County		
North Carolina	Mecklenburg County		
Ohio	Cuyahoga County		
	Franklin County		
	Hamilton County		
Pennsylvania	Philadelphia County		
Tennessee	Shelby County		
Texas	Bexar County		
	Dallas County		
	Harris County		
	Tarrant County		
	Travis County		
Washington	King County		
Washington DC			

resources. The Ryan White HIV/AIDS Program (RWHAP) remains the largest federal program focused on HIV and has been reauthorized by Congress four times since its inception in 1990.[5]

In 1993, President Bill Clinton released the first NHAS, created the Office of National AIDS Policy and appointed the nation's first AIDS Policy Coordinator. This strategy focused on prevention, treatment, and research and aimed to coordinate federal efforts to address HIV/AIDS. In addition, the first NHAS aimed to ensure that people with HIV had adequate access to health care, housing and other support services and were not subject to discrimination.[1]

In 2010, President Barack Obama released a new NHAS. This updated strategy set ambitious goals to reduce new HIV infections, increase access to care and treatment, and reduce HIV-related health disparities. The strategy also emphasized the importance of addressing social determinants of health (SDOH) and promoting comprehensive prevention efforts.[6]

Published in 2021, the NHAS for the United States 2022 to 2025 is the most recent iteration of the NHAS and as previously mentioned sets specific goals for EHE by 2023.

GOALS OF THE NATIONAL HIV/AIDS STRATEGY 2022 TO 2025

The 2022 to 2025 NHAS presents four goals aimed at achieving the strategy vision. The NHAS vision is in **Box 1** and the goals are summarized in **Fig. 1**. For each of the four goals, the strategy lays out objectives for each goal and strategies to achieve each objective.

In addition to the four specific goals, the strategy includes priority populations and core indicators. There are nine core indicators that are used to measure progress toward meeting quantitative targets. For example, an indicator of progress for preventing new HIV infections goal is to increase knowledge of HIV status to 95% from a 2017 baseline of 85.5%, by the year 2025. The 2022 to 2025 NHAS priority populations are gay, bisexual, and other men who have sex with men (MSM), in particular Black, Latino, and American Indian/Alaska Native men; Black women; transgender women; youth aged 13 to 24 years; and people who inject drugs. These are populations, based on US HIV surveillance data, disproportionately affected by HIV. Centering efforts on these populations will help reduce HIV-related disparities.

Goal 1: Prevent New HIV Infections

The first aim of the 2022 to 2025 NHAS is a 75% reduction in new HIV infection by 2025 and a 90% reduction by 2030. There are many evidence-based and effective approaches to HIV prevention that include HIV treatment as prevention (TasP), HIV

Box 1
2022 to 2025 US National HIV/AIDS strategy vision

The United States will be a place where new HIV infections are prevented, every person knows their status, and every person with HIV has high-quality care and treatment, lives free from stigma and discrimination, and can achieve their full potential for health and well-being across the lifespan.

This vision includes all people, regardless of age, sex, gender identity, sexual orientation, race, ethnicity, religion disability, geographic location, or socioeconomic circumstance.

testing and linkage to care, pre-exposure prophylaxis (PrEP), syringe service programs (SSPs), post-exposure prophylaxis (PEP), and condoms. The NHAS has specific objectives aimed at reaching this goal that include increasing awareness of HIV; increasing knowledge of HIV status; expanding access to TasP, PrEP, PEP, and SSPs; and increasing capacity of the health care system to prevent and diagnose HIV. The NHAS includes numerous strategies to prevent new infections.

The EHE plan, which is closely aligned and complementary to the 2022 to 2025 NHAS, focuses on the scale-up of access to PrEP and SSPs as the main strategy to prevent new HIV infections. PrEP is the use of medications taken by people who do not have HIV to reduce the risk of acquiring HIV.[7,8] Overall, the number of PrEP users in the United States has increased consistently since 2012. However, PrEP is not being used by some of the priority populations identified in the 2022 to 2025 NHAS. For example, youth aged 13 to 24 years have the greatest unmet need for PrEP among all age groups, and Black people represented 14% of PrEP users but 42% of new HIV diagnoses in 2021.[9] There are well-documented barriers to PrEP uptake and use including lack of awareness of PrEP, HIV risk perception, stigma, provider bias, patient distrust of the health care system, lack of access to medical care, and lack of financial assistance for PrEP and PrEP medication side effects.[10] Addressing these barriers is vital in order to achieve the goals of the 2022 to 2025 NHAS. Assuring there are a variety of health care professionals to deliver HIV prevention services is a key strategy to decreasing barriers and increasing access to services. Nurses can play a critical role in increasing access to HIV prevention services.

There are numerous examples of nurse-led models of PrEP delivery. Patrick O'Byrne and colleagues[11] established the PrEP-registered nurse (RN) referral and clinical service program managed by public health nurses to increase access to PrEP services. The program allowed for half of the high-risk eligible patients identified to start and be retained in PrEP care. Nurse scientist, Dr Schenita Randolph and her colleagues[12] have created a community-engaged intervention to improve PrEP knowledge, stigma, trust, and uptake among Black cisgender women in the Southern United States. The "Using PrEP and Doing it for Ourselves (UPDOs) Protective Styles" Web-based intervention was codeveloped with Black cisgender women and hair salon stylists. Preliminary results show improved PrEP knowledge, awareness, and trust among Black cisgender women participants.

Goal 2: Improve HIV-Related Health Outcomes of People with HIV

The second goal of the 2022 to 2025 NHAS is to improve HIV-related health outcomes of people with HIV. Antiretroviral therapy (ART) for the treatment of HIV infection has dramatically reduced HIV-related complications and morbidity. ART has made HIV a chronic, manageable condition with normal life expectancy for people with HIV who take ART consistently.[13] In addition, modern HIV treatment is highly effective a preventing sexual transmission of HIV in people who have suppressed viral loads.[14] Consistent, long-term access to ART is vital to assuring that people with HIV do not experience HIV-related complications that negatively impact their health and well-being.

The 2022 to 2025 NHAS has specific objectives to improve the HIV-related health outcomes for people with HIV. These include linking people to care immediately and providing low-barrier access to ART, identify people with HIV who are not in care and reengage them with health care services, increase retention in care and adherence to ART, increasing capacity of health care system to provide HIV treatment, expanding services to meet the needs of older persons with HIV and long-term survivors, and advance the development of the next generation of HIV treatments and HIV cure.

The EHE plan focuses on treating people with HIV rapidly and effectively to reach viral suppression and to reengage people with HIV who are not receiving care and treatment.[15] Using the US HIV care continuum, a public health model outlining the steps needed to achieve and maintain HIV suppression, shows that only 57% of people with HIV in the United States in 2019 were virally suppressed.[16] There are numerous barriers to people with HIV being retained in care and maintaining viral suppression. Some of these barriers include life circumstances such as substance use, mental health, homelessness and poverty, financial barriers, and not feeling sick enough to take medicine—all of which impede receipt of health care services. In addition, people with HIV who are not virally suppressed often report more than one barrier to care.[17] Rapid start and low-barrier access to HIV treatment and reengaging people with HIV who are not retained in health care are key issues that need to be addressed to improve health outcomes for people with HIV.

Nurse-led models that facilitate rapid ART initiation are one approach to providing treatment quickly and engaging people with HIV with health care services. Nurse Heather Alt and group at Whitman-Walker Health created a program to facilitate same-day start of ART after a positive HIV test.[18] The Health Resources and Services Administration (HRSA) has published guidelines to help with the development of rapid ART programs, and HRSA has funded 15 demonstration sites to implement rapid ART initiation.[19]

Nurse-led models that attempt to retain and reengage people with HIV in health care are also an important strategy to improve long-term outcomes. A recent review of nurse-led ART medication adherence intervention found that nurse-led and nurse-enabled medication adherence intervention was effective in promoting ART adherence in people with HIV.[20] Moen and colleagues[21] evaluated a nurse-led hospital to community transitional care program for people with HIV in Baltimore, Maryland and found increased HIV appointment attendance and viral suppression rates among participants in the program. Innovative models that include nurses, advanced practice providers, pharmacists, and community health workers are needed to address the barriers that prevent people with HIV from remaining engaged in health care over the long term.[1]

Goal 3: Reduce HIV-Related Disparities and Health Inequities

The third goal of the 2022 to 2025 NHAS is to reduce HIV-related disparities and health inequities. Although there has been some progress in decreasing the rates of new HIV infections in the US disparities still exist and must be addressed to meet the goal of ending the US HIV epidemic. Despite public health efforts to address racial and ethnic disparities in new HIV diagnosis, Black and Latino people account for the majority of new HIV diagnoses in the United States.[16] These disparities are not driven by differences in risk behaviors but by the systems and policies that affect racial and ethnic minority people.[1] For example, people from historically marginalized groups experience more barriers to health care access such as lack of transportation and childcare, lack of policies that allow for time off from work, racism, discrimination and lack of trust in health care providers secondary to being chronically underserved by the system.[22]

To meet the third goal, the 2022 to 2025 NHAS has designated four targets to be reached by 2025. These are (1) decrease stigma among people with HIV by 50%; (2) reduce homelessness among people with HIV by 50%; (3) increase the median percentage of secondary schools that implement LGBTQ-supportive policies and practices; and (4) increase viral suppression rates to 95% among MSM, Black MSM, Latino MSM, American Indian/Alaska Native MSM, Black women, transgender women, people who inject drugs, and youth aged 13 to 24 years.

Despite advances in the treatment of HIV, HIV-related stigma continues to be a common experience for people living with or at risk for HIV. Experiences of stigma negatively impact health in many ways including poorer retention in care, increased susceptibility to depression and anxiety, fear of seeking HIV prevention services, and reduced medication adherence.[23–26] In addition, HIV-specific criminal laws perpetuate HIV-related stigma and deter people from getting tested for HIV. These laws are outdated and do not align with current scientific knowledge about HIV transmission. Since 2014, nine states have repealed or updated their HIV-specific criminal laws but 21 states still have HIV-specific statutes that criminalize actions by people with HIV.[27]

The 2022 to 2025 NHAS proposes education and training on stigma, discrimination and unrecognized biases toward people with HIV for health care professionals as one strategy to decrease HIV-related stigma. A recent review of interventions to decreased HIV-related stigma and discrimination in the health care settings found that interventions addressing fear-based stigma through training on basic knowledge of HIV and universal precautions and training popular opinion leaders were effective in reducing stigma among health care workers.[28] However, the quality of studies assessed in this and other systematic reviews[29] tend to be poor and do not include validated measures of stigma and discrimination. Multilevel interventions with more rigorous designs that follow intervention participants longitudinally are needed to determine best approaches to decreasing HIV-related stigma and discrimination among health care professionals.[30]

Reducing HIV-related disparities and health inequities will require attention to the numerous SDOH that impact people with and at risk for HIV. The 2022 to 2025 NHAS target of reducing homelessness among people with HIV means addressing stable housing as a health-related need that improves health outcomes. In 2020, 17% of people diagnosed with HIV experienced homelessness or unstable housing.[31] Housing instability is a barrier to engagement in health care services and adherence to HIV treatment increasing risk for disease progression due to lack of viral suppression. Research has shown that housing stability increases retention in care and higher rates of viral suppression.[32] Multiple federal, state, and local agencies and organizations will need to collaborate to reach this goal of reducing homelessness among people with HIV. A leader in addressing this issue is the Housing Opportunities for Persons with AIDS (HOPWA), a program administered by the US Department of Housing and Urban Development (HUD). In September 2023, HUD announced $50 million to fund local governments, states, and nonprofit organizations via HOPWA to fund housing assistance and supportive services for low-income people with HIV.[33]

Goal 4: Achieve Integrated, Coordinated Efforts that Address the HIV Epidemic Among All Partners and Interested Parties

The fourth goal of the 2022 to 2025 NHAS highlights the need for coordinated and organized efforts across sectors to meet the goal of EHE. In addition, greater integration of services for people with or at risk for HIV is essential to address the syndemic of HIV, sexually transmitted infections (STIs), viral hepatitis, and substance use and mental health disorders.

Specifically, the 2022 to 2025 NHAS includes the following objectives to meet goal 4 of the plan: (1) integration of programs to address HIV, STIs, viral hepatitis, and mental health and substance use disorder syndemic with focus on addressing stigma, discrimination, and violence, (2) increase sharing of best practices from HIV programs across public and private sectors and the community; (3) enhance the quality and use of data to address HIV prevention, HIV care engagement, and SDOH; (4) promote public-private-community partnerships to identify and scale-up advances in HIV care and prevention; and (5) improve methods to measure and report progress in order to meet the NHAS goals.[1]

The previous efforts to coordinate and integrate HIV care and prevention services serve as examples of strategies that can be used to meet goal 4 of the 2022 to 2025 NHAS. The Data to Care program uses local HIV surveillance data to identify people with HIV who are not receiving regular medical care and reengaging them in HIV medical care services.[34] Two federal agencies, HOPWA and the RWHAP, partnered to determine how to improve outcomes for people with HIV and housing instability. The result was a data integration project between HOPWA, RWHAP, and four local organizations in Hartford, CT, Multnomah County, OR, Kansas City, MO, and Palm Beach County, FL, in which integrated data improved care coordination and decreased housing instability.[35] An illustration of the importance of collaborative efforts across sectors is the 2014 to 2015 HIV outbreak in Scott County, Indiana.[36] Collaboration between the Indiana State Department of Health, the CDC and Governor's office resulted in establishment of programs to prevent new HIV infections and treat those who had acquired HIV and can serve as an example to increase access to services to address substance use disorder and HIV screening and PrEP.[37]

However, challenges to coordinated and integrated approaches to addressing the HIV epidemic remain. The HIV, STI, and viral hepatitis syndemic can only be addressed if people are tested for concurrent infections. In 2019, a CDC report found that only 34% of HIV tests in both health care and non-health care settings had at least one STI of hepatitis C test conducted concurrently.[38] Another challenge is the lack of private-public-community partnerships to advance HIV care and prevention. Partnerships between communities and researchers are essential if interventions are going to be effective in communities most at risk. However, a recent study found that it is difficult to assess the extent to which to community engagement is used in HIV-related research because there are no requirements or guidelines for reporting on community engagement in HIV research.[39] To address this challenge, the CDCs Division of HIV Prevention holds regional town hall listening sessions on the barriers and facilitators to meeting the goals of the EHE initiative.[40] There are many examples of the use of community-engaged HIV research including using this strategy in the HIV Prevention Trials Network (HPTN). Using the National Institutes of Health Director's Council of Public Responsiveness Community Engagement Framework, HPTN researchers found that engagement activities with community members increased rapport, established new partnerships with community members, and led to high study participation retention rates.[41]

DISCUSSION

EHE requires concerted, organized, multi-sector, and well-funded approaches that are driven by evidence and address the various barriers that have kept this an elusive goal for so long. The 2022 to 2025 NHAS provides clear goals, objectives, and strategies to end the HIV epidemic in the United States and advances in HIV treatment and prevention that prevents sexual transmission of HIV means we have the tools to end of the HIV epidemic. However, not everyone benefits equally from these advances and until we address these inequities we will fall short of ending the HIV epidemic.[42,43]

As the United States' most trusted profession,[44] nurses must play a role in EHE. Broadening the HIV workforce by supporting nonphysician clinicians, such as nurses and nurse practitioners, to practice at the full scope of their license will allow for increased access to HIV care and prevention services.[43] Nurse-led differentiated models of care like telemedicine and community outreach could expand access to comprehensive sexual health services and integration of HIV treatment into primary care settings. Nurses, particularly nurse practitioners, are well suited to expand more integrated models of HIV care and prevention services, address comorbid conditions among people with HIV, and provide culturally sensitive care.[45] Nurses have long been advocates for advancing health and addressing health inequities and can contribute meaningfully to advocacy efforts to advance the goals of the 2022 to 2025 NHAS. The Association of Nurses in AIDS Care (ANAC) is a leading nursing organization, which aims to promote the health and well-being of people affected by HIV by advocating for effective policies and quality care for people with or at risk for HIV. In addition, ANAC provides education and professional development for nurses working with people living with HIV. School nurses can advocate for and expand access to school-based sexual health services or at a minimum create referral and linkage systems to community partners offering these services.

SUMMARY

Building on the medical and scientific advances and lessons learned since the beginning of the HIV epidemic in the United States in the 1980s, the United States now has the opportunity to end the HIV epidemic. The 2022 to 2025 NHAS provides concrete goals, objectives, and strategies to improve HIV treatment and prevention services that will end of the HIV epidemic. Although barriers exist to implementing all of the strategies in the 2022 to 2025 NHAS, nurses can play a critical role in addressing these barriers and advocating for resources to implement innovative, community-engaged interventions to end the HIV epidemic.

CLINICS CARE POINTS

- The 2022 to 2025 National HIV/AIDS Strategy outlines specific strategies to address HIV, which remains in significant health problem in the United States.
- Encouraging routine HIV testing for all individuals facilitates early diagnosis and prompt initiation of HIV treatment.
- Facilitating access to HIV prevention services, such as pre-exposure prophylaxis, can help reduce new HIV infections
- Reducing HIV-related disparities and health inequities will require attention to the numerous social determinants of health that impact people with and at risk for HIV

DISCLOSURE

No disclosures.

REFERENCES

1. The White House TW. National HIV/AIDS Strategy for the United States 2022–2025.; 2021 https://www.whitehouse.gov/wp-content/uploads/2021/11/National-HIV-AIDS-Strategy.pdf. Accessed September 28, 2023.

2. Fauci AS, Redfield RR, Sigounas G, et al. Ending the HIV Epidemic: A Plan for the United States. JAMA 2019;321(9):844–5. https://doi.org/10.1001/jama.2019.1343.

3. Surgeon General's Report On AIDS https://wonder.cdc.gov/wonder/sci_data/misc/type_txt/sgrpt.asp. Accessed September 14, 2023.

4. The AIDS Epidemic in the United States, 1981-early 1990s | David J. Sencer CDC Museum | CDC. Published April 29, 2021 https://www.cdc.gov/museum/online/story-of-cdc/aids/index.html. Accessed September 14, 2023.

5. Ryan White HIV/AIDS Program Legislation | Ryan White HIV/AIDS Program https://ryanwhite.hrsa.gov/about/legislation. Accessed September 14, 2023.

6. NHAS.pdf https://obamawhitehouse.archives.gov/sites/default/files/uploads/NHAS.pdf. Accessed September 14, 2023.

7. Grant RM, Lama JR, Anderson PL, et al. Preexposure chemoprophylaxis for HIV prevention in men who have sex with men. N Engl J Med 2010;363(27):2587–99.

8. Baeten JM, Donnell D, Ndase P, et al. Antiretroviral prophylaxis for HIV prevention in heterosexual men and women. N Engl J Med 2012;367(5):399–410.

9. AIDSVu Releases New Data Highlighting Ongoing Inequities in PrEP Use among Black and Hispanic People and across Regions of the Country. AIDSVu. Published June 21, 2023 https://aidsvu.org/aidsvu-releases-new-data-highlighting-ongoing-inequities-in-prep-use-among-black-and-hispanic-people-and-across-regions-of-the-county/. Accessed September 14, 2023.

10. Mayer KH, Agwu A, Malebranche D. Barriers to the Wider Use of Pre-exposure Prophylaxis in the United States: A Narrative Review. Adv Ther 2020;37(5):1778–811. https://doi.org/10.1007/s12325-020-01295-0.

11. O'Byrne P, Vandyk A, Orser L, et al. Nurse-led PrEP-RN clinic: a prospective cohort study exploring task-Shifting HIV prevention to public health nurses. BMJ Open 2021;11(1):e040817.

12. Randolph SD, Johnson R, Jeter E, et al. UPDOs Protective Styles, a Multilevel Intervention to Improve Pre-exposure Prophylaxis Uptake Among Black Cisgender Women: Pretest–Posttest Evaluation. J Assoc Nurses AIDS Care 2023;34(5):459.

13. Samji H, Cescon A, Hogg RS, et al. Closing the gap: increases in life expectancy among treated HIV-positive individuals in the United States and Canada. PLoS One 2013;8(12):e81355.

14. Cohen MS, Chen YQ, McCauley M, et al. Antiretroviral Therapy for the Prevention of HIV-1 Transmission. N Engl J Med 2016;375(9):830–9.

15. US Department of Health and Human Services. Overview About Ending the HIV Epidemic in the U.S. HIV.gov. Published March 23, 2021 https://www.hiv.gov/federal-response/ending-the-hiv-epidemic/overview. Accessed May 17, 2021.

16. Centers for Disease Control and Prevention. HIV Surveillance Report, 2021.; 2023 https://www.cdc.gov/hiv/library/reports/hiv-surveillance/vol-34/index.html. Accessed September 20, 2023.

17. Dasgupta S, Tie Y, Beer L, et al. Barriers to HIV Care by Viral Suppression Status Among US Adults With HIV: Findings From the Centers for Disease Control and Prevention Medical Monitoring Project. J Assoc Nurses AIDS Care JANAC 2021;32(5):561–8.

18. A Nurse-Driven Model to Facilitating Same-Day ART Initiation. ContagionLive. Published November 10, 2019 https://www.contagionlive.com/view/a-nursedriven-model-to-facilitating-sameday-art-initiation. Accessed September 18, 2023.

19. Rapid ART: An Essential Strategy for Ending the HIV Epidemic https://targethiv. org/sites/default/files/media/documents/2021-11/An_Essential_Strategy_for_ Ending_the_HIV_Epidemic.pdf. Accessed September 18, 2023.
20. Lambert CC, Galland B, Enriquez M, et al. A Systematic Review of Nurse-Led Antiretroviral Medication Adherence Intervention Trials: How Nurses Have Advanced the Science. J Assoc Nurses AIDS Care 2021;32(3):347.
21. Moen M, Doede M, Johantgen M, et al. Nurse-led hospital-to-community care, clinical outcomes for people living with HIV and health-related social needs. J Adv Nurs 2023;79(5):1949–58.
22. Social Determinants of Health - Healthy People 2030 | health.gov https://health.gov/ healthypeople/priority-areas/social-determinants-health. Accessed September 20, 2023.
23. Kalichman SC, Hernandez D, Finneran S, et al. Transgender women and HIV-related health disparities: falling off the HIV treatment cascade. Sex Health 2017;14(5):469–76.
24. Earnshaw VA, Smith LR, Chaudoir SR, et al. HIV Stigma Mechanisms and Well-Being among PLWH: A Test of the HIV Stigma Framework. AIDS Behav 2013; 17(5):1785–95.
25. Armoon B, Higgs P, Fleury MJ, et al. Socio-demographic, clinical and service use determinants associated with HIV related stigma among people living with HIV/ AIDS: a systematic review and meta-analysis. BMC Health Serv Res 2021; 21(1):1004.
26. Reif S, Wilson E, McAllaster C, et al. The Relationship of HIV-related Stigma and Health Care Outcomes in the US Deep South. AIDS Behav 2019;23(3):242–50.
27. Centers for Disease Control and Prevention. HIV Criminalization and Ending the HIV Epidemic.; 2023 https://www.cdc.gov/hiv/policies/law/criminalization-ehe. html. Accessed September 20, 2023.
28. Feyissa GT, Lockwood C, Woldie M, et al. Reducing HIV-related stigma and discrimination in healthcare settings: A systematic review of quantitative evidence. PLoS One 2019;14(1):e0211298.
29. Hill M. The effectiveness of workplace interventions to reduce HIV-related stigma amongst healthcare professionals. HIV Nurs 2016;16(3):67–72.
30. Relf MV, Holzemer W L, Holt L, et al. A Review of the State of the Science of HIV and Stigma: Context, Conceptualization, Measurement, Interventions, Gaps, and Future Priorities. J Assoc Nurses AIDS Care 2021;32(3):392–407.
31. Centers for Disease Control and Prevention. Behavioral and Clinical Characteristics of Persons with Diagnosed HIV Infection—Medical Monitoring Project, United States, 2020 Cycle (June 2020–May 2021).; 202AD 9. https://www.cdc.gov/hiv/ library/reports/hiv-surveillance.html. Accessed September 20, 2023.
32. Rajabiun S, Tryon J, Feaster M, et al. The Influence of Housing Status on the HIV Continuum of Care: Results From a Multisite Study of Patient Navigation Models to Build a Medical Home for People Living With HIV Experiencing Homelessness. Am J Publ Health 2018;108(S7):S539–45.
33. HUD Announces $50 Million Funding Opportunity to Provide Stable Housing to People with HIV and Their Families. HIV.govhttps://www.hiv.gov/blog/hud-announces-50-million-funding-opportunity-to-provide-stable-housing-to-people-with-hiv-and-their-families. Accessed September 20, 2023.
34. Sweeney P, DiNenno EA, Flores SA, et al. HIV Data to Care—Using Public Health Data to Improve HIV Care and Prevention. JAIDS J Acquir Immune Defic Syndr 2019;82:S1.

35. Towe VL, Stevens C, Fischer SH. Sharing and Integrating HIV Client Data Across Provider Organizations to Improve Service Coordination: A Toolkit. RAND Corporation; 2019 https://www.rand.org/pubs/tools/TL344.html. Accessed September 26, 2023.

36. Peters PJ, Pontones P, Hoover KW, et al. HIV Infection Linked to Injection Use of Oxymorphone in Indiana, 2014–2015. N Engl J Med 2016;375(3):229–39.

37. Haddad M, Person AK, Tookes HE. Ending the HIV Epidemic: We Have the Tools, Do We Have the Will? JAMA 2022;328(22):2207–8.

38. Centers for Disease Control and Prevention. Integrated HIV Surveillance & Prevention Programs for Health Departments (PS18-1802): Monitoring and Evaluation Report, 2019.; 2019 http://www.cdc.gov/hiv/library/reports/index.html. Accessed September 26, 2023.

39. Pantelic M, Steinert JI, Ayala G, et al. Addressing epistemic injustice in HIV research: a call for reporting guidelines on meaningful community engagement. J Int AIDS Soc 2022;25(1):e25880.

40. Community Engagement | HIV | CDC https://www.cdc.gov/hiv/capacity-building-assistance/community-engagement/index.html. Accessed September 26, 2023.

41. DeShields RD, Lucas JP, Turner M, et al. Building Partnerships and Stakeholder Relationships for HIV Prevention: Longitudinal Cohort Study Focuses on Community Engagement. Prog Community Health Partnersh Res Educ Action 2020; 14(1):29–42.

42. Supporting ambitious new goals to end the HIV epidemic https://www.myamericannurse.com/supporting-ambitious-new-goals-to-end-the-hiv-epidemic/. Accessed September 20, 2023.

43. Guilamo-Ramos V, Thimm-Kaiser M, Benzekri A. Is the USA on track to end the HIV epidemic? Lancet HIV 2023;10(8):e552–6.

44. Americans Continue to Rank Nurses Most Honest and Ethical Professionals. ANA. Published January 10, 2023 https://www.nursingworld.org/news/news-releases/2022-news-releases/americans-continue-to-rank-nurses-most-honest-and-ethical-professionals/. Accessed September 26, 2023.

45. McGee K, Bell L, Guilamo-Ramos V, et al. HIV Clinician Workforce Shortage: Nurse Practitioners Filling the Gap. J Nurse Pract 2022;18(1):58–61.

A Review of Updated Guidelines on Breastfeeding with Human Immunodeficiency Virus Using Relational Decision-Making and Intellectual Humility to Support Infant Feeding Choices

Emily A. Barr, PhD, RN, CPNP-PC, CNM, FAAN[a,*], Lisa L. Abuogi, MD, MSc[b],
Christiana Smith, MD, MSc[b]

KEYWORDS

- Breastfeeding with HIV • Perinatal HIV • Relational decision-making
- Intellectual humility • Patient–provider trust

KEY POINTS

- The updated guidelines from the Department of Health and Human Services recommend that women with HIV (WWH) who are receiving antiretroviral therapy with a sustained undetectable HIV viral load should receive evidence-based counseling on all infant feeding options. This includes the use of formula, banked donor milk, or breast milk.
- During breastfeeding, the risk of HIV transmission to the newborn is less than 1% when the mother is on antiretrovirals, and the HIV viral load is suppressed. There remain risks, including a low risk of HIV transmission, side effects from antiretroviral therapy, and challenges that accompany additional visits, blood draws, and ongoing management for 6 months after weaning.
- The relational decision-making model can support communication when providing care for birthing WWH. The model emphasizes the importance of sharing knowledge, considering internal and external factors that may impact health care decisions, and working collaboratively in interdisciplinary teams. This model recognizes that decision-making is not a one-time event, but a process that unfolds over time in the context of the ongoing patient–provider relationship.

Continued

[a] University of Texas Health Science Center at Houston, Cizik School of Nursing, 6901 Bertner Avenue, SON 5th Floor, Houston, TX 77030, USA; [b] Department of Pediatrics, University of Colorado School of Medicine, 13123 East 16th Avenue, Box 055, Aurora, CO 80045, USA
* Corresponding author.
E-mail address: Emily.Barr@uth.tmc.edu

Nurs Clin N Am 59 (2024) 309–327
https://doi.org/10.1016/j.cnur.2023.12.004
0029-6465/24/© 2023 Elsevier Inc. All rights reserved.

Continued

- Fostering intellectual humility allows us to recognize the limitations of our own knowledge and be open to the perspectives and expertise of others. When considering recent changes to the management of infant feeding in WWH, intellectual humility can build trust through fostering acceptance of alternative viewpoints and critical evaluation of one's own beliefs.
- Communication strategies should be non-stigmatizing and nonjudgmental, correcting any misinformation and presenting data in a patient-friendly way. It is important to support WWH in the feeding option that they choose and recognize that patients may not feel empowered to advocate for their decision to breastfeed if they face scrutiny from other members of the health care team. This is especially a concern among minority and disadvantaged populations.

INTRODUCTION

Recent updates to the US Department of Health and Human Services (HHS) guidelines for infant feeding in people with HIV (PWH) no longer recommend against the use of human milk for infant feeding (eg, via chest/breastfeeding or feeding of expressed human milk) for women with HIV (WWH) who are taking combination antiretroviral therapy (ART) and have a sustained undetectable human immunodeficiency virus ribonucleic acid polymerase chain reaction (HIV RNA PCR) (HIV Viral Load).[1] Significant research and expert discourse informed a major decision like this, and there continue to be mixed opinions in the medical community regarding whether to support breastfeeding in PWH. Infant feeding in PWH is interwoven with complex cultural experiences, historical racial/ethnic disparities, tension between maternal and infant benefit, and personal opinions about how and what to feed one's infant. Thus, exploring an area of health care where recommendations are in flux demands a deep examination of how nurses and providers approach health care decisions that are historically shrouded in stigma and involve elements of risk.

The purpose of this publication is to present key updates on the *Recommendations for the Use of Antiretroviral Drugs During Pregnancy and Interventions to Reduce Perinatal HIV Transmission in the United States* published by HHS.[1] Further, the authors aim to describe relational decision-making practices foundational in the midwifery care model that may benefit health care providers when discussing infant feeding recommendations with patients and colleagues.[2] The authors focus on interdisciplinary and patient-centered communication models, including tenets of intellectual humility used to build patient–provider trust, and present management strategies in caring for PWH making infant feeding decisions. In this review, the term *breastfeeding* includes breastfeeding or chestfeeding, and the term *breast milk* refers to human milk produced by a parent with HIV to feed their infant, including milk that is expressed and fed to the infant using a bottle, spoon, or cup. The authors use WWH to include women and PWH who are birthing and breastfeeding.

BACKGROUND

Before the use of ART in WWH, research studies estimated the risk of HIV transmission through breastfeeding to be about 14% to 32% in high-income settings versus 25% to 48% in low-income settings.[3] When breastfeeding WWH are not virologically suppressed, the cumulative risk of HIV transmission through breastfeeding increases gradually with extended exposure to breast milk.[4] In countries where formula and clean water were generally readily available, WWH were historically instructed to abstain from breastfeeding to prevent the risk of HIV transmission to their infants.[5] This previous infant feeding guidance from high-income countries in North America and Europe contradicted the World Health Organization's (WHO) guidelines[6] on breastfeeding among WWH. Since 2010, the WHO recommended that WWH using ART may choose to breastfeed, given evidence supporting improved infant survival in low- and middle-income countries when infants received breast milk, despite the risk of HIV transmission.[5,6] Despite this global divide in infant feeding recommendations, breastfeeding among WWH has gained traction in high-income settings.[7] WWH and some providers have argued that the noted benefits of breastfeeding (ie, increased maternal and infant health and improved health equities among disadvantaged WWH and their infants) should support a shared decision model for infant feeding.[7,8]

Yet, as the tide began to shift and high-income countries began to explore supporting WWH in their decision to breastfeed, health professionals realized that they lacked the necessary training and knowledge to medically manage breastfeeding WWH while working to prevent perinatal HIV transmission. The lack of guidance from national organizations left institutions piecing together management plans using data from research conducted in breastfeeding WWH in low-income countries.[9] Despite the changes in published US guidelines, many unanswered questions remain. For example, in WWH with viral suppression, does mixed feeding increase the risk of transmission? What antiretroviral prophylaxis, if any, should be provided to infants while breastfeeding? When is the best time to wean? How should an elevated viral load be handled during breastfeeding? Health care providers who support WWH to breastfeed must balance these remaining uncertainties against the knowledge that the risk of HIV transmission to an infant through breast milk is very low (<1%) among virologically suppressed WWH on ART with an undetectable HIV viral load and the obvious benefits of breastfeeding to the parent and child.

The benefits of breastfeeding for the child are well known, including a lower risk of disorders such as diabetes, allergies, autoimmune disorders, obesity, malignancies, sudden infant death syndrome (SIDS), and gastrointestinal and respiratory infections.[10,11] Breastfeeding has also positively impacted intelligence in some studies.[12] Breast milk contains an ideal mixture of antibodies, vitamins, and immune factors crucial for the infant's growth and development.[10,13] Breastfeeding can also benefit postpartum people, leading to faster uterine involution and a decreased risk of postpartum bleeding and depression.[14] Furthermore, breastfeeding is associated with a decreased risk of hypertension, type 2 diabetes, and breast, endometrial, and ovarian cancers in the breastfeeding parent.[13,14] Breastfeeding also reduces health care costs and avoids the monetary costs of formula.[1,13]

On the other hand, formula is a safe and acceptable alternative to breastfeeding that carries zero risk of HIV transmission. However, there may be social stigma attached to formula use in certain cultures, which may unwittingly disclose one's HIV status through the decision to bottle feed.[15,16] WWH have historically felt stigmatized and ostracized regardless of how they feed their infants. Those who formula feed have found themselves defending their decision to use formula to family and friends and in perinatal health and nutrition clinics while trying not to disclose their HIV status.[15,17]

Because WWH in high-income settings were advised not to breastfeed for so long, many health care providers, including nurses, are not aware that the recommendations have changed or that the risk of HIV transmission is very low (<1%) among virologically suppressed WWH on ART with an undetectable HIV viral load. There is room for misinformation, mistrust, and miscommunication whenever guidelines change. Here, the authors aim to present updated information within the framework of

For all pregnant women or people with HIV	• Receive evidence-based patient-centered infant feeding counseling • A shared decision making approach between WWH and their providers should be utilized regarding infant feeding • Infant feeding choices should not result in engagement of Child Protective Services • Providers are encouraged to consult the national Perinatal HIV/AIDS hotline (1-888-448-8765) with questions about infant feeding
For WWH on ART with sustained undetectable viral load	• Receive counseling on the options of formula feeding, banked or donor milk or breastfeeding • Provide support regardless of which mode of infant feeding is chosen • Providers and WWH should discuss the possible use of infant antiretroviral (ARV) prophylaxis during breastfeeding
For WWH who are not on ART or who have a detectable viral load during pregnancy	• Replacement feeding with formula or banked, pasteurized donor human milk is recommended to eliminate the risk of HIV transmission • Barriers to maintaining a supply of replacement milk should be discussed

Fig. 1. Summary of infant feeding guide for WWH.

relational decision-making and intellectual humility that directly aligns with the updated HHS guidelines for infant feeding among WWH in high-income settings.

OVERVIEW OF UPDATED RECOMMENDATIONS FOR BREASTFEEDING IN WOMEN WITH HUMAN IMMUNODEFICIENCY VIRUS
Health and Human Services Guidelines Infant Feeding Among Women with Human Immunodeficiency Virus Summary

The HHS guidelines on infant feeding note that maintaining an undetectable viral load throughout breastfeeding considerably decreases the risk of HIV transmission to infants to less than 1%.[1] However, only replacement feeding with formula or pasteurized donor milk completely eliminates the risk of transmission. **Fig. 1** provides a summary of the HHS guidance on infant feeding. All WWH should receive infant feeding counseling that includes the most recent evidence and is patient-centered, using a shared-decision making model. Infant HIV prophylaxis guidelines are available through HHS and are summarized as follows.[18]

Communication and support strategies for WWH making infant feeding decisions:

1. Open communication and shared decision-making between health care providers and families are crucial to infant feeding discussions.
2. The team should present patient-centered counseling, including providing current evidence-based recommendations with a careful discussion of risks and benefits.
3. Assess an individual's opinions and plans about infant feeding and assist them in implementing their plans for infant feeding, including providing communication with all care team members from labor and delivery to pediatrics.[9]
4. Provide supplementary materials in appropriate languages and use interpreters as needed when sharing knowledge. A patient handout, *Breastfeeding Guidance for*

people with HIV, is available to adapt or use in the supplementary materials (Appendix 1).

Recommended care for an infant of a WWH who is breastfeeding:

1. HIV nucleic acid amplification testing (NAAT) at birth, 2 and 4 weeks of age, 2 to 4 months of age, and every 3 months after that until cessation of breastfeeding.
2. After weaning, recommendations include infant HIV NAAT testing at 4 to 6 weeks, 3 months, and 6 months after the last exposure to breast milk.
3. HIV NAAT testing is also recommended if the viral load of the WWH becomes detectable during breastfeeding.
4. Weaning over 2 to 4 weeks may avoid a potential increased risk of HIV transmission during rapid or abrupt weaning.

Proposed care for Breastfeeding Women with Human Immunodeficiency Virus

1. Support from a lactation consultant may be beneficial.
2. Breastfeeding WWH should maintain an undetectable HIV viral load throughout breastfeeding, which requires sustained adherence to ART in the postpartum period. HHS guidelines acknowledge there is little evidence to support firm recommendations on viral load monitoring during breastfeeding.[18] However, obtaining the WWHs HIV viral load at delivery, 1 month postpartum, and every 1 to 2 months thereafter is a possible approach.
3. Adherence to ART should be reviewed and encouraged at every encounter.
4. If the viral load becomes detectable, take immediate action, including considering stopping breastfeeding and starting additional medications for the baby. If viral load remains detectable after immediate retesting, HHS recommends breastfeeding be discontinued and not restarted. The infant should be started on antiretroviral prophylaxis as recommended for high-risk infants until HIV testing excludes infection.[18]
5. Mastitis or cracked and bleeding nipples may require temporary discontinuation of breastfeeding due to an increased risk of transmission. Alternative feeding options may include using flash heat-treated[19,20] expressed breast milk, stored expressed breast milk from before development of the breast disorder, or giving infant formula.

Areas of Uncertainty Regarding Breastfeeding in Women with Human Immunodeficiency Virus

HHS guidelines acknowledge several areas of uncertainty regarding the care and management of WWH and their breastfeeding infants.[1]

1. As noted above, there is not firm guidance on how often to monitor the viral load of WWH who are breastfeeding.
2. There is no consensus on recommendations for infant antiretroviral (ARV) prophylaxis during breastfeeding. Some experts feel that the usual guidance of 2 to 4 weeks of infant ARV prophylaxis is sufficient, given the low risk for HIV transmission via breast milk. Others prefer extending infant prophylaxis to a minimum of 6 weeks (in harmony with the WHO recommendations[6]), whereas others recommend extended infant prophylaxis throughout breastfeeding.[9] When using extended antiretroviral prophylaxis for breastfeeding infants, consider the potential side effects related to these medications.
3. Exclusive breastfeeding (avoidance of other foods or liquids) is recommended for the first 6 months of life because mixed feeding (ie, the addition of solid foods or

other liquids, including infant formula, to breast milk) has been associated with an increased risk of HIV transmission in WWH not on ART.[21] However, HHS notes that it is uncertain whether this increased risk of transmission exists in WWH on ART with sustained undetectable HIV viral loads. In addition, although there is convincing evidence of an increased risk of transmission when introducing solid foods before 6 months of age, it is unclear whether providing liquid infant formula concurrently with breast milk increases risk.[18]

4. Prematurity is another area of uncertainty. The premature digestive system may potentially increase the risk of HIV transmission; however, premature infants are known to benefit from breast milk if enteral feeds are tolerated.[22,23]

APPROACH TO DISCUSSING INFANT FEEDING OPTIONS
Relational Decision-Making

The HHS guidelines emphasize the importance of a shared decision-making process that openly discusses breastfeeding risks and benefits without judgment.[18] The authors proposed a model that encapsulates the complex nuances present in infant feeding decisions incorporating new scientific evidence and weighing risks and benefits. The *relational decision-making model* (**Fig. 2**) has roots in the midwifery model of care—a primary care model that incorporates continuity of care, informed consumer choice, collaborative care, accountability, and evidence-based practice. This model provides a framework for complex maternity care involving the mother, child, and health care provider triad.[24] In the relational model, decision-making is not a one-time event but a process that unfolds over time in the context of the ongoing patient–provider relationship. The relational decision-making model recognizes that relationships and social contexts shape individuals' decision-making processes, which is highly relevant to the management of WWH, as HIV status and infant feeding choices are linked in certain cultures. There is an understanding that an individual's decisions are not only influenced by relationships with others but also directly impact those around them, especially their newborn infant, which can both enhance or undermine one's sense of autonomy. Finally, the relational model of decision-making

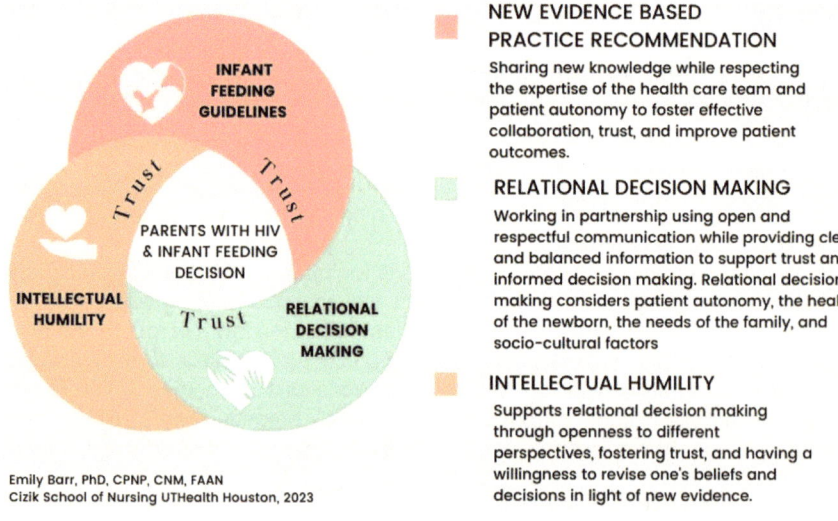

NEW EVIDENCE BASED PRACTICE RECOMMENDATION

Sharing new knowledge while respecting the expertise of the health care team and patient autonomy to foster effective collaboration, trust, and improve patient outcomes.

RELATIONAL DECISION MAKING

Working in partnership using open and respectful communication while providing clear and balanced information to support trust and informed decision making. Relational decision making considers patient autonomy, the health of the newborn, the needs of the family, and socio-cultural factors

INTELLECTUAL HUMILITY

Supports relational decision making through openness to different perspectives, fostering trust, and having a willingness to revise one's beliefs and decisions in light of new evidence.

Emily Barr, PhD, CPNP, CNM, FAAN
Cizik School of Nursing UTHealth Houston, 2023

Fig. 2. Relational decision-making model using intellectual humility and shared knowledge.

recognizes the power dynamics in the health care system and how these often reflect and reinforce similar dynamics existent in the broader social context, including historical health inequities in the care of WWH.[24]

Caring for WWH is complex and requires an interdisciplinary team of HIV experts, obstetric and midwifery team members, labor and delivery nurses, and the neonatal and pediatric health care team. The mother/parent's decision to breastfeed does not happen in a silo. Partners, extended family, and cultural norms influence infant feeding decisions. Further, for WWH, the infant feeding approaches directly impact the newborn, affect the family, and may have sociocultural implications. Successful breastfeeding among WWH requires all members of the health care team to be aware of the management plan (including the infant feeding decision), knowledgeable about the risks and benefits, and able to execute the plan in collaboration with the parents and other team members.[9] Relational decision-making is fundamental to the process of informed choice, the provision of individualized care, and the development of trusting relationships.[24] This model is especially effective when providing care for those in minority groups or marginalized settings. It emphasizes the importance of working collaboratively in interdisciplinary teams for families and navigating complications as they arise.[25]

Because this major shift in the guidelines around infant feeding has only recently occurred in high-income settings, many WWH may not be aware of the current recommendations. It is essential to recognize that the previous recommendation against breastfeeding in WWH resulted in several negative consequences for some WWH, including, in some cases, the involvement of Child Protective Services. Some infants have been removed from their home as a result of infant feeding decisions, resulting in a directive in the updated HHS guidelines specifying that child protective agencies should not be notified based on a decision to breastfeed while living with HIV.[18] There is also evidence that WWH may feel shame or guilt about not breastfeeding previous children per provider recommendations.[17] As a result, WWH may feel angry, confused, or upset about the change in guidelines, leaving health care providers trying to explain the rationale behind the previous directives against breastfeeding and evidence supporting the updated recommendations. One way to enhance relational decision-making is to use traits of intellectual humility.

Intellectual Humility

Intellectual humility in health care is a mindset, disposition, or personality trait that informs reactions to evidence as one aims to promote well-being and avoid error. It involves recognizing the limitations of one's own knowledge while being open to new ideas and, importantly, being willing to change one's beliefs in the face of new evidence.[26,27] The tenets of intellectual humility support the goals of relational decision-making and health care decisions, such as infant feeding choices in WWH, as shown in **Fig. 3**. The willingness to revise these guidelines, considering new available evidence, reflects intellectual humility on the part of health organizations. These organizations drafted the previous guidelines based on the best available evidence at the time, but they are open to changing the recommendations as new information becomes available. Furthermore, health care providers must exhibit intellectual humility when communicating these changes to patients. One may build patient–provider trust by acknowledging that previous guidelines may have been incorrect or incomplete and by providing clear and accurate current information. The challenge for the health care team lies not only in understanding the new recommendations for infant feeding and HIV but also in developing strategies for how to best share this information with patients, their families, and the wider health care team.

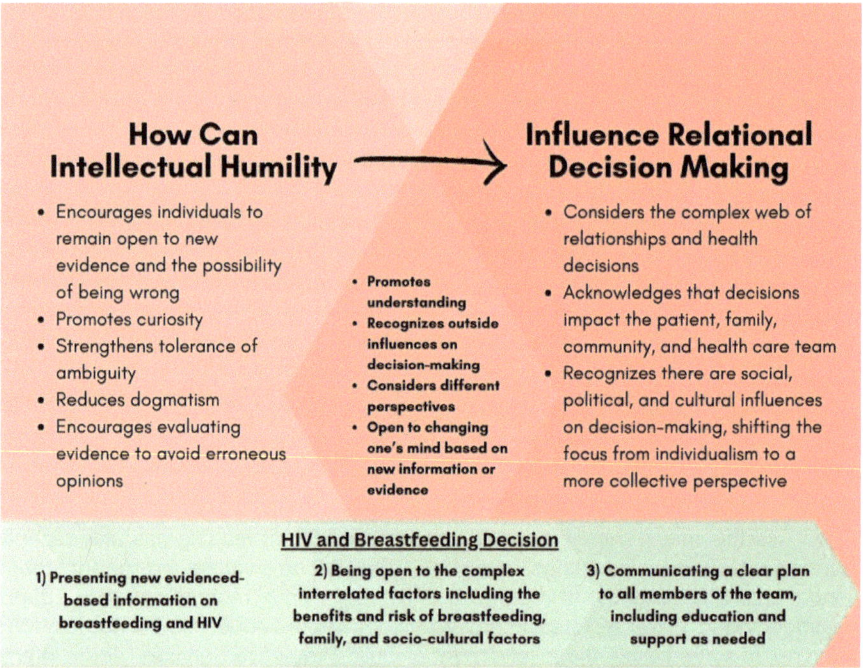

Fig. 3. How intellectual humility influences relational decision-making.

CASE STUDIES

The authors present three case studies that include challenges commonly faced in perinatal HIV care, including background information, a communication strategy based on the relational decision-making model, a consideration of internal and external factors, and the impact that the decision has on external groups, and finish with clinical management strategies for the mother and infant dyad.

Case 1

A 33-year-old woman was diagnosed with HIV at the age of 28 years. She initially elected not to start HIV medications, citing a fear of side effects and a belief that "God will cure me." She subsequently developed severe complications related to advanced HIV that required hospitalization. Her CD4 cell count at that time was 8 cells/mm^3 (7%). She began taking ART at age 30 years but had intermittent adherence struggles over the subsequent 2 years. However, when her team confirmed her pregnancy, she had an undetectable viral load and stable CD4 cell count of 270 cells/mm^3 (19%). During pregnancy, her health care team discussed possible infant feeding choices. She chose to breastfeed based on her knowledge of the benefits of breastfeeding for the infant and her belief that it was her "responsibility as a mother" to provide milk for her infant. Initially, breastfeeding was going well with no problems. However, at her 6-week postpartum checkup, her viral load was detectable at 230 copies/mL. In addition, she stated that she had a fever the day before, and her right breast was warm to the touch, tender, and mildly erythematous. Her infant was feeding and growing well with normal laboratory results and negative HIV testing at birth and 4 weeks. The 6-week HIV test results for the infant are pending.

1. Communication strategies:

    Share knowledge:

    - Explain that detectable virus in the mother's blood means there is likely to be detectable virus in her breast milk, too.
    - The risk of HIV transmission to the baby is much higher when the mother's viral load is detectable (or > 40 copies/ml).
    - Acknowledge that we are still learning about the impact of mastitis on HIV transmission but that there is a concern that mastitis could result in an increased risk of HIV transmission, even if the mother's HIV viral load was undetectable.

    Consider the internal and external factors that may impact health care decisions:

    - Ask about the mother's recent adherence to ART in a nonjudgmental way.
    - Consider how recent life events may impact her ability to adhere to ART and acknowledge that many women struggle with adherence postpartum.
    - Ask whether there are barriers to accessing or taking ART regularly (refill problems, cost, transportation, and so forth) and address them appropriately.
    - Consider whether her past beliefs about HIV and ART may be impacting her current decision to use ART (concerns about side effects, a belief that she would be cured of HIV). Ask about influences in her life that may reinforce these beliefs (family members, religious groups).
    - Ask about any pressure to either continue to breastfeed or to change to formula that may be impacting her decision. Outside influences may include religious connections, family, and/or friends.

    Consider the impact of decisions on external groups:

    - Obtain permission to communicate the final plan and the patient's decision on how she wants to proceed with her pediatric provider and lactation consultant, if she has one.

2. Management of the mother:

    - In the setting of a detectable maternal viral load and mastitis, advise the mother to pause breastfeeding immediately. Talk with the parents regarding the concern for increased risk of HIV transmission versus the benefits of ongoing breastfeeding alongside the mother's goals and desires.
    - If the mother wishes to continue breastfeeding, she can express and discard ("pump and dump") her milk until her viral load is suppressed and her mastitis has resolved.
    - Her mastitis should be treated appropriately with antibiotics, if indicated.
    - Counsel the mother about the importance of adherence to her ART. Repeat viral load testing should be arranged as soon as possible.

3. Management of the infant:

    - Discuss infant feeding options with the mother. If she has a supply of stored/frozen milk from a period before her viral load became detectable and before the onset of mastitis, she can use that to feed the infant. Alternative options may include certified banked human donor milk, mother's expressed milk that has been "flash-heated" to destroy any HIV, or infant formula.[19,20]
    - Discuss whether the infant has used a bottle for feeds in the past, as some infants struggle with switching from direct breastfeeding to use of a bottle.
    - Because of the risk that HIV transmission may have recently occurred, the infant should be tested for HIV as soon as possible and then resume follow-up testing (see "Recommended care for an infant of a WWH who is breastfeeding" above).
    - Many health care providers would advise that the infant receive empirical three-drug antiretroviral prophylaxis while awaiting the mother's and infant's test results.

Case 2

A 24-year-old woman was diagnosed with HIV during her first pregnancy. She started taking ART at 12 weeks' gestation and had an undetectable viral load beginning at 16 weeks' gestation. She fed the infant formula due to her health care team's advice at the time that WWH should not breastfeed. She has maintained an undetectable viral load since then. When she became pregnant again 2 years later, she was excited to hear from her health care team that WWH might be able to breastfeed, and she was eager to breastfeed her second child. Her partner was excited about the baby and stated that he supported her decision to breastfeed, although he expressed some concerns about the baby acquiring HIV. The mother participated in several educational sessions in the HIV clinic, but her partner did not attend. She attended educational sessions in Spanish, her native language, and took educational handouts in Spanish home with her. After these sessions, she said she felt well-informed and prepared to breastfeed. However, when she followed up in the HIV clinic a few days after delivering a full-term healthy baby girl, she stated that she had changed her mind and decided not to breastfeed. She mentioned that some of the labor and delivery unit nurses told her that it was "not a good idea." She seemed visibly upset about this decision and was tearful in the clinic.

1. Communication strategies:
   Share knowledge:
   - Use this opportunity to correct any misinformation to ensure that the parents have accurate, evidence-based information.
   - Involve the partner and any other members of the mother's support system that she would like to include in the education.
   - If possible, present data in a patient-friendly way, including using the patient's primary language.

   Consider the internal and external factors that may impact health care decisions:
   - It is important to ask how the mother feels about her decision and explore what factors led her to change her mind.
   - Recognize that the inpatient obstetrics team may have had significant concerns about the possibility of a mother transmitting HIV to her infant through breast milk, especially if those team members are unaware of the most updated data or recommendations.
   - Consider that patients may not feel empowered to advocate for their decision to breastfeed when they face scrutiny from other health care team members. This perceived lack of agency is especially a concern among minority and disadvantaged populations. This WWH identifies as a Latina who recently immigrated to the United States and understanding this aspect of her identity can be critically important to assuring she feels empowered to advocate for herself and her family.
   - Also explore whether the partner or other members of this mother's support system (family) may have expressed concerns about breastfeeding that impacted her decision.

   Consider the impact of decisions on external groups:
   - On hearing that a parent has decided not to breastfeed, health care providers may respond with a variety of emotions, including relief that the infant is at lower risk of HIV acquisition; disappointment that the mother has not managed to breastfeed despite careful preparation; and anger or frustration that a health care provider not involved in prenatal planning may have unwittingly provided misinformation about the risks of breastfeeding or made judgmental comments about the parent's decision to breastfeed.

- During the prenatal planning period, it is crucial to consider the many health care team members that will interact with a family and the importance of communicating feeding decisions to everyone involved as early as possible (obstetrics, labor and delivery, nursery, and pediatric teams).
- This communication may take the form of providing a detailed feeding plan to all parties and providing education sessions for groups unfamiliar with recent guidelines updates.

2. Management of the mother:
   - It is vital to foster autonomy in this mother's decision about how to feed her infant. It may not be too late to decide to breastfeed.
   - The mother may wish to express and store her breast milk to maintain supply while considering her options. Including a lactation consultant in the conversation and ensuring access to a breast pump, if needed, would be highly beneficial.
   - If the parents maintain their decision to feed the infant formula, then supporting them in their choice is essential. A nonjudgmental approach that involves listening and empathy builds trust and promotes engagement in care.
   - Provide all parents with ways to promote infant bonding with bottle feeding, for example, skin-to-skin contact when bottle feeding, holding the infant in the same way one would if they were breastfeeding to maintain close eye-to-eye contact, and feeding infants on demand.
   - Provide information on usual breast care when bottle feeding; for example, managing milk engorgement, comfort care, and assessing for mastitis.

3. Management of the infant:
   - Regardless of the infant feeding decision, ensure that the infant has access to a sustainable source of nutrition, whether from breast milk or formula.
   - Review the testing schedule and infant prophylaxis recommendations according to the feeding method that the parents choose.

Case 3

A 36-year-old woman was diagnosed with HIV at age 28 years. She has been taking ART continuously for several years and had an undetectable viral load before becoming pregnant. After discussing the risks and benefits of infant feeding choices, she decided to breastfeed. She expressed to her health care team her impression that breast milk was the "best" feeding choice for her baby, although she worried about the risk of HIV transmission. She also shared that she identifies as a member of a cultural group of immigrants from an African country, in which many community members equate bottle feeding with having HIV. She delivered a term male infant who received HIV prophylaxis with nevirapine beginning at birth. Initially, breastfeeding went well. The mother had an ample milk supply, and the infant had a good latch and was gaining weight appropriately. All the infant's early HIV tests were negative. At the 8-week follow-up visit, the infant presented with an erythematous sandpaper-like rash on the trunk, arms, and face. He was otherwise well-appearing and afebrile with normal vital signs. Laboratory evaluation demonstrated mild elevation of the liver enzymes (aspartate transaminase of 87 U/L and alanine transaminase of 64 U/L) and marked neutropenia (absolute neutrophil count of 500 cells/uL). The infant's 8-week HIV test is pending.

1. Communication strategies:
   Share knowledge:
   - Explain that the infant's rash is nonspecific and there are many benign causes of neonatal rashes. However, there is concern for a medication reaction in the setting of the simultaneous laboratory abnormalities.

- Acknowledge that data are lacking regarding the optimal duration of neonatal prophylaxis. Most experts recommend providing infant prophylaxis for a minimum of 4 to 6 weeks, as the early postpartum period represents the period of highest risk of HIV transmission.[18]
- There are also fewer data on antiretroviral drugs other than nevirapine for infant postnatal prophylaxis.

Consider the internal and external factors that may impact health care decisions:

- Because this parent has expressed concerns about bottle feeding potentially disclosing her HIV status within her community, it will be important to discuss how she can approach infant feeding decisions in a way that does not inadvertently disclose her diagnosis. If she decides to use formula to feed her infant, there are other medically acceptable reasons she can provide as needed to close family members, where she is unable to deflect responding due to privacy.
- Parents may struggle with competing feelings of the fear of harming their infant (through medication side effects or HIV transmission) versus fear of providing inadequate nutrition, health, or bonding experiences (by choosing formula feeding instead of breastfeeding).
- This internal struggle may result in anxiety or feelings of guilt and shame, commonly described in PWH.[15]

Consider the impact of decisions on external groups:

- Notify pediatric providers of decisions to change the feeding plan and infant antiretroviral prophylaxis.

2. Management of the mother:
   - Counsel the mother on available options, including ongoing breastfeeding or a switch to formula feeding.
   - Explore the risks and benefits of all options and support her ultimate decision.
3. Management of the infant:
   - If the infant will continue to breastfeed, options may include stopping infant antiretroviral prophylaxis altogether or switching to another medication.
   - Seek expert consultation. Follow the infant closely to ensure resolution of the clinical and laboratory abnormalities.

DISCUSSION

We have entered a new era of perinatal and newborn HIV care in which WWH living in high-income settings who are receiving ART with an undetectable viral load may elect to breastfeed with the support of their health care team. The science of preventing perinatal HIV transmission has come a long way since 1994, when studies found that zidovudine, a potent antiretroviral medication given to mothers while pregnant and in labor and to their infants, decreased the transmission rate by two-thirds.[28] When evidence emerged that HIV transmission can occur via breast milk, HIV care experts developed rigid recommendations against breastfeeding for WWH in high-income settings. Meanwhile, studies from low-income countries where breastfeeding is encouraged have taught us valuable lessons about the risks and benefits of breastfeeding among WWH.[29] These data, combined with advocacy efforts by PWH and health care providers, have led to a change in the infant feeding guidelines in many high-income countries.[30,31] However, the stigma historically associated with HIV and the complicated factors accompanying infant feeding decisions make this topic especially sensitive, requiring nuance in clinical judgment and patient–provider communication around the updated guidelines.

Providers must familiarize themselves with recent guideline changes that inform infant feeding decisions for WWH. The authors propose that nurses and health care providers caring for pregnant and postpartum WWH and their newborns update their understanding of current recommendations by contacting local or national perinatal HIV experts for the latest information on pregnancy, breastfeeding, and HIV. The US National Perinatal HIV Hotline (1–888–448–8765) is available 24 hours a day, 7 days a week, for questions related to HIV in the peripartum period, including testing, treatment, and prophylaxis for newborns. It is critical not to make assumptions about current recommendations when HIV prevention and treatment strategies are frequently updated as new evidence emerges. Health care providers should share their knowledge with staff, relevant colleagues, and trainees and explain current knowledge gaps and uncertainties. In some cases, providers may rarely care for a pregnant WWH, requiring a brief staff update on new evidence-based recommendations for all team members involved with the family's care. Finally, providers should share the information with the patient/family to enhance discussions around feeding decisions. Clearly written management plans should be shared with team members, even as the plan evolves over time. This shared knowledge is critical to establishing healthy relationships, encouraging patient autonomy, and building trust while decreasing the risk of HIV transmission to the newborn.

Intellectual humility plays a crucial role in how we approach new information, including recognizing the limitations of our own knowledge and being open to the perspectives and expertise of others.[27] Because breastfeeding can be a charged topic, applying intellectual humility may improve acceptance of alternative viewpoints and allow one to evaluate one's beliefs when considering new evidence critically. Acknowledging that we do not have all the answers makes us more open to learning from others.[27] Approaching delicate topics with humility and openness builds trust and enhances patient autonomy,[32,33] may lower stigma through less judgmental interactions, and promotes health and well-being through positive interactions with the health care team.

The authors suggest that the relational decision-making model guide provider–patient discussions around infant feeding. Applying this framework to perinatal HIV care rejects the historic paternalistic approach in which families had very little say in the obstetric and pediatric management plan and expands on the shared decision-making model proposed by HHS. As WWH have diverse cultural, religious, and ethnic backgrounds, it is essential to recognize that their infant feeding decision impacts and is impacted by their prior infant feeding experiences, relationships with family, religious communities, and society. Furthermore, WWH will interact with labor and delivery nurses, the obstetrician and midwife, the newborn medical team, and the pediatric health care team, and all these individuals will have an opinion about the decision to breastfeed or formula feed their infant. This major decision is not made in a vacuum and must consider the myriad of people involved, including, and most importantly, the WWH and their newborn infant.

SUMMARY

Current HHS guidelines recommend that WWH who are receiving ART with a sustained undetectable HIV viral load should receive evidence-based counseling on all infant feeding options, including the use of formula, banked donor milk, or breast milk and the health care providers support the chosen mode of infant feeding. As this advice represents a significant shift in the guidelines from previous versions, it is imperative that health care providers engage in conversations with WWH in an open and nonjudgmental fashion that shares current knowledge, acknowledges remaining limitations, and allows for autonomy and choice, while promoting the health and well-being of the WWH and the newborn.

CLINICS CARE POINTS

- All women with HIV who are receiving antiretroviral therapy with a sustained undetectable HIV viral load should receive evidence-based counseling on all infant feeding options including formula, banked donor, or breast milk.
- Ensure that the parents making infant feeding decisions and their health care providers understand that the risk of HIV transmission to the newborn through breastfeeding is less than 1% when the parent is on antiretroviral therapy with HIV viral suppression. However, risks remain, including a low risk of HIV transmission and medication side effects.
- Consider stopping breastfeeding and starting additional medications if the parent's viral load becomes detectable. If the viral load remains detectable after immediate retesting, discontinue breastfeeding and offer alternative feeding options. The infant should be started on antiretroviral prophylaxis as recommended for high-risk infants until HIV testing excludes infection.
- Encourage open communication with the breastfeeding family to support initiating breastfeeding, pumping and storing breast milk, managing any side effects or complications, and weaning when the family is ready.
- Use a relational decision-making model to support communication when caring for women with HIV, including sharing knowledge, considering internal and external factors that may impact health care decisions, and working collaboratively in interdisciplinary teams.

ACKNOWLEDGMENTS

The authors would like to thank Hannah Armitage, MPH, University of Texas Health Science Center at Houston Cizik School of Nursing, Houston, TX and Andrew Kim, Rice University, Houston, TX.

FUNDING

We would like to acknowledge USDA REEU NIFA Grant #2022-68018-36607, and the Sumner Roy Kates Charitable Trust for funding this work.

DISCLOSURES

The authors report no real or perceived vested interests related to this article that could be construed as a conflict of interest.

REFERENCES

1. DHHS. Infant Feeding for Individuals with HIV in the United States. 2023. Perinatal HIV Clinical Guidelines. Department of Health and Human Services. Updated January 31, 2023 https://clinicalinfo.hiv.gov/en/guidelines/perinatal/infant-feeding-individuals-hiv-united-states. Accessed September 15, 2023.
2. Noseworthy DA, Phibbs SR, Benn CA. Towards a relational model of decision-making in midwifery care. Midwifery 2013;29(7):e42–8.
3. De Cock KM, Fowler MG, Mercier E, et al. Prevention of mother-to-child HIV transmission in resource-poor countries: translating research into policy and practice. JAMA 2000;283(9):1175-1182.

4. Davis NL, Miller WC, Hudgens MG, et al. Maternal and breastmilk viral load: impacts of adherence on peripartum HIV infections averted-the breastfeeding, antiretrovirals, and nutrition Study. J Acquir Immune Defic Syndr 2016;73(5):572–80.
5. Mofenson LM, Flynn PM, Aldrovandi GM, et al. Infant Feeding and transmission of human immunodeficiency virus in the United States by the Committee on Pediatric AIDS. Pediatrics 2013;131(2):391–6.
6. WHO. Updates on HIV and Infant Feeding: The Duration of Breastfeeding, and Support from Health Services to Improve Feeding Practices Among Mothers Living with HIV. Guidelines. World Health Organization. Updated 2016 https://www.ncbi.nlm.nih.gov/books/NBK379865/. Accessed September 15, 2023.
7. Johnson G, Levison J, Malek J. Should providers discuss breastfeeding with women living with HIV in high-income countries? An ethical analysis. Clin Infect Dis 2016;63(10):1368–72.
8. Gross MS, Taylor HA, Tomori C, et al. Breastfeeding with HIV: an evidence-based case for new policy. J Law Med Ethics 2019;47(1):152–60.
9. Abuogi L, Smith C, Kinzie K, et al. Development and implementation of an interdisciplinary model for the management of breastfeeding in women with HIV in the United States: experience from the Children's Hospital Colorado Immunodeficiency Program. J Acquir Immune Defic Syndr 2023. https://doi.org/10.1097/QAI.0000000000003213.
10. Victora CG, Bahl R, Barros AJ, et al. Breastfeeding in the 21st century: epidemiology, mechanisms, and lifelong effect. Lancet 30 2016;387(10017):475–90.
11. Horta BL, Loret de Mola C, Victora CG. Long-term consequences of breastfeeding on cholesterol, obesity, systolic blood pressure and type 2 diabetes: a systematic review and meta-analysis. Acta Paediatr 2015;104(S467):30–7.
12. Horta BL, Loret de Mola C, Victora CG. Breastfeeding and intelligence: a systematic review and meta-analysis. Acta Paediatr 2015;104(S467):14–9.
13. Dieterich CM, Felice JP, O'Sullivan E, et al. Breastfeeding and health outcomes for the mother-infant dyad. Pediatr Clin 2013;60(1):31–48.
14. Chowdhury R, Sinha B, Sankar MJ, et al. Breastfeeding and maternal health outcomes: a systematic review and meta-analysis. Acta Paediatr 2015;104(S467):96–113.
15. Alvarenga WA, Nascimento LC, Leal CL, et al. Mothers living with HIV: replacing breastfeeding by infant formula. Rev Bras Enferm 2019;72(5):1153–60.
16. Griswold MK, Pagano-Therrien J. Women living with HIV in high income countries and the deeper meaning of breastfeeding avoidance: a metasynthesis. J Hum Lactation 2020;36(1):44–52.
17. Tariq S, Elford J, Tookey P, et al. "It pains me because as a woman you have to breastfeed your baby": decision-making about infant feeding among African women living with HIV in the U.K. Sex Transm Infect 2016;92(5):331–6.
18. DHHS. Antiretroviral Management of Newborns with Perinatal HIV Exposure or HIV Infection. Department of Health and Human Services. Updated April 11, 2023 https://clinicalinfo.hiv.gov/en/guidelines/pediatric-arv/antiretroviral-management-newborns-perinatal-hiv-exposure-or-hiv-infection. Accessed September 15, 2023.
19. Israel-Ballard K, Donovan R, Chantry C, et al. Flash-heat inactivation of HIV-1 in human milk: a potential method to reduce postnatal transmission in developing countries. J Acquir Immune Defic Syndr 2007;45(3):318–23.
20. Volk ML, Hanson CV, Israel-Ballard K, et al. Inactivation of cell-associated and cell-free HIV-1 by flash-heat treatment of breast milk. J Acquir Immune Defic Syndr 2010;53(5):665–6.

21. Coovadia HM, Rollins NC, Bland RM, et al. Mother-to-child transmission of HIV-1 infection during exclusive breastfeeding in the first 6 months of life: an intervention cohort study. Lancet 2007;369(9567):1107–16.

22. Fouché C, van Niekerk E, du Plessis LM. Differences in breast milk composition of HIV-infected and HIV-uninfected mothers of premature infants: effects of antiretroviral therapy. Breastfeed Med 2016;11(9):455–60.

23. Boquien CY. Human Milk: an ideal food for nutrition of preterm newborn. Front Pediatr 2018;6:295.

24. Thachuk A. Midwifery, informed choice, and reproductive autonomy: a relational approach. Fem Psychol 2007;17(1):39–56.

25. Homer CSE. Models of maternity care: evidence for midwifery continuity of care. Med J Australia 2016;205(8):370–4.

26. Leary MR. Intellectual humility as a route to more accurate knowledge, better decisions, and less conflict. Am J Health Promot 2022;36(8):1401–4.

27. Ballantyne N. Recent work on intellectual humility: a philosopher's perspective. J Posit Psychol 2023;18(2):200–20.

28. Connor EM, Sperling RS, Gelber R, et al. Reduction of maternal-infant transmission of human immunodeficiency virus type 1 with zidovudine treatment. N Engl J Med 1994;331(18):1173–80.

29. Flynn PM, Taha TE, Cababasay M, et al. Association of Maternal Viral Load and CD4 Count With Perinatal HIV-1 Transmission Risk During Breastfeeding in the PROMISE Postpartum Component. J Acquir Immune Defic Syndr 2021;88(2):206–13.

30. Gilleece DY, Tariq DS, Bamford DA, et al. British HIV Association guidelines for managing HIV in pregnancy and postpartum 2018. HIV Med 2019;20(Suppl 3):s2–85.

31. Khan S, Tsang KK, Brophy J, et al. Canadian Pediatric & Perinatal HIV/AIDS Research Group consensus recommendations for infant feeding in the HIV context. JAMMI 2023;8(1):7–17.

32. Huynh HP, Dicke-Bohmann A. Humble doctors, healthy patients? Exploring the relationships between clinician humility and patient satisfaction, trust, and health status. Patient Educ Couns 2020;103(1):173–9.

33. Schumann K, Koetke J, Ludwig JM. Intellectual humility in the health and well-being context: implications for promoting positive client relationships, client receptivity, and unbiased information gathering. Am J Health Promot 2022;36(8):1414–8.

APPENDIX 1: BREASTFEEDING GUIDANCE FOR PEOPLE WITH HIV

BREASTFEEDING GUIDANCE FOR PEOPLE WITH HIV

CONSIDERATIONS FOR BREASTFEEDING OR CHESTFEEDING

- Continue taking your HIV medication as prescribed.
- When your HIV viral load is undetectable your chances of passing HIV to your baby are very low.
- Your baby will be taking HIV medication while breastfeeding and for a short time after they wean to help prevent HIV transmission.
- You and your baby will see your medical team and have blood drawn more often while breastfeeding and after weaning to know if changes are needed in medications or feeding.

PROMOTING HEALTHY BREASTFEEDING

LATCHING

- **Meet with a lactation consultant**
- Practicing proper positioning will help your baby get a good latch
- A good latch will help your baby get the most milk and help prevent discomfort, and cracked and bleeding nipples

SELF-CARE

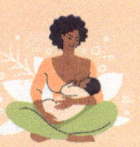

- Rest when you can
- Drink plenty of fluids
- Take your daily HIV medications

OPTIMAL POSITIONS

Cradle Position
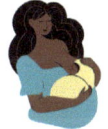

Side Lying
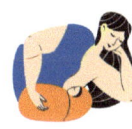

Cross-Cradle Hold
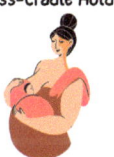

Football Hold
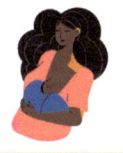

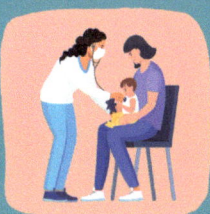

COMMUNICATION

- Talk with family and health care providers about your decision to breastfeed

- Notify your care team immediately:
  - Changes in medication
  - Changes in your HIV viral load
  - You show signs of illness, cracked nipples, or mastitis
  - Your baby starts to get sick

WHAT IS EXCLUSIVE BREASTFEEDING?

1 Your baby is getting only breast milk, and no other food, drinks, or formula

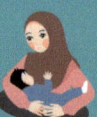

2 It is OK for your baby to take your breast milk straight from you or out of a bottle.

3 Medicine or vitamins prescribed by your doctor are allowed

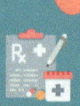

4 Start giving bottles of your own breast milk 2–4 weeks after birth to help transition to formula later

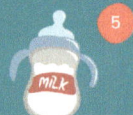

5 At 6 months, you may introduce solid foods following your child's provider's recommendations. You may continue to breastfeed until you are ready to wean.

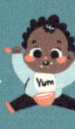

LOWERING RISK OF HIV TRANSMISSION

MIXED FEEDING

- Your health care team may ask you to try and exclusively breastfeed, but there may be times when you need to give your baby something other than breastmilk, like formula.
- Talk with your team about this if you have questions.

BABY'S SYMPTOMS

- Your child could be at higher risk of HIV transmission or have an illness that needs to be treated if there is:
  - Thrush
  - Vomitting
  - Fever
  - Rash
  - Loose poop
- Contact pediatric provider & HIV team

CRACKED NIPPLES & MASTITIS

Cracked Nipples:
- Please contact your HIV provider if this occurs
- Seek guidance from a lactation consultant to support proper positioning

Mastitis:
- An infection in the breast, which may increase the risk of HIV transmission.
- Breast pain, redness, red streaks, or fever
- If you experience any of these symptoms, contact your HIV provider immediately and switch to stored breastmilk while your mastitis is treated

NOTE: TALK WITH YOUR HIV TEAM ABOUT WHETHER HEATING BREASTMILK MAY BE A SAFE OPTION FOR YOU TO USE IN SOME CIRCUMSTANCES

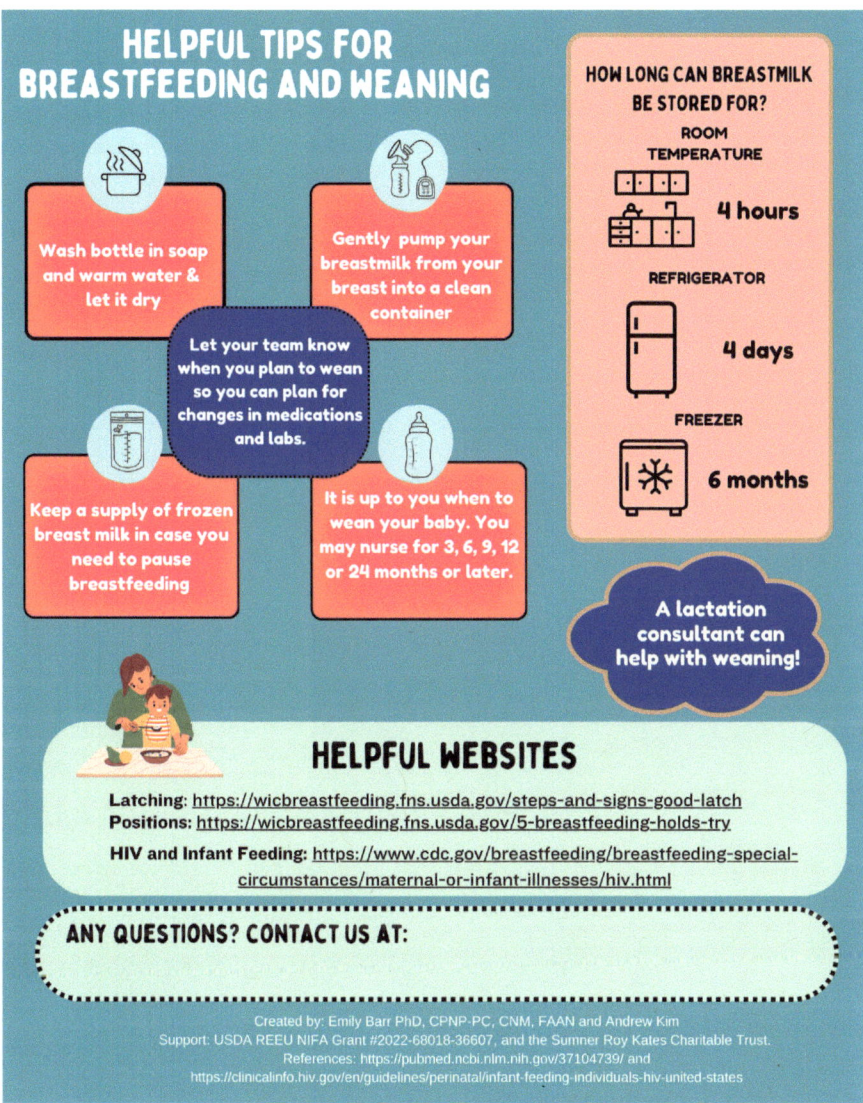

HELPFUL TIPS FOR BREASTFEEDING AND WEANING

Wash bottle in soap and warm water & let it dry

Gently pump your breastmilk from your breast into a clean container

Let your team know when you plan to wean so you can plan for changes in medications and labs.

Keep a supply of frozen breast milk in case you need to pause breastfeeding

It is up to you when to wean your baby. You may nurse for 3, 6, 9, 12 or 24 months or later.

HOW LONG CAN BREASTMILK BE STORED FOR?

ROOM TEMPERATURE — 4 hours

REFRIGERATOR — 4 days

FREEZER — 6 months

A lactation consultant can help with weaning!

HELPFUL WEBSITES

Latching: https://wicbreastfeeding.fns.usda.gov/steps-and-signs-good-latch
Positions: https://wicbreastfeeding.fns.usda.gov/5-breastfeeding-holds-try

HIV and Infant Feeding: https://www.cdc.gov/breastfeeding/breastfeeding-special-circumstances/maternal-or-infant-illnesses/hiv.html

ANY QUESTIONS? CONTACT US AT:

Created by: Emily Barr PhD, CPNP-PC, CNM, FAAN and Andrew Kim
Support: USDA REEU NIFA Grant #2022-68018-36607, and the Sumner Roy Kates Charitable Trust.
References: https://pubmed.ncbi.nlm.nih.gov/37104739/ and
https://clinicalinfo.hiv.gov/en/guidelines/perinatal/infant-feeding-individuals-hiv-united-states

Overview of the Epidemiology and Clinical Care Considerations for Adolescents and Young Adults Living with or at Risk of Human Immunodeficiency Virus

Adam Leonard, MS, MPH, CPNP-PC, AAHIVS[a,b,]*,
Brenice Duroseau, MSN, FNP-C, RNC-OB, AAHIVS[a]

KEYWORDS

• HIV • Sexual health • Adolescent • Young adult • Adolescent health services

KEY POINTS

- Adolescent and young adults (AYAs) ages 13 to 24 account for a significant proportion of new human immunodeficiency virus (HIV) infections annually in the United States.
- Developmental factors, legal and ethical constraints, and structural issues lead to disparities in HIV prevention efforts and HIV care outcomes for this age group.
- Policy changes at the legislative and health-systems level can reduce new HIV infections among youth and improve care outcomes along the HIV continuum for AYAs.

INTRODUCTION

Human immunodeficiency virus (HIV) remains a critical public health issue in the United States even after more than 40 years since cases were first reported.[1] This is especially true for adolescents and young adults (AYAs) aged 13 to 24 across the nation, who continue to be significantly impacted and have suboptimal outcomes along each step of the HIV care continuum—diagnosis, linkage to care, and retention in care.[2] Recent data indicate a disturbing trend: while overall HIV diagnoses have declined, a significant proportion of AYAs living with HIV are unaware of their status,

[a] Center for Infectious Disease and Nursing Innovation, Johns Hopkins School of Nursing, Baltimore, MD, USA; [b] Community Health Systems, University of California, San Francisco School of Nursing, San Francisco, CA, USA
* Corresponding author. 525 North Wolfe Street, Baltimore, MD 21205.
E-mail address: aleona24@jh.edu
Twitter: @ajleonard8283 (A.L.); @thenpthatcares (B.D.)

Nurs Clin N Am 59 (2024) 329–344
https://doi.org/10.1016/j.cnur.2024.03.002
0029-6465/24/© 2024 Elsevier Inc. All rights reserved.

compromising efforts to end the HIV epidemic by 2030.[3] An immediate reevaluation of public health strategies and the development of interventions are necessary due to the present state of HIV among AYAs.

The evolving landscape of HIV among AYAs necessitates a comprehensive review of current epidemiologic trends, prevention strategies, and policy environment shaping HIV vulnerabilities and access to care. This article aims to provide an updated examination of these elements, highlighting areas of progress and ongoing challenges. By integrating the latest research findings, clinical guidelines, and public health initiatives, this article seeks to identify gaps in the current approach and delineate related health and psychosocial needs for youth living with or vulnerable to HIV. Through this analysis, nursing researchers and clinical leaders will be able to develop actionable, evidence-based strategies aimed at enhancing prevention, improving diagnosis, and optimizing care—critical points along the HIV care continuum—for AYAs. Investigating the statistical trends and addressing the core challenges (overt and underlying) to effective HIV intervention and care among AYAs is not just a pressing public health priority—it is a moral imperative that requires a commitment to equitable health care access and achieving positive outcomes for all individuals affected by HIV.

EPIDEMIOLOGIC OVERVIEW OF HUMAN IMMUNODEFICIENCY VIRUS AMONG ADOLESCENTS AND YOUNG ADULTS
Human Immunodeficiency Virus Transmission

Unprotected sexual intercourse remains a significant driver of HIV transmission among AYAs. Despite a reported decline in adolescent sexual activity, the prevalence of sexually transmitted infections (STIs) among AYAs who are sexually active remains concerningly high, thus increasing biological vulnerability to HIV.[4] In 2022, AYAs had the highest reported incidence of chlamydia and gonorrhea across all age groups in the United States, with notable surges in primary and secondary syphilis.[4] Additionally, most recent data show that about half of all new STI diagnoses occur within this demographic.[4] Yet, while reported STIs are increasing and disproportionately impacting AYAs, the percentages of youth reporting condom use during their last sexual encounter and STI screening in the past year have decreased to all-time lows since 2019.[5] This underscores the critical need for enhanced STI screening, treatment, and prevention services tailored specifically to AYAs. Given their disproportionate share of new STI diagnoses, there is a pressing need to mitigate their heightened vulnerability to HIV through effective prevention and education strategies.

AYAs engaged in injection drug use or who share drug injection equipment face a heightened risk of HIV acquisition. Among people who inject drugs (PWIDs), individuals aged 13 to 34 years accounted for nearly half of the new HIV diagnoses, highlighting a pressing concern.[6] Despite 13-year-olds to 24-year-olds accounting for a smaller overall proportion of new HIV infections among PWIDs compared to the 25-to-34 age group, AYAs exhibit significantly higher rates of HIV risk behaviors associated with substance use.[6] This includes the sharing of needles, a practice reported by almost half of AYA drug users, and shared use of other injection equipment, which was endorsed by nearly three-quarters of AYA drug users, further escalating their risk for HIV as well as other infectious diseases like hepatitis C virus.[6]

Recent data indicate that among the nearly 12,000 individuals in the United States living with perinatally acquired HIV, approximately half are AYAs aged 13 to 24 years.[7] Despite the dramatic decline in perinatal HIV transmission in the United States over the last decade—with just 36 cases reported nationwide in 2020—a significant number of those with perinatally acquired HIV are now navigating the complexities of adolescence and young adulthood.[7] Perinatally impacted AYAs confront distinct medical challenges, notably antiretroviral (ARV) drug resistance, which arises both from resistance transmitted at the time of infection and from resistance developed due to ARV nonadherence. On average, individuals with perinatally acquired HIV began ARV therapy (ART) between the ages of 1 and 5, have been exposed to 3 to 3 different ART regimens, and have been on ART for at least 10 years by the time they reach adolescence.[8] Furthermore, the cumulative effects of HIV chronic inflammation contribute to risk of cardiovascular disease, neurologic dysfunction, metabolic disorders, and accelerated aging.[8,9] Shortened telomere length, a genetic indicator of accelerated aging, also correlates with impairment in working memory, executive function, and information processing speed seen among AYAs with perinatally acquired HIV.[10]

Beyond the immediate medical challenges, AYAs with perinatally acquired HIV encounter significant psychosocial barriers. The complexity of maintaining long-term adherence to demanding HIV treatment regimens is exacerbated by the personal and social challenges of disclosing their status and forming relationships with peers. These challenges are intensified in environments lacking in empathy, accurate HIV knowledge, and proper support, and where stigma and alienation are rampant.[8] Furthermore, the HIV stigma and structural inequities, such as poverty and associated trauma, play a pivotal role in not only the initial risk and acquisition of perinatal HIV but also contribute to delayed developmental milestones, psychopathology, and substance use disorders within this group.[11,12] Addressing these issues necessitates a multifaceted approach that includes enhancing support systems, providing targeted mental health services, and mitigating structural barriers to health care and social support.[11,12]

Human Immunodeficiency Virus Incidence, Prevalence, and Diagnosis

Nearly 1 in 5 estimated new HIV infections in 2021 were among AYAs, marking a notable decrease over previous years. The rate of new infections has fallen by approximately 34% since 2017, with significant reductions observed among young gay and bisexual males.[13] This downward trend is likely the result of multiple factors, including a reported decrease in sexual activity among high school–aged students and increased access to preventive measures like pre-exposure prophylaxis (PrEP).[14,15] Despite these encouraging developments, this trend may not fully capture persistent challenges in HIV prevention within this demographic, especially as percentage changes in smaller populations tend to mask intragroup disparities.[16] For instance, about 80% of new infections among AYAs were among young men who have sex with men (YMSM), predominantly within black or Latino communities.[7] Similarly, the rate of new infections among black YMSM saw a 27% decrease from 2017 to 2021, which, while significant, lags behind the reduction rates seen among their white YMSM counterparts.[7]

In 2021, prevalence estimates indicated that 41,900 AYAs were living with HIV, yet just over half were aware of their HIV status, marking the lowest awareness rate among all age groups nationally.[17] Alarmingly, HIV testing among AYAs has plummeted to only 6%, representing a drastic decline of more than 50% over the past decade.[5] This decline occurs despite longstanding, reputable guidance recommending routine HIV screening for AYAs beginning at age 13.[18,19] The repercussions of this testing deficit are significant, as many AYAs are diagnosed at a later stage of the disease, when their immune systems are already significantly compromised.[20]

Several factors contribute to this low HIV testing uptake, including restrictive state policies that limit minor consent and confidentiality protections, which pose significant barriers for AYAs at greatest risk of HIV.[21] Furthermore, the coronavirus disease 2019 pandemic has added layers of complexity to this issue, affecting sexual behavior, access to testing, and the overall incidence and diagnosis of HIV, especially among youth. The full impact of these changes is yet to be fully understood, suggesting that current HIV prevalence estimates may be underestimating true rates.[22]

Linkage and Retention in Human Immunodeficiency Virus Care

Timely linkage to HIV care after diagnosis is a priority objective of the National HIV/Acquired Immunodeficiency Syndrome (AIDS) Strategy and the Ending the HIV Epidemic (EHE) effort in the United States.[3] Delayed linkage to care prevents AYAs from initiating and benefiting from ART while also increasing risks of forward HIV transmission in the community. More than 20% of AYAs are not linked to care within the EHE stated standard of 1 month since diagnosis, the highest percentage of any age group.[23] The Centers for Disease Control and Prevention defines care retention as patients with 2 or more clusters of differentiation 4 (CD4) or viral load tests performed at least 3 months apart.[24] Retention in care improves health outcomes and reduces sexual risk behaviors and is an essential step to achieving and maintaining viral suppression. AYAs diagnosed with HIV struggle to maintain care engagement as more than 40% of this age group were lost to follow-up (LTFU) in 2019.[25] Young men had higher rates of LTFU than females and structural factors like poverty, low educational attainment, and inadequate health insurance also increase the risk of LTFU for all AYAs.[23] Targeted, high-touch interventions that provide material support and benefits navigation have been shown to improve linkage and retention in care for AYAs and should be considered for inclusion in all organizations serving AYAs living with HIV.[26]

Antiretroviral Treatment Initiation, Adherence, and Viral Suppression

The World Health Organization and US HIV treatment guidelines, as well as various professional society practice recommendations, endorse immediate initiation of ART in all patients regardless of CD4 count.[27–29] Immediate, or rapid, ART initiation is shown to increase rates of ART adherence and viral suppression at 12 months and may also improve care retention.[30] Following these recommendations, rates of ART prescription to AYAs increased to greater than 80%; however, issues with consistent daily adherence to regimens persist.[31] Estimates suggest that just over half of North American AYAs living with HIV meet thresholds for optimal ART adherence, the lowest regional proportion globally.[32] Various interventions with differing degrees of effectiveness have been implemented to improve adherence among youth, including individualized adherence counseling sessions, utilization of motivational interviewing techniques, group support meetings, family involvement, and multiple technology-based reminder modalities.[33]

As a result of adherence disparities, AYAs living with HIV are more likely to experience poor clinical outcomes, most notably, low rates of durable viral suppression. Nationally, AYAs have suboptimal viral suppression with point-in-time estimate of 68% viral suppression and rates of sustained viral suppression for 12 months ranging from 12% to 51% across studies.[25,34,35] A lack of viral suppression among people aware of their HIV status is a key driver of new HIV infections in the community. An estimated 62% of new HIV infections are attributable to transmissions from people who were aware of their status but are either not in care or in care but not virally suppressed.[36] As such, achieving high rates of durable viral suppression among youth living with HIV is a key priority of EHE.

Transition to Adult Human Immunodeficiency Virus Care

AYAs living with HIV have an additional, unique, step in the HIV care continuum: transition to adult care. As young people mature, whether HIV is acquired perinatally or during their adolescence, they must move from youth-friendly to adult models of care. This transition is often experienced as a sense of loss for both the health care teams and patients. It also is a time of stress and confusion and AYAs are at risk of falling out of care while trying to navigate an adult-oriented system that is often much less personal feeling.[37] Efforts to streamline the transition process, including formalized transition programs that assess readiness, foster self-management skills, provide detailed medical record transfer, and include case management support, may improve the process.[38] Despite this, most AYAs who do transition to an adult provider still fall out of care within the first year of transfer, suggesting sustained supports are warranted.[39]

HUMAN IMMUNODEFICIENCY VIRUS PREVENTION FOR ADOLESCENTS AND YOUNG ADULTS

HIV PrEP is a highly effective prevention tool available since 2012 and is recommended for AYAs at risk of HIV infection.[40] Leading AYA health organizations have called for the integration of routine PrEP services into existing health services for young people since PrEP was first approved for adolescent use in 2018.[41,42] Perhaps not surprisingly though, given the disparities previously noted in HIV care outcomes for youth, AYAs aged 16 to 24 have lowest PrEP coverage of any age group nationally. Only 20% of youth at increased risk for HIV infection were prescribed PrEP, once again representing the lowest proportion of PrEP uptake among all age groups nationally.[43] Various barriers for AYA PrEP initiation and persistent use across the continuum exist, from low PrEP awareness to premature discontinuation, and therefore multilevel interventions to improve HIV prevention services for AYAs are urgently needed.[44]

A 2022 meta-analysis found that only 64% of AYAs prescribed PrEP were adherent to it.[45] Several factors moderate adherence to PrEP among AYAs. Specifically, adherence to PrEP varies based on gender, with young cisgender women demonstrating lower adherence compared to YMSM and serodiscordant heterosexual couples.[45] The method of PrEP administration also influenced adherence, with daily tablet regimens associated with higher adherence compared to nondaily dosing regimens. The follow-up time point for adherence measurement was also found to be a significant moderator, with studies assessing adherence less than 6 months after PrEP initiation showing higher adherence compared to studies with a follow-up of 6 months or greater. Interest in other PrEP delivery modalities, most notably injectable, is high among AYAs yet much of the evidence is based on theoretic interest and little research has been done on acceptability and uptake of injectable options once implemented.[46] Ultimately, interventions using mobile technologies, frequent supportive follow-up, and material supports to overcome structural barriers are required to support expanded uptake and persistent use of PrEP among AYAs.[45]

COMORBID HEALTH CONCERNS

AYAs living with HIV are at increased risk compared to their HIV-negative peers for other comorbid conditions, both because of factors that predispose to HIV acquisition in the first place as well as sequelae of HIV disease. Rates of opportunistic infections and HIV-associated death have decreased significantly for AYAs since the advent of ART. However, mortality remains elevated among this group compared to youth without HIV infection.[47] AYAs living with HIV are at risk of numerous physical health concerns, including latent tuberculosis, metabolic conditions like diabetes, atypical mycobacterial infections, human papilloma virus (HPV) disease, asthma, and vitamin D deficiency, among other conditions.[47] Nurses and other health care providers working with AYAs living with HIV should be aware of these risks and screen patients appropriately. In addition to routine preventive health care surveillance, providers should be mindful of unique care guidelines for this population, including different immunization guidelines and onset and periodicity of important screenings, such as for HPV-related cancers.[48]

Psychiatric and behavioral health conditions comprise the bulk of comorbidities among AYAs living with HIV. Issues range from neurodevelopmental conditions to substance use disorders.[47] Trauma exposures and sequelae are common among this group with some community-based surveys reporting near universal endorsement of adverse childhood experiences and alarmingly high rates of post-traumatic stress disorder.[49] Harmful substance use is also common; both disordered opioid use as well as disproportionate use of psychostimulants like methamphetamine are high.[49,50] Sexual and gender minority (SGM) AYAs living with HIV report higher rates of psychiatric and behavioral health disorders, likely resulting from intersectional stigmas and discrimination.[51] Therefore, inclusion of dedicated mental health and substance use services into HIV care for AYA should be considered a standard of care.[41,52]

DEVELOPMENTAL, ETHICAL–LEGAL, AND STRUCTURAL CONSIDERATIONS
Developmental Context

Adolescence is a time of the greatest physical, psychological, social, and emotional development in life, second only to that of infancy.[53] HIV infection is implicated in delayed or altered physical and psychosocial development among AYAs. Youth living with HIV experience delays in pubertal growth, which in turn is associated with decreased virological suppression, abnormal bone health, and mortality.[54] HIV infection also impacts the psychological development trajectories of youth. Identity formation and integration is paramount during adolescence. HIV infection can be a particularly disruptive force during this period given its impact on peer relationships, stress associated with anticipated and enacted social stigma, as well as implications for one's emerging sexual life.[55] Nurses and other health care providers should be particularly mindful of the developmental needs and struggles of AYAs with HIV and provide support with the tasks of identity formation and integration, specifically as it relates to HIV status disclosure to peers and potential sexual partners.[55]

Ethical and Legal Considerations

There are multiple legal and ethical considerations to consider when working with AYAs living with or at risk of HIV infection, ranging from status disclosure to youth with perinatally acquired HIV to participation in HIV-related research. The complex web of ethical and legal constraints governing consent, confidentiality, and involvement in HIV care or research is difficult to navigate for both health care providers and AYAs. Laws regarding minor consenting ability for HIV testing and treatment vary widely by state and involvement in HIV-related research is largely a piecemeal process governed by siloed institutional review boards, which may not be consistent with current science on adolescent decisional capacity. Nurses working with AYAs must be acutely aware of state laws governing the differing legal concepts of consent and confidentiality as well as their own institution's guidance regarding AYA research participation.

The American Academy of Pediatrics suggests that children with perinatally acquired HIV should be told of their HIV status in a developmentally appropriate manner during their school-aged years.[56] Yet, health care workers and parents often find themselves at odds over timing of disclosure, having very different perspectives on harm versus benefit.[57] For youth diagnosed with community-acquired HIV, state laws vary on status disclosure to parents or caregivers. Currently, minors can consent for HIV testing and treatment in all 50 states and the District of Columbia.[58] Clear legislation endorsing minor consent for preventive care for STIs like PrEP is also lacking, leaving PrEP provision in a legal gray area in some jurisdictions.[21]

Confidentiality protections against disclosure to parents or care givers are rare in legal statutes and 18 state expressly allow for medical providers to use their discretion in parental notification, with 1 state even mandating parental notification.[59] These state laws often lack components regulating payor-related confidentiality concerns, overlooking clear privacy violations with mandated explanation of benefits mailings.[21] Inadequate minor consent and confidentiality laws are directly linked to HIV testing rates among youth, and as such, nurses should advocate for policy changes that enshrine strong minor consent and confidentiality provisions as consistent with current science.[21]

Regardless of state laws governing minor consent for HIV services, independent minor participation in HIV prevention and care research is drastically limited. PrEP was first approved for use in adults by the Food and Drug Administration in 2012, yet approval for use in adolescents was not granted until 2018. This 6-year gap in approval significantly limited roll out of highly effective PrEP to minors and was largely due to an absence of minor inclusion in initial PrEP trials. This is despite widespread pediatric use and demonstrated safety of this medication as part of a complete HIV treatment regimen.[60] Guidance supporting independent minor consent for involvement in HIV prevention research, including drug trials, with developmentally appropriate adjustments is ubiquitous.[61–63] Therefore, nurses engaged in research should advocate for inclusion of AYAs in trials as minor exclusion delays regulatory approval of biomedical prevention options for this vulnerable group and perpetuates disparities.

Social and Structural Determinants of Health

Social vulnerability and structural determinants of health heavily influence HIV risk and HIV-associated disparities. People living with HIV experience more poverty, homelessness, disability, and incarceration than other Americans.[64] These disparities impede engagement and retention in HIV care.[65] Systemic racism through redlining and economic disinvestment has led to increased social vulnerabilities in primarily African American communities.[66] These social vulnerabilities are associated with increased risk of HIV incidence and require policy-level interventions to reduce HIV racial disparities.[66] Medicaid expansion under the Affordable Care Act is 1 such policy change that can improve uptake of PrEP and improve HIV care outcomes.[67] Yet, 10 states have failed to implement this coverage expansion.[68] Seven of those non-expansion states are the South, which, as a region, accounts for more than half of all new HIV infections in the United States.[7] Modeling suggests that Medicaid expansion could be especially beneficial for YMSM, reducing new HIV infections up to 15% over time.[69]

DISCUSSION

AYAs remain vulnerable to increased rates of HIV infection and poor outcomes at each step of the HIV care continuum (**Fig. 1**). As such, they represent a priority population

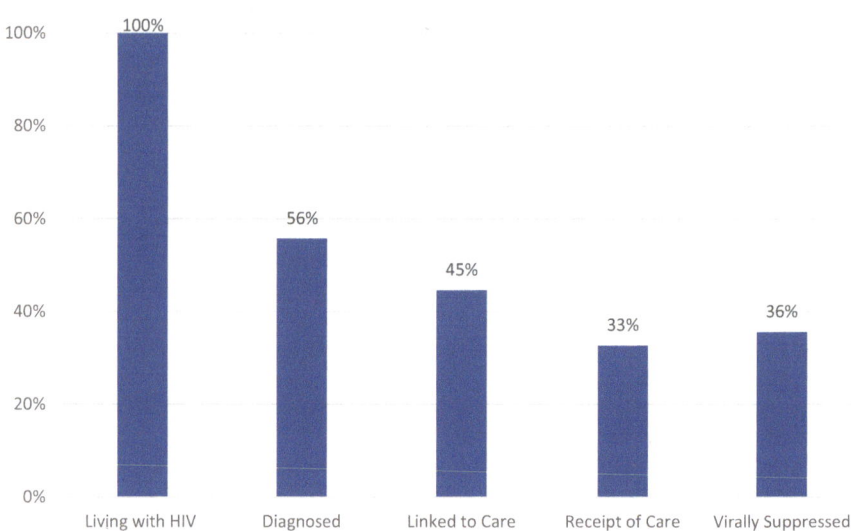

Fig. 1. Prevalance-based human immunodeficiency virus care continuum for 13-year-olds to 24-year-olds, 2019. (*Data source* Centers for Disease Control and Prevention. Monitoring selected national HIV prevention and care objectives by using HIV surveillance data—United States and 6 dependent areas, 2019. HIV Surveillance Supplemental Report 2021;26(No. 2). http://www.cdc.gov/hiv/library/reports/hiv-surveillance.html. Published May 2021. Accessed [21 February 2024].)

under the EHE strategy and need tailored clinical and public health services to meet national goals. AYAs living with or at risk of HIV are also at risk of other syndemically-related health problems, most notably harmful substance use and poor mental health. There are important developmental, legal-ethical, and structural factors that shape the context within which AYAs experience HIV vulnerability and attempt to obtain and engage with care services. This constellation of unique realities calls for focused policy changes, both at the legislative and health care system level, to reduce HIV disparities and improve care outcomes for this group.

Laws regarding minor consent and confidentiality as well as those that impede or expand health care coverage are salient determinants of AYA HIV testing, PrEP use, and care retention.[21,67] These laws also vary widely state to state, further exacerbating regional disparities in HIV outcomes for AYAs. Social and structural forces, like poverty, underpin HIV vulnerabilities and drastically impact care engagement.[65] Clinic policies represent powerful facilitators of or barriers to youth access and participation in care and prevention services.

Despite their unique developmental and social realities, most AYAs living with HIV access care in adult-oriented clinical spaces.[70] Young people often represent just a tiny fraction of HIV clinics' patient populations, and their individual needs may be over-shadowed. In these spaces, AYAs living with HIV are seen by providers with large patient panels and short visit times, which is at odds with the developmental needs and capacity of youth.[70] This translates to within clinic disparities for AYAs, including reduced rates of ART prescription compared to older patients despite meeting the same eligibility criteria, increased likelihood of initial ART regimen discontinuation, and significantly higher LTFU rates than their adult counterparts within the same practice.[70]

Table 1
Clinics care points for adolescents and young adults living with and at risk of human immunodeficiency virus

Key Focus Areas	Recommendations & Considerations
Pearls	
Early and regular screening	Initiate routine HIV screening by the age of 13 or earlier if risk behaviors are present (ie, sexually active). The US Preventive Services Task Force recommends annual screening for individuals at increased risk.
PrEP	Offer PrEP to AYAs who ask for PrEP or who are vulnerable to HIV due to sexual, substance, or social risk factors as part of a comprehensive prevention approach. Adherence is crucial for effectiveness. Moving beyond a risk centric focus, thorough sexual histories and behavior assessments can illuminate reasons for PrEP needs. In addition, if AYAs inquire about PrEP, it should be offered, regardless of assessed risk.
Youth-centered approach	Tailor care strategies to meet the unique needs of AYAs, incorporating mental health support, substance use counseling, and sexual health education.
Confidentiality and consent	Understand and respect laws regarding confidentiality and consent, especially for minors, to foster trust and encourage engagement in care.
Multidisciplinary team	Engage a multidisciplinary team including social workers, mental health professionals, and peer support specialists to address the holistic needs of AYAs living with HIV.
Cultural competence	Demonstrate cultural competence and sensitivity to the diverse backgrounds and experiences of AYAs, acknowledging the impact of stigma and discrimination on their willingness to seek and adhere to treatment.
Pitfalls	
Assuming monolithic experiences	Avoid assuming all AYAs share the same risks or experiences. Tailor interventions to individual backgrounds, preferences, and behaviors.
Neglecting mental health	Do not overlook the importance of mental health support. Depression, anxiety, and substance use are more prevalent among AYAs living with HIV and can significantly impact treatment adherence and outcomes.
Inadequate education on transmission risks	Provide comprehensive education on HIV transmission and prevention to facilitate risk reduction and PrEP uptake. Failing to provide comprehensive education on HIV transmission and prevention can lead to missed opportunities for risk reduction and PrEP uptake.

(continued on next page)

Table 1 (continued)	
Key Focus Areas	**Recommendations & Considerations**
Overlooking family and social contexts	Ignoring the role of family and social support systems can hinder engagement in care and adherence to treatment. Involving supportive family members, where appropriate, can enhance outcomes.
Underestimating the importance of adherence	Emphasize the critical role of adherence to ART and PrEP to ensure optimal control of HIV and reduce the risk of transmission. Not emphasizing the critical role of adherence to ART and PrEP can lead to suboptimal control of HIV and increase the risk of transmission.
Stigma and discrimination in health care	Combat stigma and discrimination in health care settings to ensure AYAs access necessary services and adhere to treatment plans. Allowing stigma and discrimination to manifest in health care settings can deter AYAs from accessing necessary services and adhering to treatment plans.

These clinics care points emphasize the importance of a comprehensive, individualized, and empathetic approach to human immunodeficiency virus care for adolescents and young adults, aiming to improve health outcomes and quality of life for this vulnerable population.

Abbreviations: ART, antiretroviral therapy; AYA, adolescents and young adult; HIV, human immunodeficiency virus; PrEP, pre-exposure prophylaxis.

RECOMMENDATIONS

The persistence of HIV disparities among AYAs, particularly within black and Latino communities, calls for targeted public health strategies that address the multifaceted barriers these groups face. To advance progress in reducing HIV infections, the approach must be holistic, prioritize inclusivity, and tackle the social determinants of health that disproportionately impact these communities. Collaborative efforts involving public health agencies, community-based organizations, lawmakers, and health care providers are crucial for sustaining and enhancing the achievements in HIV prevention and treatment. These partnerships are instrumental in ensuring that all individuals, regardless of their background, have equitable access to the necessary resources and support to prevent and treat HIV.

Strengthening health care access involves not only increasing the availability of services but also making these services more culturally competent and sensitive to the needs of AYAs, especially those who are black, Latino, and are SGM (**Table 1**). To do so, health care providers need to be trained on the unique challenges faced by these communities and implement practices that promote inclusivity and trust. In addition, integrating adolescent-friendly health services into our strategies to improve outcomes for AYAs living with or at risk of HIV is essential and innovative. This approach is rooted in creating youth-centric health care environments that are welcoming, accessible, and tailored to meet the unique needs of adolescents. These reimagined health care settings should be designed to feel safe and welcoming for AYAs and offer a space where they can feel comfortable seeking support and asking questions about their health. These environments should also respect their confidentiality and autonomy from parents, who may inadvertently be a barrier to truthful sexual and substance use histories. Furthermore, recognizing the busy and sometimes unpredictable schedules of AYAs and their guardians, services should offer flexible hours, including after-school and weekend appointments, and utilize digital health technologies for remote consultations when appropriate. This flexibility makes sure that logistical obstacles do not prevent access to health care.

SUMMARY

AYAs are identified as a priority group for national HIV/AIDS strategies due to their heightened vulnerability to infection and poorer health outcomes. The current epidemiology and research base underscore the necessity of developing tailored clinical and public health interventions to address the specific needs of AYAs, both those living with and at risk of HIV. Programs and policies should acknowledge the significant challenges faced by AYAs in accessing and adhering to care, including legal/ethical considerations, social determinants of health, and clinic policies. Nurses in clinical practice, research, policy analysis, and educational settings should emphasize the need for focused changes to improve access to care and, ultimately, health outcomes for AYAs.

DISCLOSURES

For Brenice Duroseau, funding should be noted as: Research reported in this publication was supported by the National Institute of Mental Health of the National Institutes of Health under award number 1R36MH135791. In addition, this publication was made possible with help from the Johns Hopkins University Center for AIDS Research, an NIH funded program (P30AI094189), which is supported by the following NIH Co-Funding and Participating Institutes and Centers: NIAID, NCI, NICHD, NHLBI, NIDA, NIMH, NIA, FIC, NIGMS, NIDDK, and OAR. The content is solely the responsibility of the authors and does not necessarily represent the official views of the NIH. Partial support towards training from Nurses Educational Funds, Inc, National League for Nurses, and International Society for the Study of Women's Sexual Health also made this publication possible.

REFERENCES

1. Pneumocystis pneumonia–Los Angeles. MMWR Morb Mortal Wkly Rep 1981; 30(21):250.
2. Zanoni BC, Mayer KH. The adolescent and young adult HIV cascade of care in the United States: Exaggerated health disparities. AIDS Patient Care STDS 2014;28(3):128–35.
3. Centers for Disease Control and Prevention. About ending the HIV epidemic in the U.S. initiative. 2021. Available at: https://www.cdc.gov/endhiv/about.html#:~:text=The%20initiative%20aims%20to%20reduce,at%20the%20heart%20of%20EHE. [Accessed 15 February 2024].
4. Kreisel KM, Spicknall IH, Gargano JW, et al. Sexually transmitted infections among US women and men: Prevalence and incidence estimates, 2018. Sex Transm Dis 2021;48(4). Available at: https://journals.lww.com/stdjournal/fulltext/2021/04000/sexually_transmitted_infections_among_us_women_and.2.aspx.
5. Centers for Disease Control and Prevention. Youth risk behavior survey data summary & trends report. 2023. Available at: https://www.cdc.gov/healthyyouth/data/yrbs/yrbs_data_summary_and_trends.htm. [Accessed 8 February 2024].

6. Centers for Disease Control and Prevention. HIV surveillance report, 2018 (updated); vol.31. 2020. Available at: https://www.cdc.gov/hiv/library/reports/hiv-surveillance/vol-31/index.html. [Accessed 19 February 2024].

7. Centers for Disease Control and Prevention. Diagnoses of HIV infection in the united states and dependent areas, 2021. HIV surveillance report 2023. 2023. Available at: https://www.cdc.gov/hiv/library/reports/hiv-surveillance/vol-34/index.html. [Accessed 19 February 2024].

8. Yusuf H, Agwu A. Adolescents and young adults with early acquired HIV infection in the United States: Unique challenges in treatment and secondary prevention. Expert Rev Anti Infect Ther 2021;19(4):457–71.

9. Cote HCF, Soudeyns H, Thorne A, et al. Leukocyte telomere length in HIV-infected and HIV-exposed uninfected children: Shorter telomeres with uncontrolled HIV viremia. PLoS One 2012;7(7):e39266.

10. Phillips N, Amos T, Kuo C, et al. HIV-associated cognitive impairment in perinatally infected children: A meta-analysis. Pediatrics 2016;138(5):e20160893.

11. Vujovic M, Struthers H, Meyersfeld S, et al. Addressing the sexual and reproductive health needs of young adolescents living with HIV in South Africa. Child Youth Serv Rev 2014;45(C):122.

12. Kang E, Mellins CA, Ng WYK, et al. Standing between two worlds in Harlem: A developmental psychopathology perspective of perinatally acquired human immunodeficiency virus and adolescence. J Appl Dev Psychol 2008; 29(3):227–37. Available at: https://www.sciencedirect.com/science/article/pii/S0193397308000105.

13. Centers for Disease Control and Prevention. Estimated HIV incidence and prevalence in the united states 2017–2021. HIV Surveillance Supplemental Report 2023;28(3).

14. Role of the COVID-19 pandemic on sexual behaviors and receipt of sexual and reproductive health services among U.S. high school students - Youth Risk Behavior Survey, United States, 2019-2021. MMWR supplements 2023;72(1):55.

15. Rodriguez A, Horvath KJ, Dowshen N, et al. Awareness and utilization of pre-exposure prophylaxis and HIV prevention services among transgender and non-binary adolescent and young adults. Front Reprod Health 2024;5:1150370.

16. Fields EL. Realizing the promise of PrEP globally for vulnerable adolescent and young adult populations. J Adolesc Health 2023;73(6):S1–3.

17. Centers for Disease Control and Prevention. Estimated HIV incidence and prevalence in the United States, 2017–2021. 2023. Available at: https://www.cdc.gov/hiv/library/reports/hiv-surveillance/vol-28-no-3/index.html. Accessed February 19, 2024.

18. Hsu KK, Rakhmanina NY, Committee on Pediatric A. Adolescents and young adults: The pediatrician's role in HIV testing and pre- and postexposure HIV prophylaxis. Pediatrics 2021;149(1). e2021055207.

19. Branson BM, Handsfield HH, Lampe MA, et al. Revised recommendations for HIV testing of adults, adolescents, and pregnant women in health-care settings. MMWR Recomm Rep (Morb Mortal Wkly Rep) 2006;55(RR-14):1–4.

20. Gutman CK, Middlebrooks L, Camacho-Gonzalez A, et al. Asymptomatic adolescent HIV: Identifying a role for universal HIV screening in the pediatric emergency department. AIDS Patient Care STDS 2020;34(9):373–9.

21. Phillips G2, Wang X, Ruprecht MM, et al. Associations between HIV testing and consent policies among sexually active adolescents: Differences by sexual behavior 2022;34(7):862–8.

22. Changes in high-risk sexual behavior, HIV and other STI testing, and PrEP use during the COVID-19 pandemic in a longitudinal cohort of adolescent men who have sex with men 13 to 18 years old in the United States. AIDS Behav 2023; 27(4):1133.

23. Gillot M, Gant Z, Hu X, et al. Linkage to HIV medical care and social determinants of health among adults with diagnosed HIV infection in 41 states and the District of Columbia, 2017. Publ Health Rep 2022;137(5):888–900.

24. U.S. Department of Health and Human Services. HIV care continuum. 2022. Available at: https://www.hiv.gov/federal-response/policies-issues/hiv-aids-care-continuum/. [Accessed 19 February 2024].

25. Centers for Disease Control and Prevention. Monitoring selected national HIV prevention and care objectives by using HIV surveillance data—United States and 6 dependent areas, 2019. HIV surveillance supplemental report 2021;26(no. 2). Updated 2021. Available at: http://www.cdc.gov/hiv/library/reports/hiv-surveillance.html. Accessed February 19, 2024.

26. Miller RL, Chiaramonte D, Strzyzykowski T, et al. Improving timely linkage to care among newly diagnosed HIV-infected youth: Results of SMILE. J Urban Health 2019;96(6):845–55.

27. Gandhi RT, Bedimo R, Hoy JF, et al. Antiretroviral drugs for treatment and prevention of HIV infection in adults: 2022 recommendations of the international antiviral Society–USA panel. JAMA 2023;329(1):63–84.

28. U.S. Department of Health and Human Services. Panel on antiretroviral guidelines for adults and adolescents. guidelines for the use of antiretroviral agents in adults and adolescents with HIV. 2023. Available at: https://www.ncbi.nlm.nih.gov/books/NBK586306/. Accessed February 19, 2024.

29. World Health Organization. Consolidated guidelines on HIV prevention, testing, treatment, service delivery and monitoring: recommendations for a public health approach. Updated 2021. Available at: https://www.who.int/publications/i/item/9789240031593. Accessed February 19, 2024.

30. Mateo-Urdiales A, Johnson S, Smith R, et al. Rapid initiation of antiretroviral therapy for people living with HIV. Cochrane Database Syst Rev 2019;6(6): CD012962.

31. Beer L, Mattson CL, Bradley H, et al. Medical Monitoring Project. Trends in ART prescription and viral suppression among HIV-positive young adults in care in the United States, 2009-2013. J Acquir Immune Defic Syndr 2017;76(1):e1–6.

32. Kim S, Gerver SM, Fidler S, et al. Adherence to antiretroviral therapy in adolescents living with HIV: Systematic review and meta-analysis. AIDS 2014;28(13): 1945–56.

33. Shaw S, Amico KR. Antiretroviral therapy adherence enhancing interventions for adolescents and young adults 13–24 years of age: A review of the evidence base. J Acquir Immune Defic Syndr 2016;72(4). Available at: https://journals.lww.com/jaids/fulltext/2016/08010/antiretroviral_therapy_adherence_enhancing.6.aspx.

34. Lally MA, van den Berg JJ, Westfall AO, et al. HIV continuum of care for youth in the United States. J Acquir Immune Defic Syndr 2018;77(1):110–7.

35. Kapogiannis BG, Koenig LJ, Xu J, et al. The HIV continuum of care for adolescents and young adults attending 13 urban US HIV care centers of the NICHD-ATN-CDC-HRSA SMILE collaborative. J Acquir Immune Defic Syndr 2020; 84(1):92–100.

36. Li Z, Purcell DW, Sansom SL, et al. Vital signs: HIV transmission along the continuum of care - United States, 2016. MMWR Morb Mortal Wkly Rep 2019;68(11): 267–72.

37. Halyard AS, Doraivelu K, Camacho-González AF, et al. Examining healthcare transition experiences among youth living with HIV in Atlanta, Georgia, USA: A longitudinal qualitative study. J Int AIDS Soc 2021;24(2):e25676.

38. Momplaisir F, McGlonn K, Grabill M, et al. Strategies to improve outcomes of youth experiencing healthcare transition from pediatric to adult HIV care in a large U.S. city. Arch Public Health 2023;81(1):49–58.

39. Ryscavage P, Macharia T, Patel D, et al. Linkage to and retention in care following healthcare transition from pediatric to adult HIV care 2016;28(5):561–5.

40. Allen E, Gordon A, Krakower D, et al. HIV preexposure prophylaxis for adolescents and young adults. Curr Opin Pediatr 2017;29(4):399–406.

41. Society for Adolescent Health and Medicine. HIV pre-exposure prophylaxis medication for adolescents and young adults: A position paper of the society for adolescent health and medicine. J Adolesc Health 2018;63(4):513–6.

42. Hosek S, Henry-Reid L. PrEP and adolescents: The role of providers in ending the AIDS epidemic 2020;145(1):e20191743.

43. Centers for Disease Control and Prevention. Centers for disease control and prevention. monitoring selected national HIV prevention and care objectives by using HIV surveillance data—United States and 6 dependent areas, 2021. HIV surveillance supplemental report. 2023. 28(no. 4). Available at: https://www.cdc.gov/hiv/library/reports/hiv-surveillance/vol-28-no-4/index.html. [Accessed 19 February 2024].

44. Fernandez MI, Harper GW, Hightow-Weidman LB, et al. Research priorities to end the adolescent HIV epidemic in the United States: Viewpoint. JMIR Res Protoc 2021;10(1):e22279.

45. Allison BA, Widman L, Stewart JL, et al. Adherence to pre-exposure prophylaxis in adolescents and young adults: A systematic review and meta-analysis. J Adolesc Health 2022;70(1):28–41. Available at: https://www.sciencedirect.com/science/article/pii/S1054139X21001695.

46. Biello KB, Hosek S, Drucker MT, et al. Preferences for injectable PrEP among young U.S. cisgender men and transgender women and men who have sex with men. Arch Sex Behav 2018;47(7):2101–7.

47. Mirani G, Williams PL, Chernoff M, et al. Changing trends in complications and mortality rates among US youth and young adults with HIV infection in the era of combination antiretroviral therapy. Clin Infect Dis 2015;61(12):1850–61.

48. Budak JZ, Sears DA, Wood BR, et al. Human immunodeficiency virus training pathways in residency: A national survey of curricula and outcomes. Clin Infect Dis 2021;72(9):1623–6.

49. Dawson-Rose C, Shehadeh D, Hao J, et al. Trauma, substance use, and mental health symptoms in transitional age youth experiencing homelessness. Public Health Nurs 2020;37(3):363–70.

50. Leonard A, Broussard J, Jain J, et al. Prevalence and correlates of methamphetamine use in transitional age youth experiencing homelessness or housing instability in San Francisco, CA. J Nurs Scholarsh 2023;55(3):711–20.

51. Hao J, Beld M, Khoddam-Khorasani L, et al. Comparing substance use and mental health among sexual and gender minority and heterosexual cisgender youth experiencing homelessness. PLoS One 2021;16(3):e0248077. https://doi.org/10.1371/journal.pone.0248077.

52. Jain JP, Santos G, Hao J, et al. The syndemic effects of adverse mental health conditions and polysubstance use on being at risk of clinical depression among marginally housed and homeless transitional age youth living in San Francisco, California. PLoS One 2022;17(3):e0265397. https://doi.org/10.1371/journal.pone.0265397.

53. National Academies of Sciences, Engineering, and medicine, health and medicine division, division of behavioral and social sciences and education, board on children Y, and families, Committee on the neurobiological and sociobehavioral science of adolescent development and its applications. No title. . 2019.

54. Williams PL, Jesson J. Growth and pubertal development in HIV-infected adolescents. Curr Opin HIV AIDS 2018;13(3):179–86.

55. De Santis JP, Garcia A, Chaparro A, et al. Integration versus disintegration: A grounded theory study of adolescent and young adult development in the context of perinatally-acquired HIV infection. J Pediatr Nurs 2014;29(5):422–35.

56. Disclosure of illness status to children and adolescents with HIV infection. American Academy of Pediatrics committee on pediatrics AIDS 1999;103(1):164–6.

57. Klitzman R, Marhefka S, Mellins C, et al. Ethical issues concerning disclosures of HIV diagnoses to perinatally infected children and adolescents. J Clin Ethics 2008;19(1):31–42.

58. Nelson KM, Skinner A, Stout CD, et al. Minor consent laws for sexually transmitted infection and human immunodeficiency virus services in the United States: A comprehensive, longitudinal survey of US state laws. Am J Public Health 2023; 113(4):397–407.

59. Guttmacher Institute. Minors' access to STI services. Updated 2023. Available at: https://www.guttmacher.org/state-policy/explore/minors-access-sti-services 29: https://www.who.int/publications/i/item/978924003159. Accessed February 19, 2024.

60. Havens PL, Hazra R. Commentary: The place of tenofovir disoproxil fumarate in pediatric antiretroviral therapy. Pediatr Infect Dis J 2015;34(4):406–8.

61. Hosek SG, Zimet GD. Behavioral considerations for engaging youth in HIV clinical research. J Acquir Immune Defic Syndr 2010;54(Suppl 1):25.

62. Shah SK, Allison SM, Kapogiannis BG, et al. Advancing independent adolescent consent for participation in HIV prevention research. J Med Ethics 2018;44(7): 431–3.

63. Zucchi EM, Ferguson L, Magno L, et al. When ethics and the law collide: A multicenter demonstration cohort study of pre-exposure prophylaxis provision to adolescent men who have sex with men and transgender women in Brazil. J Adolesc Health 2023;73(6S):S11–8.

64. Dasgupta S, McManus T, Tie Y, et al. Comparison of demographic characteristics and social determinants of health between adults with diagnosed HIV and all adults in the U.S. AJPM Focus 2023;2(3):100115. Available at: https://www.sciencedirect.com/science/article/pii/S2773065423000524.

65. Kahana SY, Jenkins RA, Bruce D, et al. Structural determinants of antiretroviral therapy use, HIV care attendance, and viral suppression among adolescents and young adults living with HIV. PLoS One 2016;11(4):e0151106. https://doi.org/10.1371/journal.pone.0151106.

66. Dailey AF, Gant Z, Hu X, et al. Association between social vulnerability and rates of HIV diagnoses among black adults, by selected characteristics and region of residence - United States, 2018. MMWR Morb Mortal Wkly Rep 2022;71(5): 167–70.

67. Fayaz Farkhad B, Holtgrave DR, Albarracín D. Effect of medicaid expansions on HIV diagnoses and pre-exposure prophylaxis use. Am J Prev Med 2021;60(3): 335–42.

68. Kaiser Family Foundation. Status of state Medicaid expansion decisions: interactive map. 2024. Available at: https://www.kff.org/medicaid/issue-brief/status-of-state-medicaid-expansion-decisions-interactive-map/. [Accessed 19 February 2024].

69. Lee F, Khanna AS, Hallmark CJ, et al. Expanding Medicaid to reduce human immunodeficiency virus transmission in Houston, Texas: Insights from a modeling study. Med Care 2023;61(1):12–9.

70. Griffith DC, Agwu AL. Caring for youth living with HIV across the continuum: Turning gaps into opportunities. AIDS Care 2017;29(10):1205–11. https://doi.org/10.1080/09540121.2017.1290211.